CW00538569

Handboo ... ic
Emergency Medicine

EDITED BY

Amina Lalani, MD, FRCPC, (PEM)
Academic Fellowship Director,
Division of Pediatric Emergency Medicine
Assistant Professor of Pediatrics, University of Toronto
Staff Physician, Division of Pediatric Emergency Medicine,
The Hospital for Sick Children, Toronto

Suzan Schneeweiss, MD, MEd, FRCPC
Director of Continuing Education, Department of Pediatrics
Assistant Professor of Pediatrics, University of Toronto
Staff Physician, Division of Pediatric Emergency Medicine,
The Hospital for Sick Children, Toronto

JONES AND BARTLETT PUBLISHERS
Sudbury, Massachusetts
BOSTON   TORONTO   LONDON   SINGAPORE

World Headquarters
Jones and Bartlett Publishers
40 Tall Pine Drive
Sudbury, MA 01776
978-443-5000
info@jbpub.com
www.jbpub.com

Jones and Bartlett Publishers
Canada
6339 Ormindale Way
Mississauga, Ontario L5V 1J2
Canada

Jones and Bartlett Publishers
International
Barb House, Barb Mews
London W6 7PA
United Kingdom

Jones and Bartlett's books and products are available through most bookstores and online booksellers. To contact Jones and Bartlett Publishers directly, call 800-832-0034, fax 978-443-8000, or visit our website www.jbpub.com.

Substantial discounts on bulk quantities of Jones and Bartlett's publications are available to corporations, professional associations, and other qualified organizations. For details and specific discount information, contact the special sales department at Jones and Bartlett via the above contact information or send an email to specialsales@jbpub.com.

6048

Production Credits
Executive Publisher: Christopher Davis
Associate Editor: Kathy Richardson
Production Director: Amy Rose
Associate Production Editor: Jamie Chase
Senior Marketing Manager: Katrina Gosek
Associate Marketing Manager: Rebecca Wasley
Composition: Paw Print Media
Cover Design: Kristin E. Ohlin
V.P., Manufacturing and Inventory Control: Therese Connell
Cover Image: © The Hospital for Sick Children
Cover Image: © Mel Curtis/Photodisc/Getty Images
Cover Image: © Photos.com
Cover Image: © Courtnee Mulroy/Shutterstock, Inc.
Printing and Binding: Malloy, Inc.
Cover Printing: Malloy, Inc.

Library of Congress Cataloging-in-Publication Data
The Hospital for Sick Children handbook of pediatric emergency medicine / The Hospital for Sick Children; edited by Amina Lalani and Suzan Schneeweiss.
    p.; cm.
Includes bibliographical references and index.
ISBN-13: 978-0-7637-5049-7
ISBN-10: 0-7637-5049-2
1. Pediatric emergencies—Handbooks, manuals, etc. I. Lalani, Amina. II. Schneeweiss, Suzan. III. Hospital for Sick Children. IV. Title: Handbook of pediatric emergency medicine.
    [DNLM: 1. Emergency Medicine—methods—Handbooks. 2. Pediatrics—methods—Handbooks. 3. Emergency Medical Services—methods—Handbooks. WS 39 H8275 2007]
RJ370.H67 2007
618.92'0025—dc22
        2007010807

Printed in the United States of America
11 10 09 08 07   10 9 8 7 6 5 4 3 2 1

Contents

Contributors

Abdullah Al-Anazi, MD, ABP
Pediatric Emergency Consultant and Traumatologist
King Abdulaziz Medical City Hospital, Saudi Arabia

Khalid Al-Ansari, MBBS, FRCPC
Fellow, Division of Pediatric Emergency Medicine,
The Hospital for Sick Children, Toronto

Sami Al-Farsi, MD, DCh, MRCP
Fellow, Division of Pediatric Emergency Medicine,
The Hospital for Sick Children, Toronto

Zaid Al-Harbash, MBBS, FRCPC
Fellow, Division of Pediatric Emergency Medicine,
The Hospital for Sick Children, Toronto

Susa Benseler, MD
Assistant Professor of Pediatrics, University of Toronto
Staff Physician, Divisions of Pediatric Emergency Medicine and
    Rheumatology,
The Hospital for Sick Children, Toronto

Carolyn Calpin, MD, FRCPC
Assistant Professor of Pediatrics, University of Toronto
Staff Physician, Division of Pediatric Emergency Medicine,
The Hospital for Sick Children, Toronto

Adam Cheng, MD, FRCPC, FAAP, (PEM)
Clinical Assistant Professor, University of British Columbia
Fellowship Director and Staff Physician, Division of Pediatric
    Emergency Medicine,
BC Children's Hospital, Vancouver

Anh Do, MD, FRCPC
Lecturer, University of Toronto
Staff Physician, Division of Pediatric Emergency Medicine,
The Hospital for Sick Children, Toronto

Stephen Freedman, MDCM, MSCI, FRCPC, FAAP, (PEM)
Assistant Professor of Pediatrics, University of Toronto
Staff Physician, Division of Pediatric Emergency Medicine,
The Hospital for Sick Children, Toronto

Leah Harrington, MD, FRCPC, FAAP, (PEM)
Assistant Professor of Pediatrics, University of Toronto
Staff Physician, Division of Pediatric Emergency Medicine,
The Hospital for Sick Children, Toronto

Shauna Jain, MD, FRCPC
Assistant Professor of Pediatrics, University of Toronto
Staff Physician, Division of Pediatric Emergency Medicine,
The Hospital for Sick Children, Toronto

D. Anna Jarvis, MBBS, FRCPC, FAAP
Associate Dean, Health Professions Student Affairs,
Faculty of Medicine, University of Toronto
Professor, Department of Pediatrics
Staff, Division of Pediatric Emergency Medicine, University of
  Toronto

Graham Jay, MBBS
Fellow, Division of Pediatric Emergency Medicine,
The Hospital for Sick Children, Toronto

Kelly Keogh, MD, FRCPC
Assistant Professor of Pediatrics, University of Toronto
Staff Physician, Division of Pediatric Emergency Medicine,
The Hospital for Sick Children, Toronto

Melanie Kirby, MBBS, FRCPC
Assistant Professor of Pediatrics, University of Toronto
Staff Physician, Division of Pediatric Hematology /Oncology,
The Hospital for Sick Children, Toronto

Luba Komar, MD, FRCPC
Assistant Professor of Pediatrics, University of Toronto
Staff Physician, Division of Pediatric Emergency Medicine,
The Hospital for Sick Children, Toronto

Amina Lalani, MD, FRCPC, (PEM)
Academic Fellowship Director, Division of Pediatric Emergency
    Medicine
Assistant Professor of Pediatrics, University of Toronto
Staff Physician, Division of Pediatric Emergency Medicine,
The Hospital for Sick Children, Toronto

Michal Maimon, MD
Staff Physician, Department of Pediatric Emergency Medicine
Soroka University Medical Center, Ben-Gurion University, Israel

Andrew Mason, MD, FRCPC, FAAP, (PEM)
Emergency Medicine
Orlando Regional Medical Center, Florida

Sanjay Mehta, MD, MEd, FRCPC, FAAP, FACEP
Assistant Professor of Pediatrics, University of Toronto
Staff Physician, Division of Pediatric Emergency Medicine,
The Hospital for Sick Children, Toronto

Angelo Mikrogianakis, MD, FRCPC
Assistant Professor of Pediatrics, University of Toronto
Staff Physician, Division of Pediatric Emergency Medicine and
    Department of Critical Care Medicine,
The Hospital for Sick Children, Toronto
Pediatric Transport Physician, Ornge (Ontario Air Ambulance)

Bruce Minnes, MD, FRCPC, FAAP, (PEM)
Associate Director—Clinical
Co-Director, Clinical Fellowship, Pediatric Emergency Medicine
Assistant Professor of Pediatrics, University of Toronto
Staff Physician, Division of Pediatric Emergency Medicine,
The Hospital for Sick Children, Toronto

William Mounstephen, MD, FRCPC, FAAP
Medical Director, Division of Pediatric Emergency Medicine
Assistant Professor of Pediatrics, University of Toronto
Staff Physician, The Hospital for Sick Children, Toronto

Jonathan Pirie, MD, MEd, FRCPC, FAAP, (PEM)
Associate Director—Education
Assistant Professor of Pediatrics, University of Toronto
Staff Physician, Division of Pediatric Emergency Medicine,
The Hospital for Sick Children, Toronto

Elena Pope, MD, MSc, FRCPC
Associate Professor of Pediatrics, University of Toronto
Section Head (Dermatology), Department of Pediatrics,
The Hospital for Sick Children, Toronto

Savithiri Ratnapalan, MBBS, MEd, MRCP, FRCPC, FAAP
Assistant Professor, University of Toronto
Staff Physician, Division of Pediatric Emergency Medicine and
    Clinical Pharmacology & Toxicology,
The Hospital for Sick Children, Toronto

Christina Ricks, MD, FAAP
Fellow, Division of Pediatric Emergency Medicine,
The Hospital for Sick Children, Toronto

Jennifer Riley, MD, FRCPC, FACEP
Assistant Professor, University of Toronto
Staff Physician, Divisions of Emergency Medicine,
The Hospital for Sick Children and St. Michael's Hospital, Toronto

Suzan Schneeweiss, MD, MEd, FRCPC
Director of Contining Education, Department of Pediatrics
Assistant Professor of Pediatrics, University of Toronto
Staff Physician, Division of Pediatric Emergency Medicine,
The Hospital for Sick Children, Toronto

Suzanne Schuh, MD, FRCPC, FAAP, (PEM)
Associate Director—Research
Professor of Pediatrics, University of Toronto
Staff Physician, Division of Pediatric Emergency Medicine,
The Hospital for Sick Children, Toronto

Dennis Scolnik, MSc, MB, ChB, DCH, FRCPC
Associate Professor of Pediatrics, University of Toronto
Staff Physician, Divisions of Pediatric Emergency Medicine and
    Clinical Pharmacology and Toxicology,
The Hospital for Sick Children, Toronto

Abdullah Shamsah, MB, BCh
Fellow, Division of Pediatric Emergency Medicine,
The Hospital for Sick Children, Toronto

Jennifer Thull-Freedman, MD, MSCI, FAAP, (PEM)
Assistant Professor of Pediatrics, University of Toronto
Staff Physician, Division of Pediatric Emergency Medicine,
The Hospital for Sick Children, Toronto

Rahim Valani, MD, CCFP-EM, PG Dip, Med ED
Associate Staff, Division of Pediatric Emergency Medicine,
The Hospital for Sick Children, Toronto

Preface

The field of pediatric emergency medicine has recently emerged as a recognized subspecialty and is constantly evolving with new evidence-based research. Keeping up to date with current information is a challenge. This book is a compilation of chapters authored by pediatric emergency staff physicians and fellows at The Hospital for Sick Children. We have included the most recent evidence-based recommendations and best practices in a handbook format that we hope you will find useful. The content can be of use to any practitioner who cares for children in an emergency setting. The chapters focus on clinical assessment and management of a wide range of medical and surgical presentations, from resuscitation of the critically ill child to system-specific problems to minor injuries.

Our hope is that this will be a widely available resource for the emergency practitioner.

Amina Lalani, MD, FRCPC, (PEM)
Academic Fellowship Director,
Division of Pediatric Emergency Medicine
Assistant Professor of Pediatrics, University of Toronto
Staff Physician, Division of Pediatric Emergency Medicine,
The Hospital for Sick Children, Toronto

Suzan Schneeweiss, MD, MEd, FRCPC
Director of Continuing Education, Department of Pediatrics
Assistant Professor of Pediatrics, University of Toronto
Staff Physician, Division of Pediatric Emergency Medicine,
The Hospital for Sick Children, Toronto

■ PART I
RESUSCITATION

1 ■ Pediatric Triage

D. Anna Jarvis

Goals of Triage

■ To rapidly identify patients with urgent, life-threatening conditions
■ To determine the most appropriate treatment area for patients presenting to the emergency department
■ To decrease congestion in emergency treatment areas
■ To provide ongoing assessment of patients
■ To provide information to patients and families regarding services, expected care, and waiting times
■ To contribute information that helps to define departmental acuity

Canadian Emergency Department Triage and Acuity Scale (CTAS)

■ Developed to enhance acute triage in the emergency department
■ Main focus is to identify patients in greatest need and prioritize care
■ Facilitates application of CTAS to younger age groups
■ Based on age-related physiological measurements encompassing developmental, family, and psychosocial issues

Triage Assignment

■ Based on "usual presentation," intuition, and experience of the provider, and objective measures such as vital signs and pain scales
■ Throughout childhood there are multiple changes in size, development, normal parameters, and significance of presenting symptom complexes

Table 1.1 Pediatric CTAS Guidelines

Triage Level	Definition	Usual Presentation	Sentinel Diagnosis
Level 1 Resuscitation Time to physician IMMEDIATE	■ Conditions that are threats to life or limb (or imminent risk of deterioration) requiring immediate aggressive interventions	■ Respiratory failure, shock, coma, or cardiopulmonary arrest ■ Requires continuous assessment and intervention to maintain physiological stability	E.g., coma, seizures, moderate to severe respiratory distress, unconscious, major burns, trauma, significant bleeding, and cardiopulmonary arrest
Level 2 Emergent Time to physician 15 min	■ Conditions that are a potential threat to life, limb, or function, requiring rapid medical intervention or delegated acts	■ Moderate to severe respiratory distress ■ Altered level of consciousness ■ Dehydration ■ Requires comprehensive assessment and multiple interventions to prevent further deterioration ■ Fever: age < 3 months and > 38.0°C	E.g., sepsis, altered LOC, ingestion, asthma, seizure (postictal), DKA, child abuse, purpuric rash, fever, open fractures, violent patients, testicular pain, lacerations, or orthopedic injuries with neurovascular compromise, dental injury with avulsed permanent tooth

Table 1.1 Pediatric CTAS Guidelines (continued)

TRIAGE LEVEL	DEFINITION	USUAL PRESENTATION	SENTINEL DIAGNOSIS
Level 3 Urgent **Time to physician 30 min**	■ Conditions that could potentially progress to a serious problem requiring emergency intervention ■ May be associated with significant discomfort or affecting ability to function at work or activities of daily living	■ Alert, oriented, well hydrated, minor alterations in vital signs Interventions include assessment and simple procedures ■ Febrile child > 3 months with T > 38.5°C ■ Mild respiratory distress ■ Infant < 1 month	E.g., simple burns, fractures, dental injuries, pneumonia without distress, history of seizure, suicidal ideation, ingestion requiring observation only, head trauma: alert/vomiting
Level 4 Semi-urgent **Time to physician 1 hour**	■ Conditions that relate to patient age, distress, or potential for deterioration or complications ■ Would benefit from intervention or reassurance within 1–2 hours	■ Vomiting/diarrhea and no dehydration age > 2 ■ Simple lacerations/sprain/strains ■ Alert with fever and simple complaints such as ear pain, sore throat, or nasal congestion ■ Head trauma: no symptoms	

(continues)

Table 1.1 Pediatric CTAS Guidelines (continued)

TRIAGE LEVEL	DEFINITION	USUAL PRESENTATION	SENTINEL DIAGNOSIS
Level 5 Non-urgent **Time to physician 2 hours**	■ Conditions that may be acute but non-urgent, may be part of a chronic problem ± evidence of deterioration ■ Investigation or interventions could be delayed/referred to other areas of the hospital or health care system	■ Afebrile, alert, oriented, well hydrated with normal vital signs ■ Interventions not usually required other than assessment/discharge instruction ■ Vomiting alone or diarrhea alone with no suspicion or signs of dehydration	

Source: Adapted from: Beveridge R, Clarke B, et al. *Implementation guidelines for the Canadian ED Triage and Acuity Scale (CTAS)*. Retrieved from: http://www.caep.ca/002.policies/002-02.CTAS/CTAS-guidelines.htm.

- Each child must be triaged according to age, developmental stage, and acuity
- Family dynamics, cultural, and social variables are also important considerations in triage decisions

Time Responses

- These are objectives, not established standard of care
- A "fractile response" is the proportion of patient visits for a given triage level where patients were seen within the recommended CTAS time frame
- Fractile response does not address whether the delay for an individual is reasonable or acceptable
- Triage levels may require upgrading if the time response has not been met
- The triage process needs to be flexible because patients' status may change while in the emergency department

References

Beveridge R, Clarke B, Janes L, et al. Canadian emergency department triage and acuity scale: implementation guidelines. *Can J Emerg Med.* 1999;1(3 suppl).

Canadian Association of Emergency Physicians. Canadian paediatric triage and acuity scale: implementation guidelines for emergency departments. *Can J Emerg Med.* 2001;3(4 suppl):1–40.

2 ▪ Pediatric Transport

ADAM CHENG

Introduction

- Critically ill children have a better clinical outcome when treated in tertiary pediatric intensive care units
- Centralization of pediatric intensive care units has increased the need for interhospital pediatric transports
- Specialized pediatric retrieval teams have been developed in many countries to undertake the stabilization and safe transfer of critically ill children

Composition of Pediatric Transport Teams

- Recommend at least two patient care providers per transport, with one being a nurse
- Other team members may be: respiratory therapists, physicians, residents, paramedics
- Aim to match the skills of the team members to the needs of the patient
- Incidence of complications is decreased with dedicated, specialized transport teams

Adverse Events During Transport

- Very common (occur up to 50–75% of the time)
- Incidence of adverse events proportional to severity of illness prior to transport
- Type of adverse events:
  - Alteration in vital signs: hypothermia/hyperthermia, hypertension/hypotension, bradycardia/tachycardia
  - Equipment related: accidental extubation, loss of oxygen supply, malfunction of ventilator, loss of intravenous catheter infusing vasoactive drugs
  - Other: drug error, respiratory arrest, cardiac arrest, death

8

- Minimize adverse events:
  - Provide adequate resuscitation prior to transfer
  - Provide appropriate monitoring during transfer
  - Anticipate potential problems during transfer
  - Team composition and equipment should reflect pretransport severity of illness and the anticipated duration of transport

Preparing for Transport: Prior to Leaving Base Hospital

Equipment

- Optimally small, lightweight, and sturdy
- Regularly check and service all transport equipment
- Bring extra batteries/power source for all equipment
- Replenish used medications and supplies after each transport

Table 2.1 Equipment Required to Transport a Critically Ill Child	
Monitors	Heart rate/rhythm
	Blood pressure
	Pulse oximetry
	Temperature
	Extra batteries
Infusion pumps	Multiple infusions
	Extra batteries
Resuscitation equipment	Airway equipment
	Central lines
	Chest tubes
	Intravenous and intraosseous needles
Drugs and fluids	Resuscitation drugs
	Infusion drugs
	Sedative/paralytic drugs
	Antibiotics
	Fluids/blood if necessary
Portable oxygen supply	Check prior to leaving
	(continues)

Table 2.1 Equipment Required to Transport a Critically Ill Child (continued)	
Ventilator	Appropriate circuit (infant vs child)
Document folder	Patient chart Transport record Information for parents Telephone numbers
Protective clothing	Warm clothes Change of clothes (for long transports) Appropriate footwear
Portable telephone	Extra batteries

Mode of Transport

■ Determined by several factors: urgency of the case, availability of air/land transport, distance required to travel, traffic conditions, and weather

Table 2.2 Selected Modes of Transport	
Road/land ambulance	
Advantages	Rapid mobilization Large working area Ability to stop for procedures
Disadvantages	Slow transit time
Helicopter	
Advantages	Rapid mobilization if service available Fast Can land directly at facility/scene
Disadvantages	Limited work area Noisy Vibration with turbulence Operation limited by weather

Table 2.2   Selected Modes of Transport (continued)

Fixed-wing aircraft

Advantages	Long distances traveled in short times
Disadvantages	Noisy
	Vibration with turbulence
	Operation limited by weather
	Additional legs of patient transport may be required (to/from airport)

Preparing for Transport: Prior to Leaving Referring Facility

General Principles

- Optimize patient condition prior to transport
- Aim to provide quality of care equivalent to that in an intensive care setting
- Follow an organized, structured approach to assessing patient
- Avoid undue delay once decision has been made to move patient
- Communicate with receiving hospital prior to departure

Airway and Ventilation

- Ensure airway is secure prior to transport
- If risk of losing airway on transport, consider intubation prior to departure
- If patient is intubated and ventilated, mechanical ventilation is preferred over hand bagging
- Confirm endotracheal tube placement prior to departure
- Securely fix endotracheal tube
- Consider a predeparture blood gas to assess adequacy of ventilation and oxygenation

- Ensure suction is working: all patients, both nonintubated and intubated, may potentially need suction
- Bring enough oxygen for transport

Circulation

- Attempt to adequately fluid resuscitate the patient prior to transport
- Consider ongoing fluid losses in fluid calculations
- For fluid–refractory shock, draw up appropriate inotrope infusions prior to departure
- Ensure sufficient fluids on board for the journey
- Secure and protect all intravenous and central lines: ensure that there is no kinking or blockage
- Use intraosseous access if unable to obtain intravenous access

Monitoring and Tubes

- Ensure that all monitors are working
- Arterial lines should be used to monitor blood pressure in cardiovascularly unstable, ventilated children
- End-tidal CO_2 monitors should be used for all intubated patients
- Foley catheter to measure urine output for long transfers
- Nasogastric tube connected to appropriate suction
- Arterial line is zeroed and functioning prior to departure

Analgesia, Sedation, and Drugs

- Assess need for analgesia, sedation, and neuromuscular blockade prior to departure
- Draw up appropriate medication that may be required prior to departure
- Consider continuous infusions of sedatives/analgesics, rather than intermittent boluses, for longer transports
- Ensure sufficient medications on board for the journey

Paperwork and Communication

- Bring all documentation and X-rays
- Inform parents of child's condition, final destination, PICU telephone number; should not follow ambulance
- Communicate with receiving facility: provide update of patient condition

Transport by Air: Special Considerations

- Patient evaluation and stabilization in the air can be affected by certain flight-imposed stresses

Boyle's Law

- Gas will expand as cabin altitude rises and barometric pressure falls
- Pneumothoraces should be drained prior to air transport; vent chest tubes into a Heimlich (flap) valve
- Fill endotracheal cuffs with water/saline instead of air
- Monitor for increased intracranial pressure in head-injured patients
- Place a nasogastric tube to prevent gastric distension

Increased Oxygen Requirements

- Oxygen requirements increase with altitude
- Provide supplemental oxygen for patients with respiratory illnesses
- Patients requiring 100% oxygen on the ground will need a change in ventilatory support in order to tolerate transport at altitude

Noise

- Difficult to communicate, and causes fatigue
- Difficulty auscultating chest, heart sounds, or blood pressure

Temperature

- Decreases with increases in altitude

- Remember to monitor patient temperature, particularly infants (use isolette)
- Bring extra clothes for transport team members

Turbulence and Vibration
- Depends on prevalent weather conditions: worse when air is warm
- Abrupt changes in altitude or aircraft position may also potentiate motion sickness
- Secure patient with belts, blankets, and restraints (if necessary)
- Ensure all equipment is secure prior to transport

Dehydration
- Lack of moisture at high altitudes
- Maintain adequate hydration for patient and team members

Acceleration/Deceleration
- Rear-load (head to rear of aircraft) hemodynamically compromised patients to prevent compromise in cerebral perfusion during takeoff
- Front-load (head to front of aircraft) head-injured patients to prevent increases in intracranial pressure during takeoff

References

Barry PW, Ralston C. Adverse events occurring during interhospital transfer of the critically ill. *Arch Dis Child.* 1994;71:8–11.

Brink LW, Neuman B, Wynn J. Air transport. *Ped Clin N Amer.* 1993; 40(2):439–455.

Macrae DJ. Paediatric intensive care transport. *Arch Dis Child.* 1994; 71:175–178.

Wallen E, Venkataraman ST, Shekhar, T, et al. Intrahospital transport of critically ill pediatric patients. *Crit Care Med.* 1995;23(9):1588–1595.

Woodward GA, Insoft RM, et al. The state of pediatric interfacility transport: consensus of the Second National Pediatric and Neonatal Interfacility Transport Medicine Leadership Conference. *Ped Emerg Care.* 2002;18(1):38–43.

3 ▪ Pediatric Cardiopulmonary Resuscitation

Suzan Schneeweiss

Introduction

- Pediatric cardiac arrest is usually caused by an underlying respiratory abnormality
- In general, the myocardium in children is normal, and the final common pathway leading to cardiac arrest is usually hypoxia
- Second most common cause of cardiac arrest is circulatory failure from hypovolemia (loss of fluid or blood) or sepsis

Airway

Open the Airway

- Similar maneuvers may be used in children and adults
- Characteristics of childhood airway:
  - Large tongue proportional to the oral cavity
  - Higher and more anterior larynx (C3–4) vs (C5–6)
  - Long, floppy epiglottis
  - Subglottic area is narrowest portion of the infant larynx
  - Large head: when lying supine on backboard, neck is relatively flexed due to the large occiput and may obstruct the airway; if there is no evidence of trauma a towel placed under the head and shoulders will help position the airway

Tracheal Intubation

- Best method for establishing and maintaining a patent airway in children who are comatose or in those with respiratory or cardiac arrest

15

- Rapid sequence intubation to facilitate intubation and reduce complications
  - Sedative, neuromuscular blocking agent and other medications to sedate and paralyze patient
  - Requires skilled personnel
- Verification of tube placement: clinical assessment and confirmatory devices
  - End-tidal CO_2 monitor; positive waveform or color change
  - Consider esophageal dectector device in children > 20 kg with a perfusing rhythm
  - Bilateral chest movement; equal breath sounds over both lung fields
  - Listen for gastric insufflation sound over stomach
  - Check oxygen saturation
  - If uncertain, perform direct laryngoscopy
  - Chest X-ray: confirm placement (not in right mainstem bronchus or high position)
- If deterioration of patient condition, consider DOPE:
  - **D**isplacement of tube from trachea
  - **O**bstruction of endotracheal tube
  - **P**neumothorax
  - **E**quipment failure

Estimation of Size of ETT in Children

- Child > 1 yr = (age/4) + 4 (uncuffed tube)
- Internal diameter of ETT = size of child's little finger (less reliable)
- Length-based resuscitation tapes (Broselow® tape)
- Consider cuffed endotracheal tube in hospital setting

Laryngeal Mask Airway (LMA)

- If endotracheal tube placement is not possible, LMA acceptable adjunct for experienced providers
- Contraindicated if intact gag reflex
- Does not protect airway from aspiration

- More difficult to maintain during patient movement than ETT
- Should not replace BVM ventilation
- LMA sizes:
  - Neonates   1–1.5
  - 7.5–10 kg   1.5
  - 10–20 kg   2
  - 20–30 kg   2.5
  - 30–50 kg   3
  - > 50 kg   3–4

Breathing

Impending Respiratory Failure

- Increased respiratory rate and effort or decreased breath sounds
- Increased work of breathing
  - Nasal flaring, use of accessory muscles
  - Head bobbing, grunting
  - Stridor and/or prolonged expiration
- Decreased level of consciousness or response to pain or stimulation
- Poor skeletal muscle control
- Slow or irregular respirations (ominous sign of impending arrest)
- Cyanosis
- Note: Tachypnea without other signs of respiratory distress quiet tachypnea is often an attempt at maintaining normal pH (compensatory respiratory alkalosis) in response to metabolic acidosis

Bag-Valve-Mask (BVM) Ventilation

- As effective as ventilation through endotracheal tube for short periods
- Caution against overventilation

- Reduced cardiac output, cerebral blood flow, and coronary perfusion
- Air-trapping and barotrauma: increased risk of stomach inflation, regurgitation, and aspiration
■ Two-person technique more effective than one-person technique
  - One person maintains open airway with jaw thrust and tight mask-to-face seal while other person compresses ventilation bag

Self-Inflating BVM Device

■ Mask should fit over mouth and nose to provide a tight seal and avoid air leak
■ Minimum volume of 450–500 mL
■ 100% oxygen with flow rate of 10–15 L/min (with reservoir bag can deliver 60–95% oxygen)
■ NG tube if bagging for more than a few minutes (gaseous distention can quickly lead to impaired ventilation)

Anesthesia Bags

■ More difficult to use, require experienced personnel
■ Should always have an attached pressure manometer

Circulation

Ventilation/Compression and Breathing

2005 guidelines from American Heart Association:
■ "Push hard" and "push fast"
■ Adequate compression rate (100 compressions/minute)
■ Adequate compression depth ($\frac{1}{3}$ to $\frac{1}{2}$ of anterior-posterior diameter) on lower third of sternum (not over xiphoid process)
■ Allow full recoil of chest after each compression
■ Coordinate chest compressions and breathing

- Compression: ventilation
  - Neonates 3:1
  - Child 15:2 (if intubated, 100 compressions/minute without pauses for ventilation and 8–10 breaths per minute)
- Rotate compressor every 2 minutes to avoid fatigue and deterioration in quality of ventilation

Initiate Cardiac Compressions

- When no palpable pulse (brachial or femoral pulse) OR
- Heart rate is < 60 bpm and evidence of poor systemic perfusion

Table 3.1 Hypotension (< 5th percentile for age)

AGE	SYSTOLIC BLOOD PRESSURE (MMHG)
Term neonates (0–28 days)	< 60
Infants 1 to 12 months	< 70
Children > 1 year	70 + (2 × age in years)
Children > 10 years	90

Volume Expansion

Fluid administration during resuscitation is used to:

- Restore effective circulating volumes in hypovolemic shock states (most common cause of shock in children)
- Restore oxygen-carrying capacity in hemorrhagic shock states
- Correct metabolic imbalances

Volume Therapy

- Signs of shock:
  - Sustained sinus tachycardia in absence of known causes such as fever or pain may be an early sign of cardiovascular compromise; bradycardia may be preterminal cardiac rhythm indicative of advanced shock, often associated with hypotension

- Mottling of the skin, cool extremities, decreased peripheral pulses, delayed capillary refill, changes in mental status, and oliguria
- *Hypotension is a late sign of shock* (often associated with high morbidity and mortality)

■ Fluid bolus consists of 20 mL/kg of an isotonic solution such as normal saline or Ringer's lactate administered as quickly as possible

■ Repeat boluses to restore circulating blood volume

■ Blood replacement for acute severe hemorrhage, if child remains in shock after 40–60 mL/kg crystalloid

■ Reassess response to each bolus of fluid

Vascular Access

Protocol for Intravenous Access

■ Peripheral IV, 2 sites: first 1.5 min

■ Intraosseous: 1.5–5 min
  Note: If intubated, many drugs can be given through ETT (LEAN—Lidocaine, Epinephrine, Atropine, Naloxone)

■ Central line: > 5 min

Intraosseous Cannulation

■ Can be quickly inserted in 30–60 seconds

■ May be used for any type of fluid (including blood) and medication

■ Rigid needle inserted through cortex of bone into medullary cavity
  - Site of choice: anterior medial aspect of tibia 1–3 cm below proximal tibial tuberosity
  - Other sites: distal tibia, distal femur, and iliac crest

■ Complications: infection, fracture, and compartment syndrome

■ Remove intraosseous line when alternate vascular site accessed

Medications (see inside front cover)

Epinephrine

- Drug of choice for cardiopulmonary arrest
- Both alpha and beta adrenergic properties; *alpha adrenergic mediated vasoconstriction* most important property acting to restore aortic diastolic pressure
- Catecholamines not as effective when patient is acidotic and hypoxemic so attention to ventilation, oxygenation, and circulation is essential

Sodium Bicarbonate

- Routine administration not shown to improve outcome
- Consider for prolonged cardiac arrest after providing effective ventilation, chest compressions, and epinephrine
- Recommended for treatment of acidosis accompanying cardiac arrest and for shock with documented significant metabolic acidosis
- May impair tissue oxygen delivery; cause hypokalemia, hypocalcemia, hypernatremia, and hyperosmolalilty; decrease threshold for VFib; and impair cardiac function

Glucose

- Infants have high glucose requirements and low glycogen stores
- Hypoglycemia is common during periods of high stress and energy needs
- Glucose monitoring is essential during resuscitation, use Dextrostix®

Atropine

- Parasympatholytic drug used to treat symptomatic bradycardia and vagally mediated bradycardia with intubation attempts
- Sinus bradycardia usually results from hypoxemia and is initially treated with oxygenation and ventilation

- Dose must be sufficient to produce vagolytic effects and avoid paradoxical bradycardia (> 0.1 mg)

Calcium

- Not routinely given during resuscitation
- Calcium may enter the cell with organ reperfusion following an ischemic event and produce toxic effects
- Indicated for treatment of hypocalcemia, hyperkalemia, and hypermagnesemia
- Administer CaCl via central line if possible due to risk of sclerosis or infiltration with a peripheral line

Amiodarone

- Antiarrhythmic drug; slows AV conduction, prolongs AV refractory period and QT interval, slows ventricular conduction
- Used in ventricular fibrillation
- Vasodilatory properties; may cause hypotension
- Monitor ECG; may cause bradycardia, heart block, torsades de pointes VTach
- Long half-life (up to 40 days)

Defibrillation

- See Figure 3.1
- Most cardiac arrests in children are asystolic or bradycardic
- Ventricular fibrillation in 5–15% of pediatric out-of-hospital arrests
- Indicated for ventricular fibrillation or pulseless ventricular tachycardia
- Paddle size: use largest paddles that will fit on chest without touching (leave 3 cm between paddles)
  - Adult paddles > 10 kg
  - Infant paddles < 10 kg
- Initial dose 2 J/kg; 4 J/kg with subsequent attempts

- Automatic electrical defibrillators safe and effective in children 1–8 yrs (pediatric attenuator)
- Sequence:
  - Give 1 shock 2 J/kg as quickly as possible
  - Resume CPR × 2 minutes
  - If shockable rhythm persists, give 1 shock 4 J/kg, then give epinephrine (repeat cycle every 3–5 minutes)
  - If persistent shockable rhythm after 2 minutes of CPR, give 1 shock 4 J/kg and amiodarone (give lidocaine if amiodarone not available)

Synchronized Cardioversion

- Timed depolarization used to treat symptomatic patients with SVT or ventricular tachycardia (with pulses) accompanied by poor perfusion, hypotension, or heart failure
- Initial dose 0.5 to 1 J/kg; increased to 2 J/kg with subsequent attempts if necessary

Medications to Maintain Cardiac Output

- Myocardial dysfunction common post cardiac arrest
- Vasoactive agents used to improve hemodynamics
- Tailor drug and dose to each patient

Dopamine

- Used for treatment of circulatory shock following resuscitation or when shock is unresponsive to fluid administration
- Endogenous catecholamine with complex cardiovascular effects
- Low dose not shown to maintain renal blood flow or improve renal function
- Higher doses (> 5 mcg/kg) stimulate β receptors and α-adrenergic vasoconstriction

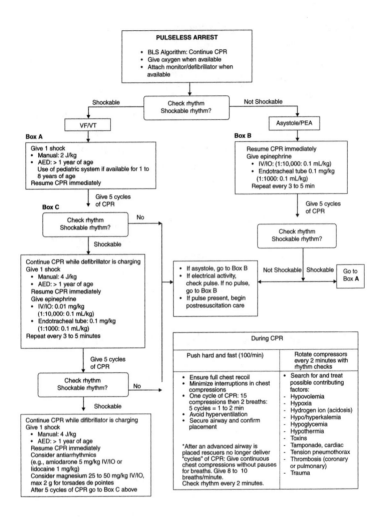

PULSELESS ARREST

- BLS Algorithm: Continue CPR
- Give oxygen when available
- Attach monitor/defibrillator when available

Shockable ← **Check rhythm Shockable rhythm?** → Not Shockable

VF/VT

Box A

Give 1 shock
- Manual: 2 J/kg
- AED: > 1 year of age
Use of pediatric system if available for 1 to 8 years of age
Resume CPR immediately

Give 5 cycles of CPR

Box C

Check rhythm Shockable rhythm? — No →

Shockable

Continue CPR while defibrillator is charging
Give 1 shock
- Manual: 4 J/kg
- AED: > 1 year of age
Resume CPR immediately
Give epinephrine
- IV/IO: 0.01 mg/kg
  (1:10,000: 0.1 mL/kg)
- Endotracheal tube: 0.1 mg/kg
  (1:1000: 0.1 mL/kg)
Repeat every 3 to 5 minutes

Give 5 cycles of CPR

Check rhythm Shockable rhythm? — No →

Shockable

Continue CPR while difibrillator is charging
Give 1 shock
- Manual: 4 J/kg
- AED: > 1 year of age
Resume CPR immediately
Consider antiarrhythmics
(e.g., amiodarone 5 mg/kg IV/IO or lidocaine 1 mg/kg)
Consider magnesium 25 to 50 mg/kg IV/IO, max 2 g for torsades de pointes
After 5 cycles of CPR go to Box C above

Asystole/PEA

Box B

Resume CPR immediately
Give epinephrine
- IV/IO: (1:10,000: 0.1 mL/kg)
- Endotracheal tube 0.1 mg/kg
  (1:1000: 0.1 mL/kg)
Repeat every 3 to 5 min

Give 5 cycles of CPR

Check rhythm Shockable rhythm?

Not Shockable | Shockable → Go to Box A

- If asystole, go to Box B
- If electrical activity, check pulse. If no pulse, go to Box B
- If pulse present, begin postresuscitation care

During CPR	
Push hard and fast (100/min)	Rotate compressors every 2 minutes with rhythm checks
• Ensure full chest recoil • Minimize interruptions in chest compressions • One cycle of CPR: 15 compressions then 2 breaths: 5 cycles = 1 to 2 min • Avoid hyperventilation • Secure airway and confirm placement *After an advanced airway is placed rescuers no longer deliver "cycles" of CPR: Give continuous chest compressions without pauses for breaths. Give 8 to 10 breaths/minute. Check rhythm every 2 minutes.	• Search for and treat possible contributing factors: - Hypovolemia - Hypoxia - Hydrogen ion (acidosis) - Hypo/hyperkalemia - Hypoglycemia - Hypothermia - Toxins - Tamponade, cardiac - Tension pneumothorax - Thrombosis (coronary or pulmonary) - Trauma

■ Figure 3.1 PALS Pulseless Arrest Algorithm

Epinephrine

- Low dose infusion (< 0.3 mcg/kg/min): β-adrenergic effect (potent inotrope and decreases systemic vascular resistance)
- High dose infusion (> 0.3 mcg/kg/min): α-adrenergic effect
- Preferable to dopamine if marked circulatory instability and decompensated shock

Dobutamine

- Affects selective β_1 and β_2 –adrenergic receptors
- Increases myocardial contractility and decreases peripheral vascular resistance
- Used to improve cardiac output and blood pressure especially if poor myocardial function

References

American Heart Association. Part 11: Pediatric basic life support. *Circulation*. 2005;112:156–166.

American Heart Association. Part 12: Pediatric advanced life support. *Circulation*. 2005;112:167–187.

American Heart Association. Part 13: Neonatal resuscitation guidelines. *Circulation*. 2005;112:188–195.

4 ▪ Shock

D. ANNA JARVIS

Introduction

- Shock is a syndrome characterized by inadequate supply of oxygen and nutrients to meet tissue needs
- Causes: hypovolemic, distributive, obstructive, cardiogenic, and dissociative
- Also classified as compensated, decompensated, and irreversible shock
- Shock is a continuum of vital organ dysfunction, from a single system problem (e.g., hemorrhage) progressing to secondary organ damage leading to multisystem failure and eventually death

  (e.g., hemorrhage → tissue hypoxia → liver dysfunction → coagulopathy + brain hypoxia → coma → death)

Table 4.1   Causes of Shock

Hypovolemic (decreased circulating blood volume)	• Dehydration • Hemorrhage • Plasma loss
Distributive (vasodilation)	• Sepsis • Anaphylaxis • Drug toxicity • Spinal cord injury
Obstructive (obstruction of cardiac filling)	• Cardiac tamponade • Tension pneumothorax • Pulmonary embolism
Cardiogenic (decreased contractility)	• Congenital heart disease • Myocarditis • Dysrhythmias
Dissociative (oxygen not released from Hg)	• Carbon monoxide poisoning • Methemoglobinemia

Classification of Shock

Compensated Shock

- Vital organ perfusion maintained
- Early signs of shock include heart rate and respiratory rate above expected
- Blood pressure is maintained via vasoconstriction with perfusion to vital organs
- Nonperfused areas of the body are hypoxic with progressive dysfunction

  Note: In young children cardiac output is dependent on heart rate

Decompensated Shock

- Hypotension and impaired tissue perfusion
- First sign may be fatigue (e.g., infant with bronchiolitis and apneic episodes)
- Slowing of the heart and/or respiratory rate to normal values without improvement in condition
- Changes in peripheral perfusion: loss of peripheral pulses, capillary refill time > 3 seconds, changes in level of consciousness, and decreased urine output
- A fall in blood pressure is a late sign and signals impending cardiopulmonary arrest

Table 4.2 Compensated vs Decompensated Shock

	COMPENSATED SHOCK	DECOMPENSATED SHOCK
Appearance	Alert, anxious	Altered mental status
Work of breathing	Tachypnea, hyperpnea	Tachypnea, bradypnea
Circulation	Tachycardia, decreased peripheral pulses, cool/pale skin	Tachycardia, absent peripheral pulses, mottled/cyanotic skin

Irreversible Shock

- Multiorgan failure leading to death
- May occur hours, days, or weeks after the episode

Clinical Spectrum of Sepsis

Bacteremia

- Presence of bacteria in the blood
- *Streptococcus pneumoniae:* most common pathogen in children age 3–36 months, often self-limiting

Systemic Inflammatory Response Syndrome (SIRS)

- Clinical presentation of the body's response to a number of insults
- May be caused by viremia, fungemia, trauma, acute respiratory distress syndrome, neoplasms, burns, pancreatitis
- SIRS is marked by presence of two or more of the following:

• Temperature	$> 38°C$ (100.4°F) *or*
	$< 36°C$ (96.9°F)
• Tachycardia-heart rate	> 160/min infants
	> 150/min children
• Tachypnea-respiratory rate	> 60/min infants
	> 50/min children
	or $PaCO_2 < 32$
• White blood cell count	$> 12,000/mm^3$ *or*
	$> 10\%$ bands

Sepsis

- Systemic inflammatory response to infection with two or more SIRS criteria
- Increased risk in young children
- Common organisms:
  - Neonates: Gram negative bacilli, group B *streptococci*

- Older infants and children: *Streptococcus pneumoniae, Neisseria meningitides, Staphylococcus aureus,* group A *streptococci*
■ Risk factors:
   - Incomplete/absent immunization
   - Infants < 3 months
   - Immunocompromised children: risk of multiple or unusual pathogens
   - Varicella
   - Travel history/contacts

Severe Sepsis

Sepsis is associated with:
■ Hypotension < 5th percentile for age
   or reduction of > 40 mm Hg from baseline with no obvious cause
■ Hypoperfusion or organ dysfunction: lactic acidosis, oliguria, hypoxemia, acute alteration in mental status (GCS 3 below baseline)

Septic Shock

■ Sepsis with hypotension and perfusion abnormalities despite adequate fluid resuscitation

Multiple Organ Dysfunction Syndrome

■ Altered organ function
■ Homeostasis cannot be maintained without intervention

Management of Shock

Airway and Breathing

■ Supplemental oxygen to maintain saturation > 95%
■ Cardiorespiratory monitoring
■ Intubation if decompensated shock and/or respiratory failure

Circulation

- Volume resuscitation with saline/Ringer's lactate 20 mL/kg rapidly (5–10 minutes), then reassess
- Repeat bolus to maintain blood pressure
- Resuscitate aggressively in first hour; may need 60–100 cc/kg in first 1–2 hours
- If venous access is not rapidly obtained ("90 seconds or 3 attempts"), consider intraosseous or central venous access
- After each 20 mL/kg crystalloid bolus, consider need for inotrope or other blood product
- Controversy regarding use of colloid: beneficial or harmful effects not yet studied in children

Hemorrhagic Shock

- If no improvement after 40 mL/kg crystalloid, give packed red blood cells (PRBCs) 10 mL/kg
- If uncontrolled brisk bleeding without stabilization after first infusion of PRBCs, consider coagulation factors, plasma, platelet infusion, AND early surgical intervention

Investigations

- CBC and differential, crossmatch, blood culture
- Coagulation screen
- Blood gas, electrolytes, glucose, calcium, urea, creatinine
- Serum lactate
- Urinalysis and culture

Consider:
- Amylase, liver function tests, albumin
- Cultures of CSF, stool, throat
- Chest X-ray, other X-rays
- Toxicology/metabolic screen
- Nasogastric tube, Foley catheter
- ECG

Note: Do not delay treatment for investigations!

Drugs

Antibiotics (consider most likely organism)

- Neonate: ampicillin plus aminoglycoside or cefotaxime
- Child: cefotaxime or ceftriaxone *plus* vancomycin
- Invasive group A *streptococci*: penicillin *and* clindamycin

Inotrope and Vasopressor Support (see inside front cover)

- Consider inotrope if inadequate heart rate or cardiac contractility
- Epinephrine is the drug of choice for symptomatic bradycardia
- Dopamine improves cardiac output and tissue perfusion; high-dose effects are similar to epinephrine
- Dopamine support is frequently the first choice in pediatric shock because dose can be titrated to clinical response

Steroids and Activated Protein C

- Ongoing studies, no definitive evidence for current use in septic shock in children
- Consider steroids if patient on steroid therapy for chronic illness or if suspect adrenal insufficiency

Secondary Assessment

- History of events
- Careful head-to-toe examination
- Reevaluation after each intervention
- Arrange appropriate consultation(s)
- Admit to critical care unit

References

American College of Surgeons. *Advanced Trauma Life Support Program for physicians: ATLS.* 7th ed. Chicago, Ill: American College of Surgeons; 2001.

Annane D, Bellissant E, Cavallon JM. Septic shock. *Lancet.* 2005;365:63–78.

Burns JP. Septic shock in the pediatric patient: pathogenesis and novel treatments. *Pediatr Emerg Care.* 2003;19:112–115.

Gausche-Hill M, Fuchs S, Yamamoto L, eds. American Academy of Pediatrics and American College of Emergency Physicians. *APLS: the Pediatric Emergency Medicine Resource.* 4th ed. Sudbury, Mass: Jones and Bartlett; 2004.

McKiernan CA, Lieberman SA. Circulatory shock in children: an overview. *Pediatr Rev.* 2005;26(12):445–453.

Schexnayder SM. Pediatric septic shock. *Peds in Review.* 1999;20:303–307.

Stoll ML, Rubin LG. Incidence of occult bacteremia among highly febrile young children in the era of the pneumococcal conjugate vaccine: a study from a children's hospital emergency department and urgent care center. *Arch Pediatr Adolesc Med.* 2004;158:671–675.

5 ▪ Anaphylaxis

CAROLYN CALPIN

Introduction

- Definition: potentially life-threatening allergic reaction
- Most commonly IgE mediated reaction
- Affected systems include skin (90%), respiratory (90%), gastrointestinal, cardiac, and CNS
- May have wide range of clinical manifestations, may be subtle
- Reliance on good history and examination is crucial
- Common causative agents: food (peanuts and shellfish) and drugs (penicillin)
- Etiologic agent may not be evident
- Biphasic form:
  - Episode appears to resolve, and then symptoms recur after several hours
  - May occur in up to 30%
  - Can occur despite appropriate treatment; therefore, observe all patients for several hours
  - Late phase can occur 8–12 hours after the initial attack
  - No reliable predictors of biphasic or protracted anaphylaxis

Clinical Presentation

- Onset of symptoms within 5–30 minutes of exposure to antigen; however, symptoms may be delayed up to an hour or more
- Early administration of intramuscular epinephrine is critical
- Delayed administration of epinephrine may increase the risk of a biphasic reaction

Table 5.1	Signs and Symptoms
Respiratory	*Upper:* hoarseness, stridor, oropharyngeal or laryngeal edema, cough, complete obstruction
	Lower: bronchospasm, tachypnea, cyanosis, use of accessory muscles, respiratory arrest
Skin	Sensation of warmth, flushing, erythema, general pruritus, urticaria, angioedema
Gastrointestinal	Nausea, vomiting, crampy abdominal pain, diarrhea
Cardiovascular	Tachycardia, hypotension, arrhythmias, cardiac arrest
Neurologic	Dizziness, weakness, syncope, seizures
Other	Conjunctival injection, lacrimation, sneezing, mouth burning, itch

Etiology

Drugs: Antibiotics, chemotherapeutic agents, radiocontrast media, blood products, aspirin, NSAIDs, gamma globulin, insulin, heparin, opiates

Food: Tree nuts (cashews, almonds, pecans, walnuts), peanuts, shellfish, milk, eggs, wheat, fish, seeds (sesame, sunflower, poppy), spices (cinnamon, nutmeg, mustard, sage), fruits (apples, bananas, peaches, oranges), chocolate, potato, corn, additives

Latex

Venoms: Hymenoptera, fire ants

Exercise

Idiopathic

Differential Diagnosis

- Severe asthma
- Hereditary angioneurotic edema
- Foreign body aspiration
- Vasovagal response

- Hyperventilation syndrome
- Pheochromocytoma
- Drug overdose

Initial Management

- Secure and maintain airway, give oxygen
- If life-threatening airway obstruction occurs, intubate; if unsuccessful, perform cricothyroidotomy
- Epinephrine 1:1,000 (0.1 mg/kg), 0.01 mL/kg up to 0.5 mL intramuscularly; may repeat every 15 minutes if necessary
  - Intramuscular epinephrine injections into the thigh have more rapid absorption and higher levels than IM or SC injections in the arm
  - IM route is preferred over subcutaneous because of more rapid absorption
- If hypotensive or unresponsive to initial dose:
  - Give epinephrine 1:10,000 IV at a dose of 0.01 mg/kg (0.1 mL/kg)
  - Give IV normal saline 20 mL/kg
  - Place patient in recumbent position with feet elevated
  - If hypotension persists, administer epinephrine infusion 2–4 mcg/kg/min or dopamine 2–10 mcg/kg/min to maintain blood pressure
- Diphenhydramine 1–2 mg/kg IM or IV up to 50 mg q 4–6 h
- Methylprednisolone 1–2 mg/kg up to 125 mg IV q 4–6 h or prednisone 1–2 mg/kg PO up to 80 mg
- Consider ranitidine 1–2 mg/kg IV q 6–8 h for severe reactions
- Salbutamol/albuterol for bronchospasm; inhaled epinephrine for stridor
- Monitor vital signs frequently

Disposition

- Observe patient for at least 6–8 hours and at least 24 hours if severe reaction or history of asthma

■ Severity of clinical presentation and distance to closest ED
should be considered when deciding on length of observation
period

Discharge patient with:

■ Counseling on avoidance of allergen
■ Referral to allergist if indicated for allergy testing
■ Medication: diphenhydramine, short course of steroids
■ EpiPen® × 2: EpiPen JR® (0.15 mg) < 15 kg, EpiPen® (0.3 mg)
  > 15 kg
■ Medic-alert bracelet information

References

Brown SG. Clinical features and severity grading of anaphylaxis. *J Allergy Clin Immunol.* 2004;114(2):371–376.

Chowdhury BA. Intramuscular versus subcutaneous injection of epinephrine in the treatment of anaphylaxis. *J Allergy Clin Immunol.* 2002;109(4):720.

Holstege CP. Proper treatment of anaphylaxis. *Ann Emerg Med.* 2003; 41(3):425–426.

Lieberman P. The diagnosis and management of anaphylaxis. *J Allergy Clin Immunol.* 2005;115(3):584–591.

6 ▪ Pediatric Trauma

ANGELO MIKROGIANAKIS

Introduction

- Leading cause of death and disability in children
- Compromise of oxygenation and ventilation is common
- Compromise of perfusion is less common but potentially lethal
- Major causes of death are airway compromise and inadequate volume resuscitation
- Blunt trauma more common than penetrating injury
  - Head injury 55%
  - Internal injuries 15%

Initial management is divided into four phases:

1. Primary survey
2. Initial resuscitation
3. Secondary survey
4. Definitive treatment

Primary Survey

Follow Advanced Trauma Life Support primary assessment algorithm:

A Airway maintenance with C-spine protection
B Breathing and ventilation
C Circulation with hemorrhage control
D Disability (neurologic status)
E Exposure and environmental control

Airway

Assess and support the airway while immobilizing the cervical spine if needed:

- Use a jaw thrust without head tilt if suspect cervical spine injury
- Have suction available at all times
- Determine need for advanced airway adjuncts (intubation)

- Treat hypoxia to prevent secondary hypoxic brain injury
- Specific indications for intubation:
  - Inability to protect airway
  - Need for positive pressure ventilation
  - Airway burn or inhalational injury
  - Severe head injury GCS < 8
  - Major maxillofacial trauma

Breathing

Identify causes of respiratory failure:

- Hypoventilation due to brain injury
- Pneumothorax or tension pneumothorax
- Hemothorax
- Flail chest
- Pulmonary contusion
- Most thoracic injuries can be diagnosed by history, examination, and chest X-ray
- Open pneumothorax

Circulation

Identify signs of shock, determine cause, and implement treatment:

- Assess for hemorrhage: assess for active external bleeding and internal bleeding (such as occurs after solid organ injury)
- Establish vascular access with two large-bore IVs and provide volume resuscitation
- Identify hemodynamic instability, which may persist despite volume resuscitation: consider occult blood loss and spinal shock
- Prevent or promptly treat potential causes of secondary brain injury, including hypovolemia, hypotension, and hypoxia

Disability

Perform a rapid neurologic assessment to identify conditions that require urgent intervention:

- Apply AVPU Pediatric Response Scale

- **A**lert
- **V**erbal—responsive to verbal stimuli
- **P**ainful—responsive to painful stimuli
- **U**nresponsive
- Determine Glasgow Coma Score (GCS): see Chapter 7, Head Injury
- Examine pupils: look for unequal size, dilation, or sluggish response to light
- Consider indications for assisted ventilation (including GCS ≤ 8)

Exposure and Environmental Control

- Remove clothing, examine for injuries, measure core temperature, and maintain a neutral thermal environment
- Prevent and treat significant hypothermia

Initial Resuscitation

- Support/protect the airway
- Treat acute breathing/thoracic issues
- Establish two large-bore IVs
- If systemic perfusion is inadequate, provide rapid volume replacement with 20 mL/kg of normal saline

Routine Investigations: "Trauma Screen"

- CBC and differential, blood type, and screen
- Electrolytes, glucose, creatinine, urea
- Liver function: ALT, AST, alkaline phosphatase
- Coagulation profile: PT, PTT, INR
- Amylase
- Blood alcohol level
- Urinalysis
- If the heart rate, level of consciousness, capillary refill, and other signs of systemic perfusion do not improve, rapidly administer a second bolus of 20 mL/kg NS or RL

- If systemic perfusion does not respond to administration of 60 mL/kg of crystalloid, then consider transfusion of 10–15 mL/kg packed red blood cells

Secondary Survey

- AMPLE history (Allergies, Medications, Past history, Last meal, Events)
- Head-to-toe examination for specific injuries

Routine X-ray Examinations

- Lateral C-spine
- AP chest
- AP pelvis

Definitive Treatment

- Transfer patient from resuscitation room to radiology, OR, or ICU
- Consider need for further imaging as indicated:
  - CT head
  - CT chest
  - CT abdomen and pelvis
- Consult other services as required

Indications for Head CT

Any severe head injury requires CT head and CT scan of C1–C2

- GCS < 15 post trauma
- Abnormal neurologic exam
- Penetrating head trauma
- Any skull fracture
- Concerning mechanism of injury (e.g., fall from height)
- Progressive/worsening headache
- Bradycardia
- More than brief LOC or unknown duration of LOC

Indications for Abdominal CT

- Suspected intra-abdominal injury but no clear indication for laparotomy
- Unstable vital signs
- GCS < 10
- Planned long extra-abdominal operation (e.g., neuro, ortho)

Specific Injuries

Thoracic Injuries

- Manifestations of chest injury may be immediate or delayed by hours or days
- Must rule out immediately life-threatening injuries
  - Tension pneumothorax
  - Open pneumothorax
  - Cardiac tamponade
- Most chest injuries can be diagnosed by history, physical examination, and chest X-ray
- Chest X-rays reveal most thoracic injuries, particularly those that can be managed conservatively
- Tension pneumothorax should be drained prior to chest X-ray
- Open pneumothorax or massive flail chest requires intubation and mechanical ventilation

Abdominal Injuries

- The two main complications of blunt abdominal trauma are:
  - Bleeding—from solid organ or vascular injury
  - Peritonitis—from hollow viscus perforation
- The two main indications for laparotomy are:
  - Intra-abdominal bleeding (> 40 mL/kg of whole blood loss)
  - Peritonitis—especially if worsening on serial examination
- Gastric dilatation is common in pediatric blunt trauma
- Gastric emptying stops at the time of injury
- Gastric dilatation results from a combination of two factors:
  - Posttraumatic ileus

- Injured or frightened children swallow air
- An orogastric or nasogastric tube should be passed to prevent vomiting, aspiration, or limiting diaphragmatic excursion

Genitourinary Injuries

- Suspect in any penetrating abdominal or pelvic trauma and in all blunt abdominal/pelvic trauma associated with hematuria
- Most upper urinary tract trauma (kidneys and ureter) is managed conservatively except major vascular or ureteral injuries
- CT scan with IV contrast is the investigation of choice
- Lower urinary tract trauma (bladder and urethra) is most often associated with pelvic fractures
- Urethral catheterization is contraindicated when there is blood at the urethral meatus or a high-riding prostate on rectal examination
- If suspect urethral injury, obtain a retrograde urethrogram

References

American Heart Association and American Academy of Pediatrics. *Pediatric Advanced Life Support Provider Manual.* Dallas: American Heart Association; 2002.

Subcommittee on Advanced Trauma Life Support of the American College of Surgeons Committee on Trauma 1993–1997. *Advanced Trauma Life Support for Doctors.* 6th ed. Chicago, Ill: American College of Surgeons; 1997.

Trauma Patient Treatment Manual, 18th ed., The Hospital for Sick Children Trauma Program. Toronto: 2005.

7 ▪ Head Injury

D. Anna Jarvis

Introduction

- Head injuries are very common throughout childhood
- Male = female < 5 years
- > 5 years: boys are injured far more frequently

Causes:

- Young children: falls and child abuse
- School age: pedestrian, motor vehicle, and bicycle injuries
- Adolescents: motorized vehicles, sports, and assault

Minor Head Injury: Definition

- Considerable controversy over definition of head injury; terminology varies
- Consider circumstances surrounding injury and estimate probable forces involved
- Low-velocity, low-impact injury may result in swelling, erythema, laceration, or pain, but child remains alert and responsive
- High-velocity injuries (e.g., motor vehicle accidents) or falls greater than patient's height require careful evaluation to rule out major life-threatening injuries

Table 7.1   Severity Classification

Mild	No loss of consciousness (LOC) Normal physical examination Initial Glasgow Coma Scale (GCS) 15 Minor soft-tissue injuries
Moderate	LOC < 5 minutes Normal physical examination Initial GCS 13–15
Severe	LOC > 5 minutes One or more high-risk criteria GCS < 13

High-Risk Criteria for Significant Brain Injury

- Altered level of consciousness:
  - Unconscious
  - Decreased level of consciousness GCS < 13
  - Irritability
- Local bony abnormalities of head:
  - Skull fracture; particularly if depressed
  - Penetrating injuries
- Evidence of basal skull fracture:
  - Hemotympanum
  - Battle's sign (mastoid hematoma): may have delayed onset
  - Raccoon's eyes (periorbital hematomas): may have delayed onset
  - CSF rhinorrhea
- Unexplained focal neurologic signs
- History of previous craniotomy with shunt in site
- Posttraumatic amnesia
- Severe and worsening headache
- Posttraumatic seizure
- Blood dyscrasia or any anticoagulant medication

Scales to Assess Neurologic Status

Glasgow Coma Scale

- GCS used in older children
- Modified GCS used in infants

AVPU Scale

- A valuable rapid quick assessment tool is the AVPU scale:
  - A = Awake and aware (alert)
  - V = Responsive to verbal stimuli
  - P = Responsive to painful stimuli
  - U = Unresponsive

Table 7.2 Glasgow Coma Scale: Standard and Modified for Infants

GLASGOW COMA SCALE			MODIFIED COMA SCALE FOR INFANTS		
ACTIVITY	BEST RESPONSE	SCORE	ACTIVITY	BEST RESPONSE	SCORE
Eye opening	Spontaneous	4	Eye opening	Spontaneous	4
	To verbal stimuli	3		To speech	3
	To pain	2		To pain	2
	None	1		None	1
Verbal	Oriented	5	Verbal	Coos, babbles	5
	Confused	4		Irritable, cries	4
	Inappropriate words	3		Cries to pain	3
	Nonspecific sounds	2		Moans to pain	2
	None	1		None	1
Motor	Follows commands	6	Motor	Normal spontaneous movements	6
	Localizes pain	5		Withdraws to touch	5
	Withdraws to pain	4		Withdraws to pain	4
	Flexion response to pain	3		Abnormal flexion	3
	Extension response to pain	2		Abnormal extension	2
	None	1		None	1

Clinical Assessment

- Obtain details of trauma and changes in condition since injury
- Consider child abuse/neglect if history does not fit child's age, developmental level, and injuries
- Ask about previous injuries, review old charts
- Rule out high-risk criteria
- Physical examination with detailed neurologic assessment

Investigations

CT Head

- CT is the diagnostic procedure of choice for head injury
- Clinical evaluation can often predict high risk of significant intracranial lesions
- Risks of CT: infants may require sedation or general anesthetic, ionizing radiation may cause permanent damage

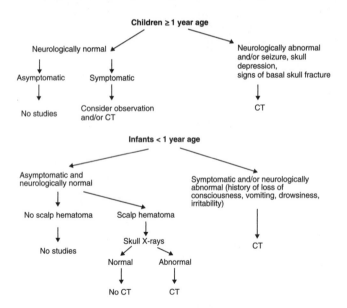

■ **Figure 7.1 Indications for Radiologic Investigation**

Other Investigations

- Shunt series: obtain if VP shunt
- Coagulation studies: if known coagulopathy or on anticoagulant treatment
- Skeletal survey and ophthalmology consult for fundoscopy if suspect child abuse
- Head circumference and CBC if infant with significant scalp swelling

Management

Mild Head Injury

- Usually no investigations indicated
  Note: Asymptomatic infants without boggy hematoma generally have no significant intracranial findings
- Safety and injury prevention education
- Assess caregiver competence to observe child at home
- Discharge with head injury instructions

Moderate Head Injury

- Observe in emergency until return to usual status and tolerating oral fluids
- Monitor neurovital signs every hour
- Consider head CT or other investigations as indicated
- Consider neurosurgical consult if symptoms persist > 4 hours or abnormal neurovitals/examination develops
- Safety and injury prevention education
- Assess caregiver competence to observe child at home
- Discharge with head injury instructions if symptoms resolve in 2–4 hours

Severe Head Injury

- ABCs
- CT head
- Consider other investigations as indicated

- Consultations as indicated:
  - Neurosurgery: abnormal CT, persistent abnormal examination findings, VP shunt
  - Hematology: coagulation disorder
- Admit

Indications for Observation in Emergency

Applies to select patients:
- Alert without focal neurologic findings
- History of brief loss of consciousness or drowsiness
- Vomiting or headache
  - Common to vomit 3–5 times following a minor head injury, or develop a nonincapacitating headache responsive to acetaminophen
- Should be observed for 4–6 hours with frequent neurovital signs

Indications for CT Head

- Presence of high-risk criteria (see above)
- Persistent vomiting
- Suspicion of abuse
- Bulging fontanelle in infant

Indications for Neurosurgical Consultation

- Loss of consciousness > 5 minutes
- Unresolving or worsening vomiting/drowsiness/headache
- Presence of high-risk criteria
- Presence/development of abnormal neurovitals or physical examination
- Potentially serious linear skull fractures (across a dural sinus, extending into foramen magnum, across path of middle meningeal artery, multiple fractures)
- Abnormal CT
- Suspicion of child maltreatment

Discharge Instructions

■ Must explicitly state that child's condition may change and symptoms/signs that indicate need for medical reevaluation:
  * Worsening headache
  * Persistent vomiting
  * Seizure
  * Weakness of extremity
  * Change in behavior or irritability

References

Berington de Gonzalez A, Darby S. Risk of cancer from diagnostic X-rays: estimates for the UK and 14 other countries. *Lancet.* 2004;363:345–351.

Hall P, Adami, HO, Trichopoulos, D, et al. Effect of low doses of ionizing radiation in infancy on cognitive function in adulthood: Swedish population based cohort study. *BMJ.* 2004;328:1–3.

Klassen TP, Reed MH, et al. Variation in utilization of computed tomography scanning for the investigation of minor head trauma in children: a Canadian experience. *Acad Emerg Med.* 2000;7(7):739–744.

National Collaborating Centre for Acute Care. Head injury: triage, assessment, investigation and early management of head injury in infants, children and adults. London (UK): National Institute for Clinical Excellence (NICE); 2003.

Quayle KS. Minor head injury in the pediatric patient. *Pediatr Clin North Am.* 1999;46(6):1189–1199.

Stein SC, O'Malley KF, Ross SE. Is routine computed tomography scanning too expensive for mild head injury? *Ann Emerg Med.* 1991; 20(12):1286–1289.

Stiell IG, et al. The Canadian CT head rule for patients with minor head injury. *Lancet.* 2001;357:1391–1396.

8 ▪ Cervical Spine Injury

CAROLYN CALPIN

Introduction

- Cervical spine injury is relatively uncommon in children
- Children more likely to sustain head trauma than cervical spine injury

Pediatric Differences

- Increased mobility of the spine in children due to:
  - Laxity of ligaments and spinous muscles
  - Anterior wedging of vertebrae
  - Shallow (horizontal) plane of facet joints, predisposes to subluxation rather than bony injury
  - Poorly formed uncinate processes (lateral superior edge of vertebral body which forms bilateral ridges): risk of SCIWORA—Spinal Cord Injury Without Radiographic Abnormality
- Larger head and weaker neck musculature in children cause 60–70% of C-spine fractures to occur in the C1/C2 range vs 16% in adults
- More room around spinal cord in children; therefore, decreased incidence of neurologic deficits
- More radiolucent cartilage in children, tapered (anterior sloped) vertebrae, multiple growth centers make X-rays difficult to interpret
- Increased incidence of physiologic subluxation in children < 8 yrs: 24% at C2/C3, 14% at C3/C4

Age	Fulcrum
< 3	C2/C3
3–8	C3/C4
9–11	C4/C5
> 12	C5/C6

- Variable interspinous distances especially between C6/C7, C1/C2

Cervical Spine Immobilization

Indications

- Trauma with severe forces (motor vehicle accident, falls > child's height)
- Trauma associated with high-risk sports (diving, football, gymnastics, hockey)
- Posttraumatic neck or back pain or tenderness
- Posttraumatic limitation of neck mobility
- Posttraumatic neurologic symptoms or signs
- Multiple system trauma
- Severe acceleration/deceleration events of the head
- Suspected cervical neck injury for any reason
- Trauma in a child with cervical spine vulnerability (Down syndrome, Klippel-Feil, Morquio, arthritis of the spine)

Immobilize with Cervical Collar and Spine Boards

Cervical Collar

- Use appropriate size collar
- If collar does not fit, use towels, other padding, or sandbags to deter movement

Spine Boards

Secure body as a unit:

- Child's neck is in relative kyphosis on hard spine board due to proportionately larger head size; can increase the risk of anterior subluxation with unstable fracture
- Place padding under torso to extend head approximately 30° (neutral)
- Align external auditory meatus with shoulders in a coronal plane
- Tape head to board to prevent additional movement of cervical spine

Radiologic Approach

ABCs: Anatomy, Alignment, Bones, Cartilage, Soft Tissues

Anatomy   Visualize entire C-spine including C7–T1 junction

Alignment   Normal lordotic curves
- Anterior vertebral line
- Posterior vertebral line
- Spinolaminar line
- Spinous process tips
- Superior tip of odontoid should align with anterior margin of foramen magnum

Bones   Anterior spinal column: vertebral bodies, intervertebral disc spaces
- Posterior spinal column: pedicles, lamina, transverse processes, articulating pillars, spinous processes
- Loss of height, abnormal wedging (> 3 mm), fractures

Cartilage   Intervertebral discs, growth plate

Soft Tissues   Predental, prevertebral spaces, anterior fat pad

Measurable Distances

Predental Space

- Dens of C2 rests posterior to anterior arch of C1 and anterior to transverse ligament permitting rotation of the neck
- Physiologic integrity of transverse ligament is reflected by predental space
- Inflammatory disorders (JRA) and other conditions (Down syndrome) can cause laxity of transverse ligament and instability at atlantoaxial level (i.e., atlantoaxial subluxation) causing an increase in the predental space
- Other causes of an increase in the predental space include Jefferson fracture or dens fracture

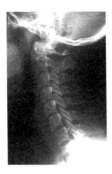

■ Figure 8.1a   Lateral View of Cervical Spine
Source: From http://www.brooksidepress.org

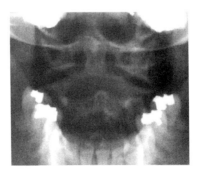

■ Figure 8.1b   Odontoid View of Cervical Spine
Source: Used with permission from Loren Yamamoto, University of Hawaii,
Kapiolani Medical Center for Women and Children. http://www.hawaii.edu/
medicine/pediatrics/pemxray/pemxray.html

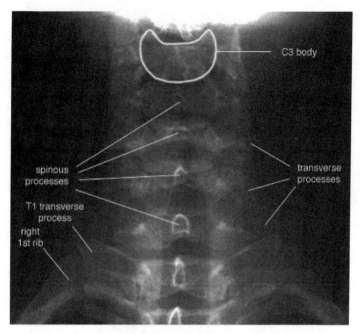

■ **Figure 8.1c   AP View of Cervical Spine**
Source: From http://www.brooksidepress.org

Posterior Cervical Line of Swischuk and Pseudosubluxation

- Pseudosubluxation with C2/C3 overrride may be a normal radiologic finding in young children
- To detect a true abnormality, draw posterior cervical line of Swischuk: if a line drawn through the cortex of spinous process of C1 to cortex of spinous process of C3 is >1–2 mm anterior to spinous process of C2, structural abnormality may be present such as a hangman's fracture

Retropharyngeal Space

- Retropharyngeal space may be widened if neck is flexed or during expiration (crying): inspiratory films should be obtained

Who Needs X-rays?

All of the following must be present to clinically clear the C-spine without radiographs:

- Age > 5 years
- Alert, interactive, no intoxication
- Normal neurologic exam at present and by history
- No neck pain, tenderness, swelling, other painful/distracting injuries (which may mask neck pain)
- No high-risk mechanism
- Normal neck mobility (observe movement)

Table 8.1   Acceptable Measurable Distances on X-ray

	ADULTS	CHILDREN
Predental space (Atlantodental interval)	3 mm	4–5 mm (to age 8)
C2/C3 override	3 mm	4–5 mm (flexion)
Retropharyngeal space (C1–C4; above glottis)	< 7 mm	Variable ($^1/_2$–$^2/_3$ vertebral body AP distance)
Retropharyngeal space (C4–C7; below glottis)	< 14 mm	2 × size of retropharyngeal space
Spinal cord size	10–13 mm	Attain adult size by age 6

Cervical Spine Radiographs

- Three-view minimum (lateral, AP, odontoid); most important initial X-ray is the cross-table lateral (identifies 75–95% of fractures, dislocations, subluxations)
- Supplemental views
  - Oblique views: greater detail of posterior spine (i.e., lamina, pedicles)
  - Flexion/extension views: ligamentous injury in stable patient
  - Swimmers view: for C7/T1 (contraindicated if high risk of abnormality)

- CT superior to MRI in delineating fractures/dislocations
- MRI superior to CT for spinal cord or soft-tissue injuries

Indications for CT Scan
- Inadequate plain film survey
- Suspicious or definite abnormalities on plain film
- If significant head trauma and patient requires CT head, CT of C1–C2 should be included

Specific Injuries
Jefferson Fracture
- Burst fracture of C1
- Caused by axial load or vertebral compression
- Often without immediate neurologic compromise
- X-ray: lateral offset of the lateral mass of C1 > 1 mm from vertebral body of C2 on odontoid view
- 1/3 associated with other C-spine fractures, most commonly C2
- Measure predental space
- Unstable, requires immediate immobilization

Hangman's Fracture
- Fracture of posterior elements of C2 due to hyperextension injury
- Hyperflexion may also occur causing subluxation of C2 on C3 and cervical cord damage
- Need to draw posterior cervical line of Swischuk to differentiate from pseudosubluxation (> 1.5–2 mm is abnormal)

Atlantoaxial Subluxation
- Due to transverse ligament laxity (severe pharyngitis, Down syndrome, arthritis, connective tissue disorder) or fracture of dens
- Widened predental space

SCIWORA (Spinal Cord Injury Without Radiographic Abnormalities)

■ Seen in children < 8 years of age
■ Accounts for 25–50% of all cervical spine injuries
■ Due to poorly formed uncinate processes (lateral superior edge of vertebral body which form bilateral ridges)
■ Displacement of vertebral elements occurs with spontaneous reduction; therefore, no bony injury seen
■ May present up to 4 days post injury
■ May have transient or delayed neurologic symptoms (paresthesias, weakness, or burning)
■ Predisposes to paraplegia and neurogenic shock

References

Betz RR. Acute evaluation and management of pediatric spinal cord injury. *J Spinal Cord Med.* 2004;27(suppl 1):S11–15.

Cirak B, Ziegfeld S, et al. Spinal injuries in children. *J Ped Surg.* 2004;39(4):607–612.

Graber MA, Kathol M. Cervical spine radiographs in the trauma patient. *Am Fam Physician.* 1999;59(2):331–349.

Martin B. Paediatric cervical spine injuries. *Injury.* 2005;36(1):14–20.

Slack SE, Clancy MJ. Clearing the cervical spine of paediatric trauma patients. *Emerg Med J.* 2004;21(2):189–193.

9 ▪ Orthopedic Injuries

SUZAN SCHNEEWEISS

Introduction
Pediatric Differences

- Bones more porous and pliable → bend, buckle, or break (greenstick fracture)
- Thick periosteum:
  - Often remains partially or entirely intact despite fracture; helps in reduction and maintenance of reduction
  - Highly vascular, role in bone formation and fracture healing
- Growth plate injuries common as growth plate (physis) cartilaginous, weaker than ligaments
- Sprains are diagnoses of exclusion
- Fractures heal more rapidly; therefore, less immobilization time

Clinical Presentation

- Children do not localize pain well, must examine entire limb
- Mechanism of injury may be difficult to obtain: need to consider common pediatric fracture patterns
- Child abuse can produce any type of fracture or injury; consider if:
  - Undisplaced avulsion fractures at metaphyses (corner or bucket handle fractures)
  - Spiral fractures in children < 2 years
  - Posterior rib fractures
  - Mechanism of injury does not fit with injury sustained
  - Delay in seeking medical attention
- Children only complain if something is wrong; immobilizing extremity should reduce pain; if persistent crying or pain, consider tight cast with nerve compression or compartment syndrome

Investigations
- Good-quality X-rays
- Selectively X-ray opposite limb if uncertainty regarding radiolucent line, growth plate, center of ossification vs avulsed fragment

Management
- Splint prior to X-ray for comfort and to minimize soft-tissue trauma
- Analgesia (see Chapter 64)
- If in doubt, immobilize extremity (see Chapter 62 for casting instructions)
- Crutches: only for children > 8 yrs
- Soft-tissue injuries
  - RICE: **R**est, **I**ce, **C**ompression, and **E**levation
  - Return to function as tolerated
  - Avoid rigorous physical activity × 3 weeks

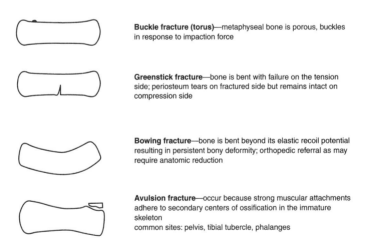

Buckle fracture (torus)—metaphyseal bone is porous, buckles in response to impaction force

Greenstick fracture—bone is bent with failure on the tension side; periosteum tears on fractured side but remains intact on compression side

Bowing fracture—bone is bent beyond its elastic recoil potential resulting in persistent bony deformity; orthopedic referral as may require anatomic reduction

Avulsion fracture—occur because strong muscular attachments adhere to secondary centers of ossification in the immature skeleton
common sites: pelvis, tibial tubercle, phalanges

▓ **Figure 9.1   Fractures Unique to Children**

Salter-Harris Fractures

- Account for 10–15% of childhood fractures
- Most heal in 3–6 weeks
- Damage to growth plate has the greatest potential for producing deformity: progressive angular deformity, limb-length discrepancy or joint incongruity

Type I: Epiphysis separates from the metaphysis
X-ray: usually appears normal; only indication of a fracture may be tenderness over the growth plate
Treatment: immobilize in a cast or backslab
Growth: unaffected

Type II: Triangular fragment of the metaphysis separates from the epiphysis; most common physeal injury
Treatment: immobilize in a cast; may require closed reduction
Growth: may cause some shortening, but rarely causes functional deformity

Type III: Intra-articular fracture extending through physis and epiphysis; tends to occur when the growth plate is partially closed
Treatment: orthopedic referral; requires accurate reduction for joint function
Growth: generally good prognosis, may have chronic sequelae

Type IV: Unstable intra-articular with fracture through metaphysis, physis, and epiphysis
Treatment: orthopedic referral; accurate reduction essential for continued growth, union, and joint function (often requires open reduction)
Growth: may lead to early fusion and growth deformity

Type V: Result of crush injury (axial force) to the growth plate; may be mistaken for a sprain or S-H type I injury
Treatment: orthopedic referral
Growth: high incidence of growth arrest

■ **Figure 9.2   Salter-Harris Fractures**
Source: The Salter-Harris classification for physical features, orthopedic trauma, *Textbook for Pediatric Emergency Medicine*, 3rd ed., 1993:1237. Used with permission from Dr. Robert Salter.

Common Injuries
Shoulder and Arm
Clavicular Fracture
- Commonly from fall onto tip of shoulder
- Treatment is supportive: immobilize in sling (figure of eight sling is *not* indicated)
  - Toddler 7–10 days, younger child 2–3 wks, older child 3–4 wks
- Consider orthopedic referral: fractures of the distal clavicle (equivalent to acromioclavicular separation), tenting of skin

Shoulder Dislocation
- Rare in children < 12 yrs
- > 95% are anterior dislocations
- Physical examination: arm held in adduction with slight internal rotation, sharp shoulder contour, prominent acromion
  - Document axillary nerve function, distal pulses
- X-ray to confirm diagnosis and post reduction films to confirm anatomic placement: AP, lateral, axillary views if possible

Treatment
- Procedural sedation
- Multiple techniques for reduction
- Traction-countertraction technique:
  - Assistant applies countertraction with a sheet wrapped around chest
  - Operator exerts linear traction on the arm, then slight lateral traction to reduce the proximal humerus
- Immobilize in sling for comfort and refer to orthopedics for follow-up
- Can resume full activity within 2–3 weeks

Complications
- Most common: recurrent instability (70–90%)
- Hills-Sachs lesion: fracture of glenoid fossa or humeral head

- Neurovascular injuries
- Osteonecrosis of humeral head

Proximal Humeral Fracture
- Most are S-H type II injuries and can be simply treated with a sling
- Large degree of angulation is generally accepted because of the tremendous remodeling potential

Humeral Shaft Fracture
- Most caused by high-energy direct blow (transverse fracture)
- If fracture with minimal trauma, consider pathologic fracture (common location for bone cysts and other benign lesions): present with localized pain, swelling, deformity
- Spiral fracture: produced by a twisting motion
  - Consider child abuse in an infant or toddler
- Treatment: Velpeau sling because most reduce themselves by gravity
- Orthopedic referral if > 15–20° angulation or rotational deformity
- Complications: radial nerve injury

Elbow

Normal X-ray Features
- Obtain two views: AP in extension and lateral in 90° flexion
- Need to consider stages of ossification: use mnemonic

	Age at ossification
C: Capitellum	1–2 years
R: Radial head	3 years
I: Internal or medial epicondyle	5 years
T: Trochlea	7 years
O: Olecranon	9 years
E: External or lateral epicondyle	11 years

Anterior Fat Pad
- Can be normal variant if narrow radiolucent strip superior to radial head and anterior to distal humerus

- If wide, also known as "sail sign" and indicative of fracture (more sensitive to small effusions and can be displaced without coexistent displacement of the posterior fat pad)

Posterior Fat Pad
- Radiolucency posterior to distal humerus and adjacent to olecranon fossa
- Not visualized on a normal lateral X-ray; if present, then abnormal

Anterior Humeral Line
- Line drawn from the anterior cortex of the humerus intersects the capitellum in its middle third
- Posteriorly displaced supracondylar fracture: anterior humeral line passes through anterior third of capitellum or may miss it entirely

Radial Axial Line
- Line drawn along the axis of the radius passes through the center of the capitellum in all projections

Figure-of-Eight
- Seen on true lateral elbow X-ray
- If disrupted, may indicate fracture

Supracondylar Fracture
- Most common between ages 3–10 years
- Most common elbow fracture (60%)
- Usually results from fall on outstretched hand with elbow hyperextended (e.g., fall from monkey bars)
- Present with localized swelling and tenderness of elbow
- Essential to ensure intact neurovascular status
- Complications include nerve injury, compartment syndrome with Volkmann's ischemia, and cubitus varus ("gunstock" deformity)

Management

Type I: nondisplaced fracture; suspect if sail sign or posterior fat pad
- Immobilize in a cast or splint with elbow at 90° flexion and forearm in neutral position for 3 weeks

Type II: angulated and displaced distal segment in which posterior cortex remains intact
- Requires orthopedic referral for reduction when capitellum is located entirely posterior to anterior border of the humerus

Type III: completely displaced distal fragment without contact between fragments and disruption of posterior periosteum
- Requires orthopedic referral for reduction +/− pin placement

Lateral Condylar Humeral Fracture
- Typically result from fall on outstretched arm
- Present with pain and decreased range of motion of elbow
- X-ray: presence of posteriorly displaced metaphyseal fragment (Thurston-Holland fragment)
- If minimally displaced, then may be difficult to diagnose; obtain oblique views

Management
- Immediate orthopedic referral
- If undisplaced, may be treated with casting alone but requires close monitoring
- Minimally displaced fractures with a large degree of soft-tissue swelling should be fixated
- Displaced fractures require open or closed reduction

Complications
- Potential for nonunion, delayed union, growth arrest, cubitus varus

Medial Condylar Humeral Fracture
- Often associated with elbow dislocation that has reduced spontaneously

- Medial epicondylar fragment visible on X-ray in older children (> 6–7 years)
- Medial epicondyle may become entirely incarcerated in the joint and have the appearance of a normal ossific nucleus
- May need comparison views

Management
- Immediate orthopedic referral
- Minimally displaced: long arm splint
- Displacement > 5 mm may need operative reduction

Complications
- Stiffness, ulnar nerve injury

Radial Head and Neck Fracture
- Radial head cartilaginous in children, resistant to fractures
- More likely to fracture radial neck, commonly associated with other injuries of the elbow
- May have localized swelling and tenderness over lateral aspect of elbow
- Pain with passive flexion and extension of elbow; increased pain with pronation and supination of forearm

Classified by Degree of Angulation
Type I: < 30° angulation, sling or posterior splint for 1–2 weeks
- If > 10 years, require closed reduction if any angulation > 15°

Type II: 30–60° angulation, orthopedic referral for open or closed reduction

Type III: > 60° angulation, orthopedic referral for open or closed reduction

Complications
- Avascular necrosis of radial head, with loss of movement

Subluxation of Radial Head (Pulled Elbow)

- "Nursemaid's elbow" caused by traction on hand with elbow extended and forearm pronated (radial head slips under annular ligament)
- Occurs in children < 6 years with peak between ages 1–3 years
- Child holds the arm pronated and partially flexed, refusing to move it voluntarily
- No visible swelling or deformity; no point tenderness
- X-rays are normal (NOT required for diagnosis with accurate history)

Management

- Reduce by supination of forearm followed by flexion of elbow to 90° with the examiner's thumb over the radial head: a click may be felt as the annular ligament slides over the radial head
- Alternate technique: hyperpronation of forearm followed by flexion of elbow
- If successful, generally child begins to use arm within 5–10 minutes; may be delayed if prolonged period of > 4–6 hrs from onset to treatment
- If maneuver does not resolve the symptoms, consider X-ray of the limb before attempting remanipulation

Forearm Fracture

- Common, 10–45% pediatric fractures
- Vary greatly; may involve one bone, both bones, and up to 50% greenstick
- Complete fractures have potential to be significantly displaced and angulated
- Most can be treated with closed reduction
- Direct trauma to forearm more likely to result in "nightstick" injury (isolated midshaft ulnar fracture); fractures of distal 1/3 present with "dinner fork" deformity

- If only one bone fractured, obtain X-rays of wrist and elbow to exclude Galeazzi or Monteggia fracture
- Monteggia fracture: fracture of proximal third of the ulna with associated radial head dislocation
- Galeazzi fracture: fracture of distal radius with associated disruption of radioulnar joint

Guidelines for Acceptable Alignment of Fractured Forearms

- < 8 years—up to 20° acceptable
- > 8 years—up to 10° acceptable

Guidelines for Acceptable Alignment of Distal Forearm Fractures

- < 5 years—up to 30° acceptable
- 5–10 years—up to 25° acceptable
- 10–12 years—up to 15° acceptable
- > 12 years—less than 15° angulation acceptable

Wrist and Hand Fractures

Scaphoid Fracture

- Most commonly fractured carpal bone
- Present with radial-side wrist pain, mild swelling in the anatomic "snuff box," and tenderness over the scaphoid
- Often have subtle findings on X-ray (should have dedicated scaphoid views)
- If suspicion, immobilize in thumb spica cast and repeat X-rays in 2–3 weeks
- If repeat films negative, may need other imaging modalities: CT, MRI, or bone scan
- If displacement or instability, open reduction and fixation are required

Hand Fractures

- Most can be treated with splinting/casting or closed reduction if necessary
- Crushed fingertips common in young children

- If significant nail trauma, look for underlying fracture distal phalanx (50%)
■ Metacarpal fractures: most commonly distal fifth metacarpal (equivalent to Boxer's fracture in adult); usually metaphyseal vs physeal injury
  - Closed reduction if > 30–40° angulation
  - Nondisplaced: gutter splint with wrist in neutral position, metacarpal phalangeal joints flexed to 70°

Indications for Immediate Surgical Referral
■ Failed closed reduction
■ Rotational deformities causing finger overlap
■ Severely angulated proximal and middle phalanx fractures
■ Displaced intra-articular fractures

Hip and Pelvis

Apophyseal Avulsion Fractures of Hip and Pelvis
■ Occur when a sudden violent concentric or eccentric contraction of the musculoskeletal unit tears an apophysis from its attachment
■ Often seen in athletes
■ Most common on the anterior inferior and anterior superior iliac spines, iliac crest, and lesser trochanter
■ Patients present acutely
■ Avulsion can often be diagnosed clinically and confirmed radiographically

Slipped Capital Femoral Epiphysis (SCFE)
■ Most important fracture of the hip (see Chapter 41)
■ Often occurs in an overweight adolescent
■ They may present with chronic thigh or knee pain or after an acute injury
■ A slipped epiphysis may not be apparent on an AP view (need a frog-legged view)

Leg and Knee

Femur Fractures

- In children under 2 years suspect child abuse
- > 2 years, caused by high-impact injuries (e.g., motor vehicle accident)
- Often associated with other injuries
- Evaluate neurovascular status
- Initial management: pain management, splinting (Thomas splint), orthopedic referral

Knee Injuries

- Meniscal and ligamentous injury are rare in children
- Hemarthrosis is often due to patellar dislocation with an osteochondral fracture or an intra-articular fracture (tibial spine fracture)
- Anterior cruciate ligament (ACL) injury becomes more common in children > 12 yrs
- X-ray with "tunnel view" to rule out small flake of bone in the intercondylar area

Tibial Spine Fracture (Fracture of Intercondylar Eminence)

- In children, often result from injuries that would cause ACL tears in adults
- Often from fall from bicycle
- Type I: Minimally displaced avulsed fragment with excellent bone apposition
- Type II: Displacement of anterior third or half (intact posterior hinge) = beak-like deformity
- Type III: Fragment completely separated from its bone bed in the intercondylar eminence with no bony apposition

Treatment

- Type I: casting with knee flexed 10–20° and refer to orthopedics
- Types II and III: immediate referral to orthopedics

Patellar Dislocation

■ Usually results from direct impact or sudden change in direction
■ Patella may reduce spontaneously or remain dislocated
■ Rule out osteochondral fracture following reduction

Patellar Apprehension Test

■ Used to detect prior dislocation or subluxation
■ Apply a laterally directed force to medial patella with knee flexed to 30°
■ If prior dislocation or subluxation, causes distress and patient becomes very apprehensive often grabbing examiner's hand to prevent further pain

Patellar Reduction

■ May require procedural sedation
■ Knee usually held in 20–30° flexion with lateral displacement of patella
■ Assistant fixes distal thigh
■ While extending the knee joint, simultaneously apply medial pressure to patella to reposition it
■ Apply knee immobilizer; restrict activity, crutches, orthopedic follow-up

Patellofemoral Pain Syndrome (PFPS)

■ Due to malalignment of the extensor mechanisms of the knee; overuse syndrome
■ May be associated with chondromalacia of patella
■ Clinical presentation: knee pain while running, sensation of knee giving way when going down stairs although does not happen, pain when sitting for a prolonged period of time with knee flexed to 90° disappears when ambulating ("movie" sign)
■ *Patellar stress test:* patient supine and knee fully extended quadriceps relaxed; move patella inferiorly and push down while asking patient to tighten quadriceps (ask patient to push knee into examining table); will elicit pain in patients with PFPS

Osgood-Schlatter Disease
- Traction apophysitis of the tibial tuberosity
- Commonly in children between ages of 10 and 15 years who participate in jumping sports
- May be asymptomatic or complain of pain at site of insertion of the distal patellar ligament
- Physical examination: tibial tuberosity tender to palpation
- X-ray: may show fragmentation of the tibial tubercle, but can be normal early on
- Rarely associated with avulsion of tibial tubercle

Management
- Rest from aggravating activities
- NSAIDs
- Often improves over time

Toddler's Fracture
- Spiral or oblique fracture through the distal third of the tibia
- Often present in children 9–36 months refusing to weight bear or limp
- May have history of minor injury
- Physical findings often subtle: minimal swelling, tenderness; passive twisting motion may elicit pain
- An internal oblique film is sometimes necessary to make the diagnosis if plain radiographs normal
- If the initial X-ray is normal, repeat X-ray in 7–10 days and consider bone scan if symptoms persist
- Treatment: immobilize for symptomatic relief

Ankle and Foot Injuries

Ankle Fractures
- In preadolescents, inversion injuries with S-H type I fractures most common
- Patient presents with swelling and tenderness over distal fibular physis

- X-rays often normal
- Treatment: immobilize in lower leg backslab

Tillaux Fracture

- Salter-Harris type III injury to distal lateral tibia
- Mechanism: lateral rotation of foot or medial rotation of leg on fixed foot
- Usually occurs as growth plate is closing in adolescents (12–14 years typically)
- Physical examination: tenderness and swelling anterolaterally, unable to weight bear
- X-ray, may need CT scan
- Treatment: closed reduction < 2 mm displacement, open reduction > 2 mm displacement

Triplanar Fracture

- Salter-Harris type IV fracture of distal tibia; three major fragments
- CT scan often required to determine degree of displacement
- Treatment: orthopedic referral for cast vs open reduction/fixation

Ankle Sprains

- More common in older children (> 12 years)
- Children usually injure distal fibular physis whereas adolescents sustain lateral sprains
- Management: functional treatment for most children
    - Aircast stirrup, ankle brace
    - Weight-bearing with crutches
    - Ice
    - Nonsteroidal antiinflammatory
    - Physiotherapy

Treatment

- *Grade 1*: most common, minor ligamentous injury, little swelling and no instability; return to sports in 1–2 weeks

- *Grade 2*: more swelling and tenderness, near complete ligamentous rupture with some ligamentous laxity, ambulate with difficulty; may require up to 2 months for return to sports
- *Grade 3*: gross instability with complete ligamentous rupture, marked swelling, tenderness, and severe pain, inability to weight bear; immobilize in cast × 3 weeks, followed by intense physiotherapy

Metatarsal Fracture
- Most common injury to foot
- Exam: swelling, pain, and bruising of forefoot, careful examination of neurovascular status
- X-ray: most fractures undisplaced or minimally displaced
- Avulsion fracture at base of 5th metatarsal
  - Common isolated foot injury resulting from eversion or adduction forces
  - May be confused with apophyseal center or accessory ossicles
  - Apophyseal center appears 8 yrs; fusion complete 12 yrs in girls, 15 yrs boys

Phalangeal Fracture: Foot
- Usually resulting from object fall onto the foot or stubbing a toe
- Heals rapidly in 3–4 weeks
- Treatment: buddy tape injured toe to its neighbor

Sever's Disease
- Calcaneal apophysitis
- Often seen in preadolescents involved in running and jumping sports
- Patient complains of heel pain, often bilateral, aggravated by activity
- Physical examination: localized tenderness of the posterior heel at the site of the insertion of the Achilles tendon
- X-rays: +/– sclerosis of secondary ossification center

Management
- Rest from aggravating activities
- NSAIDs
- Achilles tendon-stretching exercises, heel cups

References

Bachman D, Santora S. Orthopedic trauma. In: Fleisher G, Ludwig S, eds. *Textbook of Pediatric Emergency Medicine.* 4th ed. Philadelphia: Lippincott Williams & Wilkins; 2000:1435–1478.

Carson S, Woolridge DP, et al. Pediatric upper extremity fractures. *Pediatr Clin North Am.* 2006;53:41–67.

Conrad EU, Rang MC. Fractures and sprains. *Pediatr Clin North Am.* 1986;33(6):1523–1541.

Huurman WW, Ginsburg GM. Musculoskeletal injury in children. *Pediatr Rev.* 1997;18(12):429–440.

Rodriguez-Merchan CE, Radomisli TE, eds. Symposium: pediatric skeletal trauma. *Clin Orthop.* 2005;432:8–131.

10 ▪ Apparent Life-Threatening Event

GRAHAM JAY

Introduction

- An apparent life-threatening event (ALTE) in an infant is difficult to define precisely
- Presents as an acute event that is:
  - Frightening to the observer
  - Has a defined onset and offset
  - Occurs suddenly and unexpectedly
  - A combination of apnea, color change, marked change in muscle tone, choking, and/or gagging
- Often the infant will recover and appear normal when seen by prehospital providers or the physician
- The description will often be given by frightened caregivers and may not be observed by hospital staff

Occurrence

- 0.6–0.8% of all emergency visits < 1 year age
- ~ 2.5 per 1,000 live births
- Most infants are under 12 months; mean age 13 weeks
- Peak incidence 1 week–2 months of age
- No seasonal variation

ALTE vs SIDS

- Link between ALTE and subsequent SIDS (sudden infant death syndrome) is weak
- Consider ALTE and SIDS as manifestations of different disease processes
- The only prominent risk factor for both ALTE and SIDS is maternal smoking during pregnancy

■ In one retrospective study 15% of infants with SIDS had a history of ALTE
■ In a prospective study of infants with episodes of ALTE, 0% subsequently developed SIDS

History

■ Smoking: 60% of infants have a smoker within the home
■ GERD symptoms (32%), respiratory symptoms since birth (25%), recent fever (23%)
■ Two-thirds present with one of the following in the first few weeks of life: cyanotic episode, repeated apneas, pallor, difficulty feeding
■ Obtain history of:
  • Details of the event
  • Who was present? What resuscitation was given? Time to recovery?
  • Past medical and antenatal history
  • Recent health
  • Family history and social history
  • Consider fictitious illness/child abuse

Examination

■ Pay particular attention to respiratory and cardiovascular systems
■ Look for signs of nonaccidental injury
■ Plot height, weight, and head circumference on growth chart
■ Obtain oxygen saturation and glucose
■ Urine for toxicology and metabolic screen and culture if evidence of infection

Etiology

■ 40% idiopathic
■ Presence of a subsequent diagnosis may not imply causality

- Most frequent diagnoses:
  - Gastroesophageal reflux (31%)
  - Lower respiratory infection (21%)
  - Upper respiratory infection (13%)
  - Seizure (11%)
  - Pertussis (11%)
  - RSV (10%)
  - Metabolic disease (1.5%)
  - Ingestion of toxins (1.5%)
  - Urinary tract infection (1.1%)
  - Structural heart lesion (1%)
- Induced or fabricated illness or child abuse is an important although rare diagnosis

Recurrence of ALTEs

- Vary between 0–24%
- More concerning, may warrant more extensive investigation

Emergency Management

- ABCs
- Admit for investigation and monitoring

Investigations

Should be guided by history and examination, and most common diagnoses

Consider:
- GERD: pH monitoring
- Airway infection: nasopharyngeal aspirate, chest X-ray
- Seizure: cranial ultrasound, EEG, CT, MRI
- Cardiac: ECG, ECHO, Holter monitoring
- Metabolic: serum amino acids and urine organic acids, lactate, ammonia

- Infection: CBC, blood and urine cultures, septic workup
- Toxins/nonaccidental injury: urine toxicology screen, skeletal survey, CT head

Disposition

- Admit all infants
- Observe for a minimum of 24 hours
- Consider resuscitation training for parents
- Often much panic, fear, guilt, concerns about repeat episodes, risk of SIDS, and need for observation: need to address

References

Gibb SM. The management of apparent life-threatening events. *Curr Paediatr.* 1998;8:152–156.

Kiechl-Kohlendorf U. Epidemiology of apparent life-threatening events. *Arch Dis Child.* 2005;90:297–300.

McGovern MC. Causes of apparent life-threatening events in infants: a systematic review. *Arch Dis Child.* 2004;89:1043–1048.

11 ▪ Newborn Emergencies

SUZAN SCHNEEWEISS

Introduction

- Need to distinguish between benign conditions/normal variants and critical neonatal illness
- Signs and symptoms of critical neonatal illness often nonspecific
  - Red flags: poor feeding, vomiting, lethargy, cyanosis, apnea, seizures, hypo/hyperthermia, excessive weight loss

Table 11.1 Normal Variants	
Uric acid crystals in diaper	• Appearance: red brick dust • Differentiate from blood: negative urine dipstick or guaiac test
Harlequin sign	• 5% of newborns; upper half of body appears pale and dependent half turns deep red • Transient phenomenon lasting seconds to minutes and is altered by changing position of baby • If episodes beyond 4 wks, consider CV abnormalities
Transient cutis marmorata	• Mottling or marbling of skin accompanies acrocyanosis and occurs when infant is cold
Breast tissue hypertrophy	• May be seen in both males and females during first postnatal week; may remain enlarged well into first year • Do not squeeze as this often leads to abscess formation

Table 11.2   Benign Conditions

Cephalohematoma	• Becomes more apparent and increases in size several days after birth; resolves spontaneously
Nasal congestion or stuffiness	• Mucous membrane swelling from repetitive suctioning of nose • Unilateral usually associated with deformity of nose which resolves spontaneously • Consider an acute viral infection and congenital syphilis: "snuffles"
Fractured clavicle	• Superficial swelling and loss of normal distinct edge of clavicle
Torticollis	• Fibrotic shortening of sternocleidomastoid muscle resulting from hemorrhage within muscle belly at time of birth • Infant holds head to one side; 1–3 cm swelling on contralateral side of neck • Treatment: range of motion exercises
Umbilical granulomas	• Hypertrophic granulation tissue at base of stump • May have serosanguinous drainage • Differential diagnosis: umbilical polyp (urachal or omphalomesenteric duct anomaly) • Treat with cauterization with silver nitrate stick or double ligature technique to surgically remove

Table 11.3   Transient Benign Cutaneous Lesions

Milia	• Common; due to retention of keratin and sebaceous material in pilosebaceous unit • 1–3 mm whitish papules on nose, cheeks, upper lip, and forehead; disappear spontaneously in first month of life

Table 11.3   Transient Benign Cutaneous Lesions (continued)

Sucking blisters	• Bullae found on thumb, index finger, dorsum of hand or wrist; secondary to continued sucking in utero
Neonatal acne	• 20% of infants; appears after 1–2 weeks, resolves spontaneously within 6 months • Inflammatory papules and pustules
Erythema toxicum neonatorum	• 20–60% newborns; onset 24–72 hours of life • Erythematous macules, papules, wheals, vesicles, and pustules; evanescent waxing and waning appearance; disappear within 2 weeks
Transient neonatal pustular melanosis	• Vesiculopustular lesions that rupture in a few days leaving well demarcated 2–3 mm hyperpigmented lesions with a collarette of scale that fades to hyperpigmented macules; disappear within weeks to months • More common in African-American newborns (2–5%) • No treatment required
Miliaria	• Due to obstruction of sweat glands • Miliaria crystalline: 1–2 mm grouped flaccid vesicular lesions with no associated erythema • Miliaria rubra (prickly heat): confluent tiny, scaly, erythematous papules or papulovesicular lesions • Avoid excessive heat, occlusive clothing or devices

Cutaneous Lesions Requiring Treatment

Staphylococcal pyoderma

- Due to *Staphylococcus aureus* colonization in first few weeks of life
- Vesicles, pustules, and bullae arising on normal or slightly erythematous skin; bullae rupture easily to leave superficial erosion with a collarette of scale
- Common sites: periumbilical region, neck folds, axillae, and diaper area
- Diagnosis: Gram stain and culture of contents of bullae or pustule
- Treatment: topical antibiotic ointment if localized, but most infants require oral therapy with cloxacillin or a cephalosporin

Staphylococcal Scalded Skin Syndrome

- Due to endotoxin from certain *Staphylococcus aureus* strains
- Onset between 3–7 days with fever, irritability, cutaneous tenderness and erythema; flaccid bullae that rapidly denude on erythematous base
- Nikolsky sign: rubbing of skin causes skin separation
- Treatment: intravenous cloxacillin

Neonatal Candidiasis

- Due to *C. albicans* often in first weeks of life; often involves diaper area and oral mucosa (thrush)
- Erythematous scaly patches with characteristic satellite papules and pustules
- Topical therapy with an imidazole cream for skin rash

Herpes Neonatorum

- HSV 1 or 2; 80% due to HSV 2—poorer prognosis
- Route of transmission usually occurs during delivery (85%), but may occur in utero (5%) or postnatally (10%)
- Highest risk of transmission in pregnant women with primary infection in third trimester (50%)

- May occur in absence of skin lesions; need high index of suspicion
- 60–80% of infected infants born to mothers with no history of genital herpes

Clinical Manifestations

SEM: skin, eye, mouth

- Presents at ~ day 10–11
- Discrete vesicles and keratoconjunctivitis
- Risk of neurologic impairment 30–40% if do not receive antiviral therapy
- 75% progress to either CNS or disseminated disease without antiviral treatment; therefore, all require aggressive treatment

CNS disease (encephalitis)

- May present with seizures (50%), lethargy, irritability, tremors, poor feeding, temperature instability, bulging fontanelle, and pyramidal tract signs
- CSF culture positive in 25–40%; generally have proteinosis and pleocytosis (50–100 WBC/mm^3) with predominantly mononuclear cells
- 40% do not have cutaneous vesicles at presentation
- High incidence of morbidity and mortality despite treatment

Disseminated disease

- Present generally at day 9–11 of life
- Multiple organ involvement and signs: irritability, seizures, respiratory distress, jaundice, bleeding diatheses, shock, and often vesicular rash
- 22% of HSV-infected neonates
- 70% survival with treatment; 15% neurologic abnormalities

Investigations

- Look for disseminated infection (visceral) and CNS disease
  - CBC, LFTs, LP with CSF (including PCR), CXR (respiratory symptoms)

- Viral culture from skin, conjunctiva, mouth and throat, rectum, urine
- PCR assays more sensitive than culture for neurologic infection

Treatment

- Intravenous acyclovir for 14–21 days (21 days if CNS involvement or disseminated disease)
- Monitor neutrophil count if receiving IV acyclovir (neutropenia)

Infantile seborrheic dermatitis

- Self-limited inflammatory condition, usually appears within 3–8 weeks of life
- Well-demarcated areas of erythema covered by greasy scale over scalp (cradle cap), face, diaper area, trunk, and proximal flexures
- Treatment: olive oil to loosen scales on scalp and mild topical hydrocortisone cream or ointment to involved areas

Jaundice

- Imbalance between production and elimination of bilirubin
- Occurs in 60–70% of term infants and most premature infants
- Visual estimation of degree of jaundice poor
- Severe jaundice and kernicterus can occur in full-term healthy newborns with no apparent hemolysis or any cause other than breastfeeding
- Increased risk of kernicterus with G6PD deficiency

Clinical Evaluation

- Assess adequacy of breastfeeding
  - Weight loss (average 6.1% by day 3)
  - Urine output (4–6 wet diapers) and 3–4 stools/day
- Acute bilirubin encephalopathy
  - Clinical neurologic findings caused by bilirubin toxicity

- Early phase: lethargy, hypotonia, poor feeding
- Intermediate phase: stupor, irritability, and hypertonia; fever, high-pitched cry; may alternate with drowsiness and hypotonia
- Late phase: pronounced *retrocollis-opisthotonos,* shrill cry, no feeding, apnea, fever, deep stupor to coma, seizures → death

Major Risk Factors for Jaundice
- Predischarge total serum bilirubin in high-risk zone
- Jaundice in first 24 hours
- Gestational age 35–36 weeks
- Previous sibling requiring phototherapy
- ABO incompatibility with positive Coombs or other hemolytic disease
- Cephalohematoma or significant bruising
- Adequacy of breastfeeding
- East Asian race

Investigations
- Total and direct bilirubin
- Coombs test, blood type, and Rh
- G6PD screen
- If direct hyperbilirubinemia, evaluate for UTI, sepsis if indicated
- Check newborn screening—thyroid function and galactosemia screen

Management
- See guidelines for phototherapy
- Total serum bilirubin (TSB) > 428 mol/L: immediate admission to NICU for intensive phototherapy
- IV gamma globulin for isoimmune disease if TSB level rising despite phototherapy

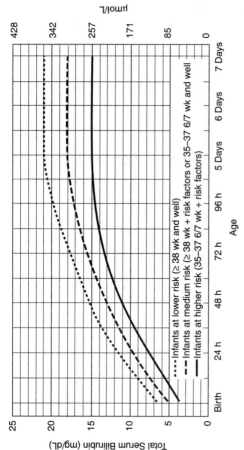

■ **Figure 11.1 Guidelines for Phototherapy for Infants > 35 Weeks Gestation**
Source: With permission from AAP. *Pediatrics.* 2004;114:1:304.

Guidelines for Exchange Transfusion

Immediate exchange:
- Signs of bilirubin encephalopathy
- TSB > 85 μmol/L above curve

Fever

Definition: temperature > 38°C (100.4°F) rectally

Serious Bacterial Infection in Febrile Infants

- Bacteremia, meningitis, UTI, pneumonia, gastroenteritis, osteomyelitis, suppurative arthritis, or skin and soft-tissue infection
- Infants < 28 days:
  - Higher incidence of *E. coli* and group B *Streptococcus* (67%)
  - *H. influenza* and *Strept. pneumoniae* (10%)
- Other organisms: *Salmonella* species, *Staphylococcus aureus*, *Listeria monocytogenes*, *Enterococcus*, *Neisseria meningitidis*

Evaluation and Treatment of Fever

Infants < 28 days: full septic workup (FSWU), admit, parenteral antibiotics

Infants < 60 days:
- If fail to meet Rochester criteria: FSWU—CBC, blood culture, urine culture, LP ± CXR admit, parenteral antibiotics
- If meet Rochester criteria: CBC, blood culture, urinalysis + culture ± LP, admit, antibiotics
- IV ampicillin + cefotaxime (meningitis/sepsis)
- IV ampicillin + gentamicin (sepsis–neonate)

Vomiting

- Bilious vomiting in the neonate indicates malrotation until proven otherwise
- Delay in passage of meconium for > 24 hrs in a term baby or > 48 hrs in a preterm baby requires investigation

Table 11.4 Causes of Vomiting in the Newborn	
NONBILIOUS VOMITING	BILIOUS VOMITING
GE reflux	Malrotation
Infection: pneumonia, UTI, meningitis, gastroenteritis	Intestinal atresias
	Hirschsprung's disease
Metabolic	Meconium ileus
Uremia	Meconium plug syndrome
Increased intracranial pressure	Necrotizing enterocolitis
Surgical: pyloric stenosis, proximal duodenal atresia, esophageal atresia ± tracheoesophageal fistula	

Pyloric Stenosis

- Most common in whites of North European descent, less in African-American, rare in Asian or Indian race
- M:F 4:1, first-born males more common
- Genetic predisposition

Clinical Presentation

- Occurs between 1–10 weeks of age
- History of projectile, nonbilious vomiting often 30–60 min after feeding
- Jaundice in 2%
- Dehydration, weight loss
- May see visible gastric contractions in a wave-like manner from left to right
- "Olive"
  - Smooth, hard, oblong mass 1–2 cm palpated in epigastrium or just to right of midline
  - Feed sugar water during exam to relax baby or NG tube to suction

Diagnostic Findings
- Hypochloremic hypokalemic metabolic alkalosis
- Ultrasound criteria: pyloric diameter ≥ 15 mm, pyloric length ≥ 4 mm

Management
- Correction of metabolic abnormalities and dehydration, surgical referral

Hirschsprung's Disease
- Congenital absence of ganglion cells in submucosal and myenteric plexus of distal bowel
- Variable loss of ganglion cells above anorectal junction
- Aganglionic segment lacks normal bowel motility → results in dilatation of upstream bowel with functional obstruction

Clinical Presentation
- Suspect in newborn if delayed passage of meconium > 48 hrs
- Refusal to feed, vomiting, abdominal distention, failure to thrive
- Severe constipation from birth
- Rectal examination: tight anus, empty rectal ampulla

Investigations
- Abdominal X-ray: dilated bowel loops, lack of stool, or gas in pelvic rim
- Barium enema: 80% accuracy
  - Transitional zone: funnel-shaped dilatation of bowel at junction of aganglionic and ganglionic gut
- Consult surgery for rectal manometry and biopsy

Complications
- May have long-term constipation after surgical pull-through operation

- Enterocolitis:
  - Up to 33% after surgical correction
  - Proliferation of bacteria secondary to stasis
  - Abdominal distension and tenderness, explosive diarrhea, fever, vomiting, lethargy, hematochezia, shock
  - Abdominal X-ray: distended bowel loop along left flank, with abrupt termination in the pelvis ("intestinal cut off sign")
  - Management: NPO, NG, IV fluids, bowel rest, rectal tube drainage, antibiotics (ampicillin, gentamicin, metronidazole)
  - Urgent surgical referral

Gastroesophageal Reflux

- Involuntary passage of stomach contents into esophagus
- Common; most resolve by 1 year age
- Physiologic vs pathologic

Complications

- Esophagitis: irritability, chronic crying, feeding resistance, dysphagia
- Anemia, hematemesis
- Failure to thrive
- Respiratory symptoms
- ALTE

Investigations

- None routinely recommended
- If concern of pathologic reflux, consider upper GI series and pH monitoring

Management

- Parental reassurance
- Thickening feeds: does not improve reflux index scores, but clinically may result in decrease in number of vomiting episodes

- Formula-fed infants: 1- to 2-week trial of hypoallergenic formula
- Prone position improves reflux but higher risk of SIDS; NOT recommended
- Prokinetic agents controversial, not routinely recommended
- Trial of ranitidine may be helpful for esophagitis

Congenital Heart Disease (CHD)

- One-third develop symptoms in first few days of life
- Presence or absence of murmur is not a reliable sign for diagnosis of CHD
- Intensity of murmur may not be related to significance of defect
- Often divided into cyanotic vs acyanotic heart disease

Cyanotic Congenital Heart Disease

- Normal O_2 saturation: right heart 70–75%; left heart 95–98%
- Some lesions are duct-dependent → develop cyanosis when duct closes
- 5 Ts: **T**etralogy of fallot (TOF), **T**ransposition of the great arteries (TGA), **T**ricuspid atresia (TA), **T**otal anomalous pulmonary venous drainage (TAPVD), **T**runcus arteriosus
- Severe left-sided outflow obstruction: critical aortic stenosis, hypoplastic left heart, and severe coarctation of the aorta

Clinical Presentation

- Generalized or central cyanosis (differentiate from acrocyanosis)
- Signs of shock: poor distal perfusion, cool extremities, weak cry, tachycardia
- Quiet tachypnea ± respiratory distress

Initial Evaluation

- Central vs peripheral cyanosis
- O_2 challenge (hyperoxia test): 100% oxygen by face mask; in cyanotic heart disease PaO_2 will only increase slightly (< 100 mm Hg)

- CXR
  - Look for abnormally shaped heart (e.g., boot shaped: Tetralogy of Fallot)
  - Increased pulmonary vascularity: TAPVD, Truncus, TGA
  - Decreased pulmonary vascularity: TOF, Ebstein's anomaly, hypoplastic right heart
- ECG
- Arterial blood gas
- Echocardiogram

Management
- ABCs
- 100% oxygen 10–15 L/min; consider elective intubation if significant respiratory distress
- Baseline bloodwork: CBC, electrolytes, arterial blood gas
- Prostaglandin E1: to maintain open ductus
  - 0.05–0.1 mcg/kg/min and increase to 0.2 mcg/kg/min over several minutes
  - Side effects: apnea, pulmonary congestion, fever, hypotension, seizures, diarrhea
  - Consider elective intubation if apnea or to decrease work of breathing
- If shock, give normal saline fluid bolus 10 mL/kg; reevaluate for cardiac overload
- Consider diuretics to treat fluid retention
- Consider dobutamine 2–20 mcg/kg/min to augment cardiac contractility

Cardiovascular Collapse

- Consider cardiac (hypoplastic left heart, coarctation of aorta, critical aortic stenosis, interrupted aortic arch), sepsis, intracranial bleed, metabolic/genetic
- History of poor feeding, poor output, tachypnea, poor color, lethargy
- Evaluation

- Initial stabilization—ABCs
- CXR, ECG, 4 limb BP
- Prostaglandin E1
- Inotropes
- Antibiotics

Acyanotic Congenital Heart Disease

- May present with congestive heart failure or heart murmur
- Lesions with increased pulmonary vascularity: ASD, VSD, PDA, AVSD
- Lesions with normal pulmonary vascularity: aortic stenosis, pulmonary stenosis, coarctation

Congestive Heart Failure

Clinical Presentation

- Signs and symptoms more insidious
- Murmur may not appear until 2 weeks to 2 months of life
- Excessive pulmonary circulation (left to right shunt): tachypnea, tachycardia, diaphoresis, irritability, poor weight gain, murmur, gallop rhythm, poor feeding, palpable liver
- Ventricular failure
  - More acute presentation
  - Myocarditis, dilated cardiomyopathy, anomalous left coronary artery from pulmonary artery (may present with myocardial infarction)

Evaluation

- Chest X-ray: cardiomegaly, increased pulmonary flow
- ECG
- Echocardiogram

Initial Management

- Oxygen, monitors
- Consider elective intubation if significant distress without improvement with initial management

- IV access with baseline bloodwork—CBC, electrolytes
- Diuretics: furosemide 0.5–2 mg/kg
- Consult cardiology

Arrhythmia (see Chapter 21, Cardiac Emergencies)

Most common: supraventricular tachycardia
- 25% have congenital heart defects
- 60% present in the first 4 months of life
- Many outgrow by 1 year
- Treatment: adenosine 80–90% successful

Neonatal Seizures

- Differentiate from jitteriness or benign sleep myoclonus
- Few idiopathic seizures in neonates; search for etiology
- Focal seizures may be due to metabolic disturbance, not focal structural lesion

Classification

- May be difficult to identify
- EEG may not be abnormal as may be brain stem or subcortically mediated
- Newborns rarely have generalized tonic-clonic seizures
- Clonic: focal or multifocal, tonic, myoclonic, subtle, motor automatisms
- Subtle: bicycling, lip smacking, roving eye movements, ocular fixation or deviation, apnea, mouthing movements, stereotypical limb movements

Etiology

- Most common: hypoxic ischemic encephalopathy
- Others: intracranial hemorrhage, infections, cerebral malformations, inborn errors of metabolism, metabolic disturbances, toxins
- Benign idiopathic neonatal seizures, benign familial neonatal convulsion are diagnoses of exclusion

- *Fifth-day fits:* term infants, seizures in first week of life, often clonic, duration < 24 hours
- *Familial neonatal seizures:* onset day 2 or 3 of life, partial or generalized; family history of similar events

Investigations

- Dextrostix and blood glucose STAT
- CBC and diff; electrolytes, calcium, blood cultures
- Full septic workup
- Metabolic workup (see section below)
- Head ultrasound/CT head
- EEG

Treatment

- ABCs
- Correction of acute metabolic abnormalities
  - Hypoglycemia: 10% glucose 2–4 mL/kg IV
  - Hypocalcemia: 50–200 mg/kg 10% Ca gluconate IV over 30 min
  - Hyponatremia: if Na < 125 mg/dL and actively seizing, 3% saline 5 mL/kg
- Anticonvulsants
  - Lorazepam 0.05–0.1 mg/kg IV
  - Phenobarbital 20 mg/kg IV followed by boluses of 5 mg/kg to maximum of 40 mg/kg
  - Phenytoin (fosphenytoin) 20 mg/kg IV
- Broad spectrum antibiotics
  - Treatment for possible meningitis/sepsis should not be delayed for LP
- Consider antiviral therapy (acyclovir)
- Consider IV pyridoxine for prolonged seizure with EEG monitoring
- Consider continuous EEG monitoring

Metabolic Disease of the Newborn

- Initial symptoms often nonspecific: poor feeding, poor weight gain, vomiting, altered mental status, irritability, tachypnea, tachycardia, seizures
- Uncommon, but early recognition may significantly affect long-term morbidity
- Newborn screening may only test for select diseases (such as, phenylketonuria, hypothyroidism, galactosemia (check local screening programs)
- Suspect if:
  - Acidosis or altered mental status out of proportion to systemic findings
  - Unusual odor
  - Hypertonia or abnormal tone
  - Hiccups
  - Family history—consanguinity, neonatal deaths in siblings, or affected males on mother's side of the family
  - Persistent hypoglycemia
  - Ketones in urine

Metabolic Signs

- Hypoglycemia—especially if associated with metabolic acidosis, ketonuria, or both
- Hyperammonemia—look for urea cycle disorders, organic acidemias, and transient hyperammonemia of the newborn
  - Acidosis + urinary ketones: consider organic acidemia
  - Acidosis, no urinary ketones: consider fatty-acid oxidation defect
  - No acidosis: consider urea cycle defect
- Acidosis—estimation of anion gap
  - Normal anion gap does not exclude metabolic disease

Investigations

Critical Blood Sample:
- Serum electrolytes, urea, creatinine, glucose
- Venous/arterial blood gas
- Liver function tests, ammonium
- Lactate, pyruvate (arterial sample best)
- Quantitative plasma amino acids
- Free fatty acids/3-hydroxybutyrate
- Ketones
- Insulin

Other Tests:
- Urine: organic acids, amino acids, ketones
- Specialized tests: total and free carnitine, plasma acylcarnitine, urine acylcarnitines
- CSF glycine, lactate
- Galactosemia screen, PKU screen—if not done at birth
- Urine clinitest: reducing substances

Emergency Management

- ABCs
- Stop oral feeds
- IV D10W + 0.2 NS at 150% maintenance after obtaining critical blood sample
- Metabolic consult

References

American Academy of Pediatrics. Subcommittee on Hyperbilirubinemia. Management of hyperbilirubinemia in the newborn infant 35 or more weeks of gestation. *Pediatrics*. 2004;114:1:297–316.

Brousseau T, Sharieff GQ. Newborn emergencies: the first 30 days of life. *Pediatr Clin N Am*. 2006;53:69–84.

Burton DA, Cabalka AK. Cardiac evaluation of infants, the first year of life. *Pediatr Clin N Am*. 1994;41(4):991–1015.

Gerdes JS. Diagnosis and management of bacterial infections in the neonate. *Pediatr Clin North Am.* 2004;51:939–959.

Goodman SI, Greene CL. Metabolic disease of the newborn. *Peds in Review.* 1994;15(9):359–365.

Hulka F, Campbell TJ, Campbell JR. Evolution in the recognition of infantile hypertrophic pyloric stenosis. *Pediatrics.* 1997;100:E9.

Kimberlin D. Herpes simplex virus, meningitis and encephalitis in neonates. *Herpes.* 2004;11(suppl 2):65A–76A.

Orenstein SR, Izadnia F, Khan S. Gastroesophageal reflux in children. *Gastroenterol Clin of North Am.* 1999;28:947–969.

Ross AJ. Intestinal obstruction in the newborn. *Pediatr Rev.* 1994;15(9):338–347.

Swenson O. Hirschsprung's disease: a review. *Pediatrics.* 2002;109:914–918.

Zip C, Singhal N. Skin lesions in neonates. *Paediatrics Child Health.* 1996;1(1):25–32.

Zupanc ML. Neonatal seizures. *Pediatr Clin North Am.* 2004;961–978.

■ PART II
HEAD AND NECK EMERGENCIES

12 ▪ Eye Emergencies

Carolyn Calpin

Definitions

- Globe: the eye
- Anterior segment: cornea; anterior chamber: iris, and lens
- Posterior segment: vitreous body, retina, and optic nerve
- Closed globe injury: no full thickness eye wall injury
- Open globe injury (ruptures, perforating, penetrating injury): full thickness eye wall injury
- Anterior iritis: WBC in anterior chamber
- Microhyphema: blood in anterior chamber without settling or layering out (slit lamp diagnosis)
- Hyphema: blood in anterior chamber that has settled or layered
- Eight ball hyphema: blood filling entire anterior chamber (eye looks like an "eight ball")
- Leukocoria: white pupil (traumatic cataract)
- Ciliary flush: conjunctival redness at sclera-corneal junction

Eye Injury History

- When, where, and how did the incident occur
- Mechanism of injury: blunt, penetrating, foreign body
- Initial intervention at scene
- Does patient wear glasses or contacts
- Vision now compared to previous
- Pain, photophobia, foreign body sensation, discharge, tearing
- Headache, nausea, vomiting, lethargy
- Pertinent past medical and ocular history

General Eye Examination

Visual Acuity

- First and most important component of eye exam
- Many preschool children do not have 20/20 acuity
- A difference of more than 2 lines on the chart between the eyes is more significant than absolute acuity
- Pinhole exam will help decipher if preexisting refractive error (i.e., if VA improves with pinhole, then refractive error)

External Eye Examination

- Position of globe: exophthalmos, enophthalmos
- Lids: laceration, integrity of lid margin, function
- Cornea: clarity (clouding)
- Sclera or conjunctival laceration, foreign body, or hemorrhage
- Anterior chamber: depth and clarity
- Pupil: shape, size, reactivity to light
- Red reflex: symmetry
- Ocular motility: nine positions
- Visual fields

Fundoscopic Examination

- Papilledema
- Retinal or vitreous hemorrhage

Fluorescein Stains

- Only detects corneal epithelial defects (i.e., 3 layers to cornea: epithelium, stroma, endometrium; therefore, will not detect deeper stromal endometrium defects)

Procedure
- Use fluorescein strip moistened with saline and touch lightly to bulbar conjunctiva while patient looks up; use blue light on ophthalmoscope to assess corneal integrity
- Corneal defect will stain green

X-ray Studies
■ Water's view orbital rim (fracture)
■ CT scan: localization of a foreign body or facial fracture

Eye Injuries (See Table 12.1)
■ Intraocular
■ Perforating: cornea, sclera, lens, retina, intraocular foreign body
■ Nonperforating: hyphema, vitreous hemorrhage, retinal detachment, traumatic cataract, corneal abrasion
■ Extraocular: lid laceration, foreign body of lid

References

Friedman LS, Kaufman LM. Guidelines for pediatrician referrals to the ophthalmologist. *Pediatr Clin North Am.* 2003;50(1):41–53.

Tomazzoli L, Renzi G, Mansoldo C. Eye injuries in childhood. *Eur J Opthalmol.* 2003;13(8):710–713.

Table 12.1   Eye Injuries

CONDITION	PERTINENT FINDINGS	MANAGEMENT
Perforated/ruptured globe	• Common sources of injury: guns (pellet, BB gun, paintball), tree branches • History of significant trauma to eye or seemingly benign trauma caused by a high-velocity object • Symptoms of increased intraocular pressure: eye pain, nausea/vomiting (sensitive indicator), decreased vision, corneal clouding	• Have patient lie supine and stabilize head • Ask patient to open eyes, do not touch lids • Look for: prolapse of brown uveal tissue through wound, peaked tear-shaped pupil (i.e, key hole pupil) pointing to wound • Assess visual acuity—decreased visual acuity suggestive of significant injury • Shield eye, keep in bed with head elevated 40° • Immediate ophthalmologic consult
Posterior globe rupture	• Severe, blunt trauma • Symptoms of increased intraocular pressure	• Normal pupil, decreased vision, abnormal red reflex
Intraocular foreign body	• Striking metal on metal, high-speed missile • Suspect intracranial penetration with long objects, or high speed • Retained organic material increases risk of infection because delayed repair is associated with much higher risk of enophthalmitis	• Must consider possibility of intraocular foreign body, can be present with little evidence on external exam • No blood supply in the eye; therefore high risk of enophthalmitis once globe integrity is breached • Refer to ophthalmology • CT scan • Admit for intravenous antibiotics +/− surgery

Table 12.1 Eye Injuries (continued)

CONDITION	PERTINENT FINDINGS	MANAGEMENT
Retinal detachment	• Spontaneous sudden monocular loss of vision, painless, flashes and floaters • Curtain across vision, pupil—normal, red to grayish visual reflex—field defects	• Refer to ophthalmology
Hyphema	• Usually follows blunt trauma • May complicate a penetrating injury • Traumatic forces can tear iris vessels, resulting in bleeding into anterior chamber of eye • Most damage caused by hyphema is secondary to increased intraocular pressure	Associated injuries: 1. Increased intraocular pressure 2. Secondary hemorrhage: highest risk in first 5 days 3. Ischemic optic neuropathy • Refer to ophthalmology Admission: 1. Increased IOP 2. Eight ball hyphema Outpatient: 1. Bedrest 40° 2. Daily follow-up for 5 days • Topical steroids, cycloplegics
Traumatic iritis/cataract	• Iritis: commonly associated with hyphema • Photophobia, tearing • Ciliary flush • Cataract—lens subluxation or penetration	• Diagnosed by slit lamp exam; WBCs in anterior chamber • Leukocoria (white pupil) • Refer to ophthalmology *(continues)*

Table 12.1 Eye Injuries (continued)

Condition	Pertinent findings	Management
Chemical burns	• Most exposures are mild and caused by accidental splashing of household chemicals into the eyes • Alkali burns penetrate rapidly and deeper into tissues, more damaging than acids	• Copious irrigation—saline: continuous flow using IV tubing attached to 1L saline bag, held over eye × 20 min
Corneal abrasion	• Corneal epithelial defect (i.e., superficial) • Most common eye injury in the emergency department • Minor trauma to the eye, pain, photophobia, tearing	• Fluorescein positive and normal vision • Important to search for a foreign body and perform complete eye exam to rule out associated injuries (evert lid) • Eye patching does not affect rate of healing, discomfort, or daily activities • Normally heals in 1–2 days
Subconjunctival hemorrhage	• Associated with trauma (birth), coughing, valsalva maneuver, or coagulation disorder	• Vision is normal • Blood surrounding pupil • Resolves within 1–2 weeks • Refer to ophthalmology if 360°
Foreign body lid	• Difficult to open eye, tearing, photophobia, FB sensation	• Eversion of lid and sweep • Fluorescein stain may show corneal abrasions with repetitive linear patterns

Table 12.1 Eye Injuries (continued)

CONDITION	PERTINENT FINDINGS	MANAGEMENT
Eyelid lacerations	• Careful examination of lacerations of eyelid because may involve globe	Ophthalmology consult if: • Laceration involves eyelid margin • Involvement of lacrimal system • Significant exposure of ocular surfaces

13 ■ Dental Emergencies

Introduction

- Treatment often delayed because parents may not be able to detect seriousness of injury
- Over one third of preschool children suffer trauma that affects their primary teeth
- Maxillary anterior primary teeth are affected most often

Assessment

- Systematic approach to soft tissues and teeth is required
- Knowledge of normal sequence of primary and permanent tooth eruption is essential

History

- Mechanism and time of injury, where injury occurred
- Immunization status as dental trauma may coexist with soft-tissue injury; tetanus prophylaxis may be required
- Temperature sensitivity, pain, mobility of teeth
- Consider nonaccidental trauma if injuries inconsistent
- Child abuse may present with maxillofacial or dental injury
- Past dental problems and treatment

Extraoral Examination

Inspection

- Symmetry of face, both frontal, profile, and with neck extended: asymmetry may indicate fracture of mandible or abscess
- Skin: hematoma, bruising, lacerations
- Mouth: range and symmetry of mandibular movement
- Lips: color, swelling, ulceration, laceration

Palpation

- Palpate TMJ joints as patient opens and closes mouth: look for pain and tenderness over condyles: may indicate subcondylar fracture
- Equal movement of jaw on both sides without deviation
- Palpate along entire mandible
- Palpate orbital rim, zygoma, nose
- Palpate neck for nodes/swellings/abscesses/masses
- Test for sensation over facial skin: deficits or numbness may indicate trigeminal nerve disruption

Intraoral Examination

Good light source necessary

Inspection

- Swelling, bleeding, inflammation, ulcers
- Sign of foreign bodies
- Gums, mucosa, palate, tongue, floor of mouth, teeth (hematomas or discoloration of floor of mouth may indicate fracture of mandible)
- Subjective sensation of malalignment after traumatic displacement of teeth when mouth is closed
- Chipped, displaced, or fractured teeth
- Bloody socket indicates traumatic injury
- Prior loss/loose primary tooth vs traumatic injury

Palpation

- All teeth should be palpated for mobility, tenderness, fragmentation
- Palpate alveolar bone: loose or floppy alveolar bone indicates fracture
- Palpate the palate for crepitations; may indicate maxillary fracture

Percussion
- Tap each tooth using end of tongue depressor or dental instrument
- Pain on percussion may indicate abscessed, fractured, or traumatized tooth

Initial Assessment
- ABCs: rule out airway obstruction secondary to bleeding, aspiration of tooth or fracture of mandible with posterior displacement of the tongue
- Control bleeding with direct pressure
- Determine tetanus immunization status
- Congenital or acquired heart disease or immunocompromised patient: consider endocarditis prophylaxis

Types of Dental Trauma
Tooth Fractures

Uncomplicated tooth fracture
- Involves hard dental tissue (enamel, dentin, cementum) but does not extend into pulp
- Usually jagged edge, no sign of bleeding from pulp (central core)
- Refer to dentist within 48 hours for temporization to protect pulp from exposure and necrosis

Complicated tooth fracture
- Involves pulp and presents with bleeding from the pulp (central core)
- Immediate referral to dentistry to initiate treatment to preserve pulp viability

Concussion
- Dental trauma resulting in mild injury to periodontal ligament without tooth mobility or displacement

- Bleeding usually seen at gingival margin, sensitive to percussion
- Soft diet, no treatment necessary; refer to dentist for follow-up

Subluxation

- Dental trauma resulting in excessive mobility in vertical and/or horizontal direction but no displacement within the dental arch
- Often tooth very sensitive to percussion
- May see bleeding at the gingival margin
- Soft diet; refer to dentist immediately if permanent tooth and > 2 mm mobility

Luxation

- Displacement of tooth in a labial, lingual, or lateral direction
- Most common displacement of primary tooth is crown pushed toward palate
- Displacement injuries should be referred to dentist as soon as possible for treatment
- *Primary teeth* labially luxated need to be extracted to prevent further damage to permanent tooth bud; other luxation injuries may be splinted to stabilize
- *Permanent teeth* may be repositioned and referred to dentist for splinting to stabilize

Intrusion

- Tooth pushed up into socket
- X-rays required
- Refer to dentist immediately
- *Intrusion of primary tooth:* must be evaluated for proximity to developing permanent tooth—severely intruded primary tooth requires extraction
- *Intrusion of permanent tooth:* if severe, may require immediate (surgical) repositioning; otherwise, requires monitoring and possible future orthodontic extrusion

Extrusion

- Tooth is displaced vertically out of socket
- Refer to dentist immediately
- *Primary tooth:* usually extracted unless extrusion is minimal
- *Permanent tooth:* requires repositioning and likely splinting by dentist

Avulsion

- Tooth completely displaced from socket

Primary Tooth

- Usually not reimplanted due to significant risk of injury to developing permanent tooth bud or ankylosis (fusion of tooth root with adjacent alveolar bone)

Permanent Tooth

- Best prognosis if therapy occurs within 30 minutes of avulsion
- Rinse off tooth only if dirty; do not scrub
- Attempt to reimplant tooth gently into socket; hold by crown; do not handle root area; gently irrigate socket with saline only if clot in socket prevents reimplementation
- If cannot reimplant, keep tooth moist by submersing in milk, saliva, water, saline (Hanks Balanced Salt Solution preferred)
- Do not allow tooth to dry; tooth should not be wrapped in tissue or cloth
- X-ray (foreign body survey) if tooth cannot be found (may be intruded, ingested, or aspirated)
- See dentist immediately

Root Fractures

- Trauma usually results in horizontal fractures of anterior teeth
- Classification of horizontal root fractures based upon location of fracture on root: apical, middle, or coronal third of root
- The more coronal (near the crown) the fracture, the poorer the prognosis

- X-ray needed for diagnosis
- Tooth mobility or dislocation may be a sign of root fracture
- *Primary teeth:* if coronal fragment is dislocated or loose, extraction of coronal fragment is required; otherwise, only monitoring is needed
- *Permanent teeth:* treatment consists of reduction of fracture and rigid immobilization of crown of tooth
- See dentist within 24 hours

Soft-Tissue Lacerations

- Any intraoral soft-tissue laceration needs to be cleaned and examined for foreign bodies
- Foreign bodies such as tooth fragments or gravel must be debrided from tissue
- Lacerations of the frenulum will heal without suturing
- Tongue lacerations
  - Often caused by teeth
  - Only require suturing if severe

References

Belanger G. Dental injuries. In: Barkin R, Rosen P, eds. *Emergency Pediatrics.* 6th ed. Philadelphia: Mosby; 2003:449–455.

Mistry GJ, Kraus S. Dental emergencies. In: Crain E, Gershel J, eds. *Clinical Manual of Emergency Pediatrics.* 4th ed. New York, NY: McGraw-Hill; 2003:67–71.

Nowak AJ, Slayton RL. Trauma to primary teeth: setting a steady management course for the office. *Contemp Ped.* 2002;11:99.

Robert D. Dentoalveolar trauma. In: Rutkansloas J, ed. *Emer Med Clin North Am, Oral-Facial Emer.* 2000;18(3):521–538.

14 ▪ Otitis Media

AMINA LALANI

Introduction

- Otitis media is an inflammatory process in the middle ear cavity
- One of the most frequent infections in childhood
- Most frequent reason for antibiotics in developed countries
- Very common in children in daycare
- Peak incidence 6–12 months age when infants have lost maternal antibodies
- Typical pathogens: *Streptococcus pneumoniae, Moraxella catarrhalis*, nontypable *Haemophilus influenzae*

Clinical Practice Guidelines

- Revised American Academy of Pediatrics guidelines (2004)
- Include delaying treatment of otitis media in specific cases due to concerns about increasing antibiotic resistance
- Rate of penicillin-resistant *S. pneumoniae* up to 12–14% in Canada
- Need to know local rates of resistance
- AAP recommendations to observe children with acute uncomplicated OM are controversial

Table 14.1 Risk Factors for Antibiotic Resistance

PENICILLIN RESISTANCE	MACROLIDE RESISTANCE
Daycare	Previous antibiotics
Antibiotics in preceding month	Age < 5 yrs
Age < 3 yrs	Nosocomial infection
	Penicillin resistance

Table 14.2   Otitis Media Subtypes

Acute otitis media	Diagnosis requires all three signs:
	1. Acute onset of signs and symptoms of middle ear effusion and inflammation
	2. Presence of middle ear effusion indicated by:
	• Bulging of the tympanic membrane
	• Limited or absent mobility of the tympanic membrane
	• Air fluid level behind the tympanic membrane
	• Otorrhea
	3. Signs and symptoms of middle ear inflammation indicated by:
	• Erythema of the tympanic membrane OR
	• Otalgia (interferes/prevents normal activity or sleep)
	Middle ear effusion with constitutional signs of illness is not sufficient for a diagnosis of AOM.
	In case of doubt, wait and reassess.
Otitis media with effusion	• Presence of middle ear effusion without signs or symptoms of acute infection
	• Very common after an episode of otitis media
	• Usually no pain or fever
	• May be difficult to differentiate from acute OM
Chronic otitis media	Infection persists > 2–3 weeks

■ Three different meta-analyses showed up to 80% of children recover without antibiotics, but may have included children with otitis media with effusion

AAP 2004 Clinical Practice Guidelines

Treatment

■ Amoxicillin is first-line treatment, high dose 80–90 mg/kg/d
■ Optimal duration of treatment is unknown
■ For younger children or severe disease: treat for 10 days
■ Healthy children with uncomplicated AOM: treat for 5 days
■ Management of AOM should include an assessment of pain

Table 14.3   Criteria for Initial Antibiotics vs Observation in Acute Otitis Media

AGE	CERTAIN DIAGNOSIS	UNCERTAIN DIAGNOSIS
< 6 months	Antibiotics	Antibiotics
6 months to 2 yrs	Antibiotics	Observation option if nonsevere* Antibiotics if severe** illness
> 2 yrs	Antibiotics if severe illness Observation option if nonsevere	Observation option

*Nonsevere illness is mild otalgia and fever < 39°C in last 24 hrs
**Severe illness is moderate to severe otalgia or fever > 39°C

Observation (48–72 hours) is only appropriate if:
• Follow-up ensured
• Analgesia provided, and
• Antibiotics can be started if symptoms persist or worsen

Table 14.4   Second-line Agents

ANTIBIOTIC	DOSE	INTERVAL
Amoxicillin/clav (Clavulin®)	80–90 mg/kg/d	bid to tid
Cefprozil (Cefzil®)	30 mg/kg/d	bid
Cefuroxime axetil (Ceftin®)	40 mg/kg/d	tid
Clarithromycin (Biaxin®)	15 mg/kg/d	bid
Azithromycin (Zithromax®)	10 then 5 mg/kg/d Or 10 mg/kg/d	qd x 4 qd x 3
Clindamycin (Dalacin®)	30 mg/kg/d	tid
Ceftriaxone (Rocephin®)	50 mg/kg/d IM/IV	qd x 1 or 3 days

Complications

- Most common acute complication is perforation and drainage
- Up to 40% may have residual fluid for 3–6 weeks after treatment: can cause transient hearing loss and speech delay
- Mastoiditis presents with fever, tenderness over mastoid bone, +/– anterior displacement of pinna; rare, requires intravenous antibiotics
- Other rare complications: bacteremia, meningitis, cerebral abscess

Indications for Tympanostomy Tubes

- No clinical practice guidelines, controversial
  - Recurrent infections: > 3 infections in 6 months, or > 4 infections in 1 year
  - Persistent middle ear fluid > 3–6 months with hearing loss
- Tubes remain in situ for 6 months to 2 yrs and fall out spontaneously

References

American Academy of Family Physicians, American Academy of Otolaryngology-Head and Neck Surgery, American Academy of Pediatrics. Otitis media with effusion. *Pediatrics.* 2004;113:1412–1429.

American Academy of Pediatrics and American Academy of Family Physicians Clinical Practice Guideline: diagnosis and management of acute otitis media. *Pediatrics.* 2004;113:1451–1465.

Finkelstein JA, Stille CJ, Rifas-Shiman SL, et al. Watchful waiting for acute otitis media: are parents and physicians ready? *Pediatrics.* 2005;115:1466–1473.

Glasziou PP, Del Mar CB, Sanders SL, et al. Antibiotics for acute otitis media in children. *Coch Data Syst Rev.* 2006;3.

Kozyrskyj AL, Hildes-Ripstein GE et al. Short course antibiotics for acute otitis media. *Coch Data Syst Rev.* 2006;3.

McCormick DP, Chonmaitree T, Pittman C, et al. Nonsevere acute otitis media: a clinical trial comparing outcomes of watchful waiting versus immediate antibiotic treatment. *Pediatrics.* 2005;115:1455–1465.

Rovers MM, et al. Otitis media. *Lancet.* 2004;363:465–473.

15 ▪ Sinusitis

SUZAN SCHNEEWEISS

Introduction

- Often underdiagnosed because it presents as a spectrum of nonspecific symptoms
- Unlike adults, children do not complain of sinus congestion, pain, or headache
- Complicates 5–13% of upper respiratory tract infections in children (viral URTI usually lasts 5–7 days); less commonly allergic rhinitis
- Up to 50% gradually resolve spontaneously (usually within 4 weeks) without use of antimicrobials
- Peak age 3–6 years

Sinus Development

- Maxillary and ethmoid sinuses present at birth and continue to grow until adolescence; the most frequently infected sinuses
- Sphenoid sinuses develop during first few years of life (by 5 years) and are rarely affected without involvement of other sinuses
- Frontal sinuses appear by 7–8 yrs and continue to develop until late adolescence; isolated frontal sinusitis rare, but may be a focus of spread to orbit or CNS

Clinical Presentations

Persistent

- Persistent respiratory symptoms that last > 10 days and < 30 days and have not begun to improve

Severe

- Cold that seems more severe than usual
- High fever (temp > 39°C) and purulent nasal discharge for 3–4 days

Clinical Criteria for Diagnosing Acute Sinusitis

Symptoms present > 10 days

Common

- Nasal congestion
- Purulent nasal discharge or pharyngeal discharge
- Cough: wet or dry; must be present in the daytime
- Periorbital edema

Less Common

- Ear or throat pain
- Throat clearing
- Halitosis
- Fever (often low grade)
- Fatigue

Older Children/Teens

- Headache/facial pain, tooth pain, hyposmia

Diagnosis

- Diagnostic imaging *not* necessary to confirm diagnosis in children
- Laboratory or radiologic evaluation only supportive
- Plain sinus X-rays: diffuse opacification, air-fluid levels, or mucosal thickening (at least 4 mm)
- CT scan:
  - Limited scan ("screening"): lacks sensitivity
  - CT scan abnormalities with URI persist for up to 2 weeks following clinical improvement
  - Indications: children with sinusitis and suspected subperiosteal or orbital abscess or intracranial complication

Complications of Acute Sinusitis

Periorbital/Orbital

- Preseptal cellulitis (periorbital cellulitis), orbital cellulitis/abscess, osteomyelitis, subperiosteal orbital abscess

Intracranial Complications

- More common in older children and adolescent males
- Subdural or epidural empyema, meningitis, brain abscess, cortical thrombophlebitis, and cavernous or sagittal sinus thrombosis

Pott's Puffy Tumor

- Complication of frontal sinusitis
- Osteomyelitis and subsequent subperiosteal abscess of frontal bone
- Presents as a forehead mass: soft, fluctuant swelling; often erythematous, warm, and tender
- Patient complains of headache, photophobia, and fever (often low grade)
- Admit for IV antibiotics, consult ENT

Treatment of Acute Sinusitis

- If history and physical exam are consistent with sinusitis, treatment can be initiated *without* confirmatory radiology testing
- Symptoms resolve with therapy, no further evaluation
- Most common organisms: *Streptococcus pneumoniae,* nontypable *Haemophilus influenzae,* and *Moraxella catarrhalis*

Antibiotics

- Amoxicillin—reasonable first-line drug (45 mg/kg/day) PO if not attending daycare, no recent antibiotics, and < 2 years
- Amoxicillin—high dose 80–90 mg/kg/day PO

- • Penicillin allergy—clarithromycin, cefuroxime axetil, cefixime, clindamycin
- • If no response in 48–72 hours, change to amoxicillin-clavulinic acid (with high-dose amoxicillin component)
- ■ Duration of therapy: 10–14 days (continue antibiotics for 7 days after resolution of symptoms)
- ■ If toxic appearing child or poor oral intake, consider parenteral therapy
- ■ Adjuvant therapies (antihistamines, inhaled corticosteroid, decongestants, saline washes): data limited and controversial; not currently recommended
- ■ Children with complications or suspected complications require aggressive treatment (parenteral antibiotics) and referral to subspecialist

Subacute Sinusitis

- ■ Symptoms for 30–90 days, but less intensity than that of preceding acute process
- ■ Chronic cough that is worse at night, nasal congestion, and sniffling
- ■ Fever, headache, and malaise are uncommon
- ■ Mucopurulent material may be visible in the nasal vault or in the posterior nasal drainage
- ■ Treatment with antimicrobial for minimum 14 days ± oral/topical decongestants

Recurrent Acute Bacterial Sinusitis

- ■ Three episodes of acute bacterial sinusitis in 6 months or four episodes in 12 months
- ■ Response to antibiotics is brisk and patients completely free of symptoms between episodes

Chronic Sinusitis

- Episodes of inflammation lasting > 90 days
- Chronic cough, nasal congestion, and sometimes headache
- Mouth breathing with snoring, sore throat, and occasionally reactive adenoidal hypertrophy
- Requires antimicrobials for 3–4 weeks, ± nasal decongestant, ± oral/topical corticosteroid

References

American Academy of Pediatrics. Clinical practice guideline: management of sinusitis. *Pediatrics.* 2001;108(3):798–808.

Conrad DA, Jenson HB. Management of acute bacterial rhinosinusitis. *Curr Opin Pediatr.* 2002;14(1):86–90.

Jacobs RF. Judicious use of antibiotics for common pediatric respiratory infections. *Pediatr Infect Dis.* 2000;19:938–943.

Zacharisen MC, Kelly KJ. Allergic and infectious pediatric sinusitis. *Pediatr Ann.* 1998;27(11):759–766.

16 ▪ Oropharyngeal Infections

Jonathan Pirie

Introduction

- Most infections are viral but need to consider other causes
- Strep throat uncommon in children < 2 years age
- Consider infectious mononucleosis in older children, but may also present in young children

Pharyngitis

- Acute pharyngitis can be caused by numerous viral and bacterial agents
- Viruses predominate, while group A streptococcus is the predominant bacterial cause
- *Chlamydia trachomatis* and *Mycoplasma pneumoniae* may be responsible for pharyngitis in adolescence
- Candida may present in infants, immunosuppressed children, and children taking antibiotics

Clinical Presentation

- Coryza, hoarseness, cough, diarrhea, conjunctivitis, anterior stomatitis, and discrete ulcerative lesions suggest a viral etiology
- Epstein-Barr virus and cytomegalovirus typically have pharyngeal inflammation, diffuse lymphadenopathy, and hepatosplenomegaly
- Streptococcal pharyngitis typically has an abrupt onset, fever, sore throat, ± headache, vomiting, abdominal pain, and a scarlatiniform rash
- Other clinical findings: tonsillopharyngeal erythema ± tonsillar exudates, tender cervical adenopathy, a beefy red

swollen uvula, petechiae of the palate, and excoriated nares in infants

Investigations

- Throat culture remains the gold standard for streptococcus
- Decision to obtain a throat swab should be based on age, signs and symptoms, season, and family and community epidemiology
- Clinical decision rules have been used but poor positive predictive value
- Rapid streptococcus by latex agglutination or immunoassay is useful if positive but does not rule out streptococcal infection
- Obtain CBC, EBV titres, monospot and other bacterial isolates (*Chlamydia, N. gonorrhoeae, Mycoplasma*) on a case-by-case basis
- Monospot commonly negative in children < 5 years; may need EBV serology

Management

- Penicillin is the drug of choice for treatment of acute streptococcal pharyngitis
- 10-day course recommended for maximal eradication of group A streptococci
- Treatment should be reserved until positive throat culture or rapid strep test
- Penicillin, amoxicillin, and erythromycin are equally effective whether divided bid, tid, or qid when used for 10 days
- Other antibiotics (azithromycin, cefixime, cefuroxime axetil) have been shown to be equally effective when used for shorter duration (≤ 5 days)
  - Should not be routinely used as first-line therapy because of limited studies or concerns regarding broad spectrum of antimicrobial activity

Complications

- Suppurative spread may cause:
  - **Peritonsillar abscess** (quinsy)
  - **Ludwig's angina** (submandibular abscess):
    - Inflammation of submandibular and sublingual space may lead to airway compromise
    - Potentially life-threatening, rapidly expanding inflammation
    - May be caused by multiple organisms including staph, strep, Gram negatives, and anaerobes
    - Treat with high-dose IV penicillin
  - **Lemierre's postanginal sepsis**:
    - Acute oropharyngeal infection followed by unilateral jugular vein septic thrombophlebitis and neck pain, due to infection with *Fusobacterium*
    - Risk of pulmonary abscesses from septic emboli
- Hematologic spread may cause cervical or mesenteric adenitis, meningitis, cavernous sinus thrombosis, endocarditis, osteomyelitis, suppurative arthritis, or sepsis
- Nonsuppurative complications of streptococcal infection include scarlet fever, glomerulonephritis, and rheumatic fever

Peritonsillar Abscess

- Most common ENT deep space infection
- Typically occurs after streptococcal infection, but may occur with EBV
- Uncommon in children < 12 years
- Abscesses typically grow multiple organisms such as group A streptococcus, *Peptostreptococcus, Peptococcus*, anaerobes, *H. influenzae, S. pneumoniae*, and *S. aureus*

Clinical Presentation

- Typically increasing ipsilateral dysphagia
- Drooling, trismus, dysarthria, and odynophagia

- Voice may have a muffled, "hot potato" quality (as in EBV infections)
- May appear toxic
- Oral findings include cellulitis with diffuse peritonsillar swelling or abscess formation with trismus, soft palate, and uvula displacement

Investigations and Diagnosis

- Nonspecific findings; elevated WBC
- Streptococcal culture is often positive
- Tonsillar aspirates are useful for patients not responding to initial therapy
- CT may be indicated for patients not improving with therapy as may be extension to the parapharyngeal spaces

Differential Diagnosis

- Parapharyngeal infections
- Cervical adenitis and abscess
- Dental abscess
- Salivary gland infections

Management

- Most patients require hospitalization for IV hydration, IV antibiotics, and analgesia
- Patients with fluctuant masses or increasing in size despite IV antibiotics are candidates for surgical drainage
- A number of antibiotic regimens have been recommended:
  - Clindamycin
  - Cefoxitin
  - Combination of a penicillin and a beta-lactamase inhibitor (i.e., clavulanate)
- Patients with recurrent episodes may ultimately require tonsillectomy

Complications

- Parapharyngeal extension
- Necrotizing fasciitis
- Airway obstruction
- Aspiration pneumonia
- Sepsis

Retropharyngeal Infections

- Retropharyngeal abscess (RPA) and parapharyngeal infections are rare but carry significant potential mortality and morbidity
- Diagnosis is challenging due to low incidence, variable symptoms, and lack of physical findings
- Two-thirds of patients are male, < 6 years old; more frequent in winter
- Predominantly streptococci, occasionally anaerobes, and *S. aureus*

Clinical Presentation

- Signs and symptoms are variable and require high index of suspicion
- Typically signs and symptoms evolve following a URTI or pharyngitis
- Common symptoms at presentation include fever, sore throat, torticollis, neck pain/mass
- Less commonly presents with dysphagia, trismus, drooling, stridor, neck stiffness

Differential Diagnosis

- Epiglottitis
- Croup
- Peritonsillar abscess
- Mononucleosis

Investigations and Diagnosis

- Nonspecific findings: elevated WBC
- Gram stain and culture from incision and drainage
- Soft-tissue lateral neck X-ray demonstrates soft-tissue mass in prevertebral space (PVS):
  - Must be performed in extension, during inspiration, and without the child crying to avoid false increase in PVS
  - Normally PVS is < 7 mm at C2 and 5 mm at C3–C4 or less than 50% of the adjacent vertebrae. There is debate when to call the PVS abnormal; > 100% of the adjacent vertebrae is highly suspicious for RPA
  - Normally "step-off" between posterior wall of pharynx and posterior wall of trachea at level of the larynx (approximately at level of C4): loss of step-off suggests RPA
  - Parapharyngeal infections are not visible on lateral X-rays
- CT scan:
  - Used to confirm retropharyngeal space enlargement
  - Features suggestive of an abscess vs retropharyngeal cellulitis (RPC) include complete rim enhancement and lucency with respect to CSF
  - Does not always accurately predict pus at surgery

Management

- Controversial because clinical, X-ray, or CT scan does not accurately predict pus at surgery
- Generally patients with RPC on CT are managed with IV antibiotics
- Patients with evidence of RPA on CT can be managed initially with IV antibiotics and operated on if not improving or repeat CT shows deterioration
- If respiratory compromise, need immediate surgery
- Antibiotic choices:
  - Clindamycin (first choice)
  - Alternative: third-generation cephalosporin, cloxacillin, and metronidazole

Complications

- Airway obstruction
- Aspiration pneumonia
- Rupture into esophagus, mediastinum, or lungs
- Blood vessels can erode and hemorrhage
- Abscess reformation (0–5%)

References

Abrunzo T, et al. Emergencies of the oral cavity and neck. In: Strange GR, ed. *Pediatric Emergency Medicine: Just the Facts.* New York, NY: McGraw-Hill Companies; 2004:309–311.

Bisno AL, Gerber MA, Gwaltney JM, et al. Diagnosis and management of group A streptococcal pharyngitis: a practice guideline. *Clin Infect Dis.* 1997;25:574–583.

Brook I. Microbiology and management of peritonsillar, retropharyngeal, and parapharyngeal abscesses. *J Oral Maxillofac Surg.* 2004;62:1545–1550.

Craig FW, Schunk JE. Retropharyngeal abscess in children: clinical presentation, utility of imaging, and current management. *Pediatrics.* 2003;111;1394–1398.

Dajani A, Taubert K, Ferrieri P, et al. Treatment of acute streptococcal pharyngitis and prevention of rheumatic fever: a statement for health professionals. *Pediatrics.* 1995;96:758–764.

Daya H, et al. Retropharyngeal and parapharyngeal infections in children: the Toronto experience. *Int J Pediatr Otorhinolaryngol.* 2005;69(1):81–86.

Dawes LC, Bova R, Carter P. Retropharyngeal abscess in children. *ANZ J Surg.* 2002;72:417–420.

Ebell, MD, Mark, H, Mindy, A, et al. Does this patient have strep throat? *JAMA.* 2000;284:2912–2918.

Rimoin AW, et al. Evaluation of the WHO clinical decision rule for streptococcal pharyngitis. *Arch Dis Child.* 2005;90:1066–1070.

■ PART III

RESPIRATORY EMERGENCIES

17 ▪ Bronchiolitis

Introduction

- Viral infection of the lower respiratory tract, usually from November to April
- Usually in children < 2 years of age
- Bronchiolitis, viral induced reactive airways disease, and the first episode of asthma are clinically indistinguishable
- Children with atopy or family history of atopy or severe bronchiolitis requiring hospitalization have increased probability of developing asthma

Clinical Presentation

- Characterized by preceding coryza and cough, followed by respiratory distress
- Respiratory distress is associated with tachypnea, chest retractions, and expiratory wheezing
- Fever may or may not be present and crepitations are often heard
- Severe bronchiolitis: may see grunting, nasal flaring, and poor air entry
- Associated agitation, lethargy, pallor, cyanosis, apnea accompany impending respiratory failure

Practice Points: Diagnosis

- Wheezing may be absent, especially at initial presentation
- Wheezing may appear after a trial of inhaled bronchodilators
- Although persistent absence of wheezing should prompt consideration of other diagnoses, it does not rule out bronchiolitis
- Wheezing in bronchiolitis is often a low-pitched, rhonchi-like quality

Red flags suggesting an alternate diagnosis:
- Toxic appearance (sepsis, bacterial infection)
- Preexisting chronic feeding problems
- Poor weight gain
- Chronic respiratory symptoms (congestive heart failure, congenital lung anomaly, cystic fibrosis, chronic aspiration)

History

- Antecedent coryza and worsening cough
- Cough may be severe and at times paroxysmal and suggest pertussis
- Occasional vomiting after cough is common
- Bronchiolitis vs pertussis:

  Bronchiolitis: Respiratory distress is usually present between coughing episodes

  Pertussis: Usually no respiratory distress between coughing

- Decreased oral intake is common, even in mild bronchiolitis
- Symptoms usually abate in 2–3 weeks, rarely last 3–4 weeks or longer
- High-risk history that may be associated with more severe disease or need for hospitalization: age < 6–8 weeks, prematurity, neonatal ventilation, coexistent chronic lung disease, hemodynamically significant heart disease, neuromuscular disease, immunodeficiency

Examination

- Nontoxic appearance (fever may be high)
- Absence of agitation/pathologic lethargy
- Normal level of consciousness for time of day
- Dehydration is *rare* despite decreased oral intake
- Degree of tachypnea is highly variable: persistent RR ≥ 80 is usually associated with severe disease

- Suprasternal and supraclavicular retractions may be difficult to see due to the short neck
- Marked chest wall retractions (especially laterally and posterior) may be more helpful
- Crepitations are common in bronchiolitis and do not signal a need for further investigations
- Wheezing before or after bronchodilator therapy is common but not universal

Investigations

- Pulse oximetry
- Bloodwork and X-rays usually unnecessary
- Chest X-ray: chest radiographs may show airspace disease (consolidation) in addition to usual airway disease
  - This finding is compatible with bronchiolitis and usually does not warrant antibiotic therapy
- In contrast, isolated consolidation *without* airway disease points to diagnosis of bacterial pneumonia and away from diagnosis of bronchiolitis
  - These children do not exhibit typical presentation of bronchiolitis (usually no wheeze)
- Chest radiographs are only indicated in infants if alternative diagnosis is suspected (see "red flags" above)
- Viral cultures or rapid antigen tests do not aid in routine patient management

Emergency Care

- Supplemental oxygen if pulse oximetry persistently < 90%
  - Avoid unnecessary agitation: blow-by oxygen often adequate
  - Nonrebreather mask necessary for providing reliable oxygen concentrations > 60%
- Frequent small oral feedings usually necessary; IV insertion only in critically ill infants and those with dehydration (rare)

Salbutamol/Albuterol

A trial of inhaled salbutamol is indicated in all infants with bron-chiolitis with moderate to severe respiratory distress

- Deposition of inhaled drugs is lower for young infants than for older children
- Airway edema and mucus with debris compromise drug deposition further
- Therefore, a relatively high dose of salbutamol is needed in infants
- Minimum dose: 0.5 mL (2.5 mg) via nebulizer or 4–5 inhalations via MDI (metered dose inhaler)/spacer q 20–30 min for 3 doses
- Discontinue if poor or no response

Epinephrine

- 1:1,000 solution 2.5–5 mL q 1–4 h
- Effect often starts to wane after 1–2 hours
- Indicated in severe distress, especially if poor response to salbutamol
- Cannot be given in outpatients or by MDI

Dexamethasone

- Preliminary evidence suggests that oral dexamethasone may be effective in infants with severe bronchiolitis
- Consider dexamethasone 0.3–1 mg/kg PO in infants with moderate to severe distress (optimal dose not known)
- Takes at least 3–4 hours for effect
- Optimal duration of corticosteroid therapy unknown

Practice Point: Treatment

- No evidence that inhaled corticosteroids are effective in bronchiolitis
- Inhaled steroids should not be given in acute management of bronchiolitis

- Ribavirin plays no role in emergency management of bronchiolitis
- Antibiotics not indicated unless likely source of bacterial infection present (e.g., otitis media)
- Most patients with bronchiolitis with radiographic signs of pneumonia do not require antibiotics

Hospitalization

Absolute

- Severe respiratory distress after 2–3 doses of inhaled salbutamol and/or 4 hrs post corticosteroids
- Need for supplemental oxygen
- Objective signs of dehydration
- History of apnea

Relative

- Age < 8 weeks
- Comorbidities
- Psychosocial factors
- Recurrent emergency department visits

Discharge Instructions

- Inform parents that resolution of bronchiolitis is slow and symptoms may persist up to 3–4 weeks
- Danger signs include inability to feed, lethargy, increasing respiratory distress
- Frequent follow-up may be necessary
- Small, frequent feeds
- Nebulized salbutamol (Ventolin®) 0.5 mL in 3 mL saline < 6 months of age or
- Salbutamol 2–3 puffs q 4 h × 5–7 days in infants > 6 months of age if good response to emergency therapy
- Medical reassessment in 24–48 hrs

■ Educate caretakers about signs of deterioration: worsening chest retractions, apnea, and/or feeding difficulty

References

Dawson KP, Long A, Kennedy J, et al. The chest radiograph in acute bronchiolitis. *J Paediatr Child Health.* 1990;26:290–311.

Gadomski AM, Lichensttein R, Horton L, et al. Efficacy of albuterol in the management of bronchiolitis. *Pediatrics.* 1994;93:907–912.

Kellner JD, Ohlsson A, Gadomski AM, et al. Efficacy of bronchodilator therapy in bronchiolitis: a meta-analysis. *Arch Pediatr Adolesc Med.* 1996;150(11):1166–1167.

Menon K, Sutcliffe T, Klassen TP. A randomized trial comparing the efficacy of epinephrine with salbutamol in the treatment of acute bronchiolitis. *J Pediatr.* 1995;126:1004–1007.

Reionen T, Korppi M, Pitkakangas S, et al. The clinical efficacy of nebulized racemic epinephrine and albuterol in acute bronchitis. *Arch Pediatr Adolesc Med.* 1995;149:686–692.

Roosevelt G, Sheehan K, Grupp-Phelan J, et al. Dexamethasone in bronchiolitis: a randomized controlled trial. *Lancet.* 1996;348:292–295.

Schuh S, Coates AL, Binnie R, et al. Efficacy of oral dexamethasone in outpatients with acute bronchiolitis. *J Pediatr.* 2002;140:27–32.

18 ▪ Croup

SUZANNE SCHUH

Introduction
- Croup is a viral infection of the upper airway
- Most commonly caused by parainfluenza virus
- Most frequent in infants 6 months to 3 years of age but can occur up to 15 years of age

Clinical Presentation
- Abrupt onset of barky cough frequently associated with stridor on inspiration, hoarseness, and respiratory distress

History
- Onset usually during the night
- Dog- or seal-like barking cough
- Hoarse voice/cry
- Respiratory distress and noisy breathing often improve upon exposure to cool night air en route to the emergency department
- Duration of symptoms: 48 hours to 7 days

Practice Point
- Consider epiglottitis if toxic appearance, drooling, and anxiety
- Consider bacterial tracheitis if preexisting croup with sudden deterioration, toxic appearance, poor response to inhaled epinephrine

Examination
- Hoarse cry/voice
- Seal-like cough
- Inspiratory stridor (with agitation or at rest), no change with position

- Chest wall retractions
- Fever common but nontoxic
- No drooling

Investigations

- Usually unnecessary
- Only after stabilization of respiratory distress
- Lateral and AP neck X-ray for atypical presentation to rule out other diagnoses

Emergency Management

- Upright position
- Avoid unnecessary interventions
- Humidity has been shown to be of *no* benefit and should not be given
- Blow-by oxygen if saturation < 90%
- Dexamethasone in *all* cases (even if no distress)
  - 0.6 mg/kg PO as a single dose, improve in 2–4 hours
- Epinephrine in severe cases
  - Half-life 45 minutes
  - Observe for 2 hours to detect deterioration
  - 1:1,000 solution, 5 mL via nebulizer
  - Give 2–3 consecutive doses in children with severe distress

Hospitalization

- Stridor at rest and/or significant respiratory distress 4 hours after dexamethasone
- Need for more than 1–2 doses of epinephrine
- Psychosocial issues

References

Bjornson CL, Klassen TP, Williamson J, et al. A randomized trial of a single dose of oral dexamethasone for mild croup. *N Engl J Med.* 2004;351:1306–1313.

Johnson DW, Jacobson S, Edney PC, et al. A comparison of nebulized budesonide, intramuscular dexamethasone, and placebo for moderately severe croup. *N Engl J Med.* 1998;339:498–503.

Kairys S, Olmstead EM, O'Connor GT. Steroid treatment of laryngotracheitis: a meta-analysis of the evidence from randomized trials. *Pediatrics.* 1989;83:683–693.

Neto GM, Kentab O, Klassen TP, Osmond MH. A randomized controlled trial of mist in the acute treatment of moderate croup. *Acad Emerg Med.* 2002;9:873–879.

19 ▪ Asthma

SUZANNE SCHUH

Introduction

- True asthma and viral-induced infant wheezing (usually temporary, few progress to asthma) are difficult to distinguish; acute treatment is identical
- Occasionally, even asthmatics may develop respiratory distress due to other conditions such as allergic reaction, pneumonia, salicylate intoxication: exclude via careful history and physical exam

History

- Majority of attacks are viral-induced with history of URTI
- Current asthma medications, doses, and frequency
- Frequency of acute exacerbations in the past 6–12 months
- Hospitalizations for the past 6–12 months
- Previous ICU admission for asthma
- Atypical presentation (e.g., persistent high fever, wet cough: often signal pneumonia)

Examination

- Usual findings: tachypnea, intercostal/suprasternal retractions, expiratory ± inspiratory wheeze
- Fever (especially low-grade) and crepitations are common
- Red flags:
  - Nasal flaring, grunting, poor air entry
  - Pallor, duskiness
  - Agitation/persistent lethargy
  - Difficulty talking in sentences/feeding in infants/playing

Investigations

- Majority require no investigations

- Pulse oximetry
- FEV1 may be indicated if uncertain diagnosis or to document response to therapy:
  FEV1 < 50% predicted: Severe asthma
  FEV1 50–70%: Moderate asthma
  FEV1 71–80%: Mild asthma

However, some patients with significant symptoms have FEV1 > 80% predicted and others with relatively mild symptoms have FEV1 < 70%

- Chest X-ray only indicated in atypical presentation, toxic appearance, chronic symptoms, critically ill patients
- Arterial blood gas only indicated in critically ill children, abnormal level of consciousness, or increasing oxygen requirements

Emergency Management

- Supplemental oxygen if SaO_2 < 90%

Salbutamol/Albuterol

- *Nebulizer:* 2.5–5 mg (0.5–1.0 mL) in 2–3 mL NS q 20 mins × 3 in first hour in severe disease
  - Repeat if poor response
  - Reevaluate hourly and prolong intervals to q 1–2 h if good response
  - If no or minimal respiratory distress 1–2 hrs past last inhalation, can usually discharge
- *MDI:* 4–8 puffs (400–800 mcg/dose) per dose as above
  - Use mask aerochamber in young patients—mouth piece (aerochamber) in children > 6 years of age
- Supplemental potassium if > 10 frequent inhalations in ED

Ipratropium

- 250–500 mcg per dose, mixed with salbutamol via nebulizer

- MDI: 100 mcg per dose via MDI with aerochamber
- Consider at least 3 doses with severe asthma

Corticosteroids

- Indicated in all but the mildest acute asthma exacerbations
- Give as soon as possible as takes 3–6 hours for effect
- Usually given orally
- IV route only if unable to take oral medications, persistent vomiting, dehydration, critically ill
- Efficacy of IV comparable to PO

Options

- Dexamethasone 0.3 mg/kg PO in emergency department and prednisolone 1 mg/kg q 24 h × 4–5 further doses *OR*
- Prednisolone 2 mg/kg in emergency department and 4–5 further daily doses of 1 mg/kg

Advantages of Dexamethasone

- Lower volume
- Better taste than prednisolone
- Longer half-life (50 hours) than prednisolone (24–30 hrs)

Practice Point

- Inhaled corticosteroids should not be used in stabilization of children with acute asthma exacerbations, regardless of severity status
- Evidence suggests that recurrent courses of oral steroids are not associated with side effects

Inhaled Corticosteroids (ICS)

- All children with acute asthma treated in emergency require 8–12 weeks of ICS to prevent subsequent exacerbations
- Option: Fluticasone (Flovent®) 100–200 mcg bid via MDI and spacer

- ICS dose may have to be temporarily increased if the child relapsed on a lower dose
- ICS must be taken regularly, even if child is asymptomatic

Magnesium Sulphate

- For critically ill children, ICU candidates
- Depending on clinical severity, give on arrival or after intensive bronchodilator therapy and corticosteroids
- Dose: 25–75 mg/kg IV infusion over 30 mins
- Response usually within minutes
- May have to repeat in 1–2 hours
- Side effects rare, monitor BP for hypotension

Hospitalization

Absolute

- Need for supplemental oxygen
- Significant respiratory distress 4–6 hours post corticosteroid therapy (salbutamol q 1–2 h at 4 hrs)

Relative

- Significant comorbidities
- Repeat visits for same episode, lack of asthma education
- Major social/asthma control problems

Discharge

- Teach correct technique for MDI and aerochamber
- All patients should use aerochamber, regardless of age (use spacer with mouthpiece in children > 6–7 years old)
- Advise patients to notify their physician if contact with varicella while on steroid therapy
- Mandatory immediate reassessment if greater or more frequent doses used at home
- Advise all patients to be reassessed in 24–48 hours

Salbutamol/Albuterol

- Moderate to severe disease: inhaled 0.2–0.3 puffs/kg/dose (maximum 8 puffs) qid × 24 hrs, then 2–3 puffs qid × 7 days, via MDI and aerochamber
- Mild to moderate exacerbation: 2 puffs qid × 7 days via MDI and aerochamber

Oral Corticosteroids

- Prednisone/prednisolone 1 mg/kg daily for 5 days (optimal length of therapy unknown)
- Do not substitute inhaled for oral corticosteroids at this stage
- Tapering is not necessary

Inhaled Corticosteroids

- For example, fluticasone propionate (Flovent®) 100–200 mcg/day × 4–8 weeks in all but the mildest exacerbations because inflammation takes several weeks to subside
- May require prolonged treatment if frequent exacerbations (> 5) in the past year or > 3 attacks/year and suboptimal chronic control
- Consider temporarily augmenting dose if relapse occurs while on inhaled steroids

References

Edmonds ML, Camargo CA, Pollack CV, Rowe BH. The effectiveness of inhaled corticosteroids in the emergency department treatment of acute asthma: a meta-analysis. *Ann Emerg Med.* 2002;40:145–154.

Johnson D, Jacobson S, Edney P, et al. A comparison of nebulized budesonide, intramuscular dexamethasone, and placebo for moderately severe croup. *NEJM.* 1998;339(8):498–503.

Kellner J, Ohlsson A, Gadomski AM, Wang EEL. Efficacy of bronchodilator therapy in bronchiolitis, a meta-analysis. *Arch Adol Med.* 1996;50:1166–1172.

Klassen T, Feldman M, Watters L, et al. Nebulized budesonide for children with mild to moderate croup. *NEJM.* 1994;331(5):285–289.

Klassen TP, Rower PC, Sutcliffe T, et al. Randomized trial of salbutamol in acute bronchiolitis. *J Pediatr.* 1991;118:807–811.

Menon K, Sutcliffe T, Klassen T. A randomized trial comparing the efficacy of epinephrine with salbutamol in the treatment of acute bronchiolitis. *J. Pediatr.* 1995;126(6):1004–1007.

Scarfone RJ, Fuchs SM, Nager AL, Shane SA. Controlled trial of oral prednisone in the emergency department: treatment of children with acute asthma. *Pediatrics.* 1993;92:513–518.

Schuh S, Canny G, Kerem E, et al. Nebulized albuterol in acute bronchiolitis. *J Pediatr.* 1990;117(4):633–637.

Schuh S, Johnson D, Callahan S, et al. Efficacy of continuous nebulized ipratropium bromide in severe asthma. *J Pediatr.* 1995;126(4):639–644.

Schuh S, Parkin P, Rajan A, et al. High vs low dose continuous nebulized albuterol in severe childhood asthma. *Pediatrics.* 1989;83(4):513–519.

Schuh S, Reisman J, Alshehri M, et al. A comparison of inhaled fluticasone and oral prednisone for children with severe acute asthma. *N Engl J Med.* 2000;343:689–694.

20 ▪ Pneumonia

SAMI AL-FARSI

Introduction

- Viruses are a common cause of pneumonia in younger children
- Most children can be treated as outpatients with full recovery

Community-Acquired Pneumonia

- Definition: Fever and acute respiratory symptoms and signs, plus parenchymal infiltrate on chest X-ray in a previously healthy child due to a community-acquired infection
- Risk factors for increased incidence and severity: prematurity, malnutrition, low socioeconomic status, passive exposure to smoke, daycare attendance, overcrowding, previous pneumonia or wheeze

Etiology

- Age is a good predictor of the likely causative agent
- In neonates < 3 weeks, pneumonia is usually due to maternally acquired infection
- In young infants, consider *Chlamydia trachomatis:* afebrile, nontoxic, dry cough, peripheral eosinophilia
- Consider pertussis especially if immunizations are not current
- In children > 5 yrs and adolescents, *Streptococcus pneumoniae* is the most common cause followed by *Mycoplasma pneumoniae* and *Chlamydia pneumoniae (TWAR)*
- Other bacterial causes especially in ill infants and toddlers are *Staphylococcus aureus, Streptococcus pyogenes, Haemophilus influenzae,* and *Moraxella catarrhalis*

Clinical Presentation

- Fever, difficulty breathing, and > 1 of the following: tachypnea, cough, nasal flaring, retractions, crackles, decreased breath sounds
- May also present with lethargy, poor feeding, or localized pain to chest or abdomen
- Fever, tachypnea, and intercostal retractions are more reliable than auscultation in diagnosing pneumonia in children
- Tachypnea (RR > 50 breaths/min) is the most sensitive indicator of pneumonia in infants
- Wheeze and hyperinflation suggest viral cause in younger children, and *Mycoplasma* in older children
- In older children, a history of difficulty breathing is more helpful in identifying pneumonia than actual retractions
- Older children may present with classic signs such as dullness to percussion, crackles, bronchial breath sounds, increased tactile fremitus

Presentations

- Typical: Fever, chills, pleuritic chest pain, and productive cough
- Atypical: Gradual onset over several days to weeks, dominated by symptoms of headache and malaise, nonproductive cough, and low-grade fever

Investigations

- Assessment of oxygenation is a good indication of severity of disease
- Increased WBC with left shift may indicate bacterial cause
- CRP and ESR do not distinguish between bacterial and viral and are not routinely recommended
- Blood cultures are recommended in all *hospitalized* patients
- Blood cultures only positive in 10–30% of cases

- Nasopharyngeal aspirate (NPA) for viral antigen detection is not routinely recommended
- Cultures for mycoplasmas, and chlamydia are not routinely recommended
- Adolescents and some older children may be able to produce sputum for Gram stain

Chest Radiograph
- Consider chest radiograph to confirm diagnosis
- Not useful in differentiating bacterial and nonbacterial causes
- Round or lobar infiltrates seen in young children, due to prevalence of pneumococcus
- Interstitial infiltrates are more common in viral and mycoplasma infections
- Both lobar and interstitial infiltrates can be seen in all types of infection

Pleural Effusions
- Small pleural effusions are commonly seen in pneumococcal and mycoplasma infections and less commonly with viral infections
- Large effusions and empyemas seen with *Staph. aureus* pneumonia particularly in infants
- Indications for thoracentesis: hypoxia, dyspnea, large effusions with shifting of fluid on lateral decubitus film
- Pleural fluid should be sent for microscopy and culture
- Place chest tube if foul-smelling fluid, purulent, organisms on Gram stain, or pH < 7.3
- Consider ultrasound for diagnosis of pneumonia vs pleural effusion if CXR findings are ambiguous
- Consider ultrasound guidance for thoracentesis and chest tube placement if small or loculated effusion

Consider Admission If:
- Toxic appearance
- Age < 6 months

- Oxygen saturation < 92%
- Respiratory rate > 70 breaths/min in infants, > 50 breaths/min in older children
- Respiratory distress
- Vomiting, decreased oral intake, or signs of dehydration
- Noncompliant parents
- Intermittent apnea, grunting
- Failed initial oral therapy
- Large pleural effusion

Consider Intensive Care Unit Admission If:
- > 60% oxygen requirement
- Shock
- Increasing respiratory and heart rates with evidence of severe respiratory distress and exhaustion
- Recurrent apnea or irregular breathing

Management
- Empiric management is based on age of child and likely causative organism

Aspiration Pneumonia
- Aspiration of gastric or oral contents, mainly in children with neuromuscular impairment
- May also be seen in abnormalities of airway or GI tract, recent sedation or anesthesia, CNS impairment, or history of substance abuse
- Aspiration causes a chemical pneumonitis
- True incidence of bacterial pneumonia after aspiration is unclear, but injured lung is susceptible to infection
- > 90% are symptomatic within 1 hour
- Usually present with fever, tachypnea, cough, and hypoxia
- May be delay of several hours before positive X-ray findings
- Often require close observation and supportive therapy

Table 20.1 Antibiotic Management by Age

AGE	ORGANISMS	OUTPATIENTS		IN HOSPITAL	
		Agents of choice	Alternative agents	Agents of choice	Alternative agents
1–3 months	S. pneumoniae C. trachomatis B. pertussis S. aureus H. influenzae	Initial outpatient treatment not recommended		Cefuroxime +/- erythromycin or clarithromycin	Ampicillin +/- erythromycin or clarithromycin
3 months to 5 years	S. pneumoniae S. aureus H. influenzae Mycoplasma	Amoxicillin	Cefuroxime or amoxicillin-clavulanic acid	Ampicillin	Cefuroxime or amoxicillin-clavulanic acid
> 5 years	S. pneumoniae S. aureus H. influenzae Mycoplasma C. pneumoniae	Clarithromycin/ erythromycin	Amoxicillin or amoxicillin-clavulanic acid or Cefuroxime	Ampicillin + erythromycin or clarithromycin	Cefuroxime or amoxicillin-clavulanic acid + erythromycin or clarithromycin

Note: Use cloxacillin if suspect Staphylococcus aureus pneumonia/sepsis in critically ill infants. Macrolides or clindamycin are alternatives for beta-lactam allergic patients.

Source: Adapted from: Kowalczyk A, ed. The 2005–2006 Formulary of Drugs, The Hospital for Sick Children. 24th ed. Toronto: The Graphic Centre, HSC; 2005.

- Consider antibiotics (penicillin) in medically complex patients or children with foul sputum
- Use of steroids controversial, not indicated in emergency department

References

Allen U, Baron T, MacLusky I. Emergency guidelines for the treatment of community-acquired bacterial pneumonia. *Pediatr Infect Rep, HSC.* 2005;8(13).

Gaston B. Pneumonia. *Pediatr Rev.* 2002;23(4):132–140.

Jadavji T, Law B, Lebel M, et al. A practical guide for the diagnosis and treatment of pediatric pneumonia. *CMAJ.* 1997;156:S703–11.

Kowalczyk A, ed. *The 2005–2006 Formulary of Drugs, The Hospital for Sick Children.* 24th ed. Toronto: The Graphic Centre, HSC; 2005.

Kumar P, McKean M. Evidence based paediatrics: review of BTS guidelines for the management of community acquired pneumonia in children. *J Infect.* 2000;48:134–138.

McCracken G. Diagnosis and management of pneumonia in children. *Pediatr Infect Dis J.* 2000;19:924–928.

McIntosh K. Pneumonia in children. *NEJM.* 2002;346:429–437.

Ostapchuk, M, et al. Community-acquired pneumonia in infants and children. *Am Fam Physician.* 2004;70(5):899–908.

■ PART IV

CARDIAC EMERGENCIES

21 ▪ Cardiac Emergencies

LUBA KOMAR

Introduction

- Congenital cardiac diseases often present in the newborn period and may require emergency management (see Chapter 11)
- Other cardiac emergencies include arrhythmias, myocarditis, and pericarditis
- Chest pain is uncommonly due to cardiac disease in children (< 5%)

Dysrhythmias

- Tachyarrhythmias: heart rate faster than accepted normal range
- Heart Rates in Normal Ranges

Age	Normal Range (bpm)	Mean (bpm)
0–3 mos.	90–180	140
3–6 mos.	80–160	130
6 mos to 1 yr	80–140	115
1–3 yrs	75–130	105
6 yrs	70–110	95
10 yrs	60–90	80

- Narrow vs wide complex
- Mechanisms: reentry, automaticity, or triggers

Narrow Complex Tachyarrhythmia

- Most common tachyarrhythmia

Sinus Tachycardia

- Most common tachycardia in children

Electrocardiographic Features

- Heart rate above normal range for age

- Heart rate
  - Usually < 220 bpm in infants
  - < 180 bpm in children
- Normal P wave axis
- Normal AV conduction
- Normal QRS duration
- Beat to beat variability
- Variable RR interval BUT constant PR interval

Causes of Sinus Tachycardia

- Fever, hypovolemia (dehydration, blood loss), pain, sepsis, stress, poisoning, anemia, hyperthyroidism

Treatment of Sinus Tachycardia

- Treat underlying cause—antipyretic, fluids, pain medication, etc.

Supraventricular Tachycardia (SVT)

Rapid, regular rhythm

- Often sudden onset
- Most often caused by reentry mechanism that involves an accessory pathway
- Usually well tolerated in most infants and children
- May lead to congestive heart failure and cardiovascular collapse

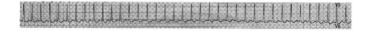

■ **Figure 21.1   Supraventricular Tachycardia (SVT)**

Electrocardiographic Features

- Heart rate > 220 in 60% of infants
- Heart rate > 180 in children
- P waves may be difficult to identify, P wave axis is abnormal
- No beat to beat variability

Causes of Supraventicular Tachycardia
- Wolff-Parkinson-White (22%)
- Congenital heart disease (23%): corrected TGA, Ebstein's anomaly, mitral valve prolapse, asplenia-polysplenia syndromes, post Mustard, Fontan, or ASD repair
- Hyperthyroidism
- Myocarditis
- Drugs: sympathomimetics, caffeine, digitalis toxicity

Treatment of Hemodynamically Stable SVT
- Resuscitation room, cardiac and saturation monitors
- Initial 12-lead ECG, and continuous 12-lead ECG during cardiac conversion
- Vagal maneuvers (62% successful, less successful in infants and younger children):
  - Ice (diving reflex): ice/water mixture in bag applied over forehead and eyes only for 15–20 seconds
  - Gag, carotid sinus massage, abdominal pressure, or Valsalva: ask older child to blow through straw, rectal stimulus (do not apply pressure to eyeballs)
- IV access
- Adenosine: 0.05–0.25 mg/kg IV/IO quick push, increase by 0.05 mg/kg q 2 min or 6 mg max first dose
- Cardiology consultation to consider other medications including phenylephrine, neostigmine, verapamil, propranolol, esmolol, procainamide, digoxin
- Esophageal overdrive pacing
- ECG post conversion

Treatment of Hemodynamically Unstable SVT
- ABCs
- Synchronized cardioversion 0.25–1 J/kg, then 0.5–2 J/kg, max 10 J/kg
  Note: cardioversion may not be successful in presence of hypoxia or acid-base imbalance

Cardioversion

■ Successful cardioversion or defibrillation requires passage of sufficient electric current through the heart
■ Energy dose: the optimal dose has not been established
■ Paddle size: the larger the size, the lower the impedance; use largest size that allows good chest contact
■ Infant paddles (4.5 cm) should be used on infants up to 1 yr or 10 kg
■ Electrode interface: use defibrillation pads, not ultrasound gel or saline-soaked gauze
■ Ensure bridging does not occur because this can cause a short circuit
■ Electrode pad position:
  Anterior-posterior (chest and back) up to 1 yr
  Standard position > 1 yr: position one pad over right upper chest and second pad to left of left nipple line
■ Safety: One–I'm clear Two–You're clear
  Three–Everybody clear Four–Oxygen clear

Wide Complex Tachycardia

■ Tachycardia with wide QRS complex
■ Assume ventricular tachycardia until proven otherwise
■ Differential diagnosis:
  • SVT with aberrancy (8% of pt with SVT)
  • Atrial flutter with aberrancy
  • Antidromic WPW
  Note: if bundle branch block morphology present, > 90% are ventricular tachycardia

Ventricular Tachycardia (VT)

  • Uncommon in children

Electrocardiographic Features

■ Three successive beats of ventricular origin
■ Heart rate > 120 beats per minute

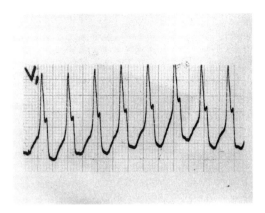

■ **Figure 21.2   Ventricular Tachycardia (VT)**

- QRS morphology different from normal sinus rhythm
- Infants: QRS duration may be normal (0.06–0.11 sec)
- Children > 3 yrs: QRS > 0.09 sec
- Nonsustained VT: 3–30 beats
- Sustained VT: > 30 beats
- Uniform morphology vs multiform morphology
- AV dissociation
- Fusion or sinus capture beats

Torsades de Pointes: "twisting of the peaks"

- QRS gradually changes from one morphology to another
- QRS morphology changes every 5–10 beats, appearing to twist around the isoelectric line
- Usually in patients with prolonged QT interval

Measurement of QTc

- Should measure in Lead II
- **Bazett's Formula: QTc =** $\dfrac{\text{QT}}{\text{preceding RR interval}}$

- Normal: < 0.45 sec in infants, < 0.44 sec in children, < 0.43 sec in adolescents

Congenital Causes of Ventricular Tachycardia

- Ventricular hamartoma
- Prolonged QT Syndrome (Jervell-Lange-Neilsen, Romano-Ward)
- Mitral valve prolapse
- Ebstein's anomaly
- Hypertrophic cardiomyopathy
- Post tetralogy of fallot repair

Acquired Causes of Ventricular Tachycardia

- Cardiac
  - Bacterial endocarditis
  - Myocarditis (including rheumatic fever)
  - Myocardial infarction (hyperlipidemias, Kawasaki disease)
- Metabolic disturbances: acidosis, hypoxia, electrolyte imbalance, liquid protein/starvation diet
- Drug toxicity/sensitivity: anesthetics, antidysrhythmic agents, digitalis, sympathomimetics, phenothiazines, tricyclic antidepressants, organophosphates
- Recreational drugs
- Environmental: electrical injuries
- Plants: foxglove, lily of the valley, yew, blue squill, oleander

Treatment of Hemodynamically Stable VT

- ABCs
- Bloodwork and IV access
- ECG

Initial Management

- Amiodarone: 5 mg/kg IV over 20–60 min *or*
- Procainamide: 15 mg/kg IV over 30–60 min
- Do not administer amiodarone and procainamide together

- Synchronized DC cardioversion: 0.5–1 J/kg, then 2 J/kg
- Overdrive pacing: through atrium or ventricle 30–50 bpm faster than the tachycardia for 5–10 minutes and then stop

Specific Management
- Electrolyte: treat electrolyte disturbance
- Drugs:
  - Digitalis toxicity: Fab antidigoxin antibodies, phenytoin 15 mg/kg IV over 1 hr
  - Tricyclic antidepressant: sodium bicarbonate
  - Organophosphate poisoning: atropine and pralidoxime

Treatment of Hemodynamically Unstable VT
See algorithm in Chapter 3, Cardiopulmonary Resuscitation

Ventricular Fibrillation
- Uncommon as terminal cardiac activity in children (6–19%)
- Uncoordinated ventricular depolarization with no cardiac output

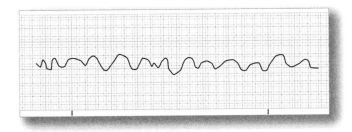

■ **Figure 21.3   Ventricular Fibrillation**

Electrocardiographic Features

- Low amplitude, rapid, irregular ventricular contractions
- No identifiable P waves, QRS complexes or T waves
- Fine: very low amplitude (may appear similar to asystole)
- Coarse: higher amplitude
- Similar pattern may be due to loose electrocardiographic lead connection

Causes

- Hypoxia, hypothermia, electrical shock, chest trauma, long QT syndrome, severe myocardial hypertrophy, Wolff-Parkinson-White

Treatment

2005 American Heart Association Guidelines—See Figure 21.4

Myocarditis

- Inflammation of muscle wall of the heart
- Most common viral cause is coxsackie B
- Presents with fever, tachycardia out of proportion to degree of fever, pallor, cyanosis, respiratory distress from pulmonary edema
- Muffled heart sounds with gallop rhythm
- Hepatomegaly from right-sided heart failure

Investigations

- Chest X-ray
- ECG: nonspecific signs, low-voltage QRS complexes (< 5 mm in limb leads), deep Q waves, poor R wave progression in precordial leads, S-T changes, AV conduction disturbances, ventricular arrhythmias

Management

- If clinical or ECG findings of myocarditis, need intensive monitoring, urgent cardiology consult and echocardiogram, ICU admission

Pericarditis

- Inflammation of pericardium: membranous lining of heart
- Multiple causes: infectious, collagen vascular, malignancy, metabolic disease, postpericardiotomy syndrome
- Main bacterial causes: *S. aureus, H. influenzae, N. meningitidis, S. pneumoniae*
- Viral: enteroviruses—*group B coxsackievirus*
- Presents with fever, chest pain, dyspnea (worse in supine position), friction rub, tachycardia, distant heart sounds
- Pain improves with leaning forward
- Pain usually sharp and sternal/parasternal
- Signs of tamponade: tachycardia, hypotension, weak pulse, elevated jugular venous pressure, hepatomegaly, pulsus paradoxus > 20 mm Hg
- Friction rub may disappear if large effusion

Investigations

- Chest X-ray: cardiomegaly
- ECG: low voltages, ST elevation, PR depression, followed by T wave inversion
- Echocardiogram
- CBC, ESR

Treatment

- Collagen vascular or inflammatory cause: NSAIDs, steroids
- Bacterial: antibiotics
- Pericardiocentesis if signs of cardiac tamponade

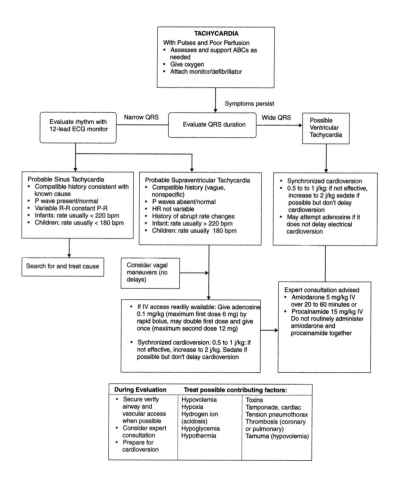

■ **Figure 21.4   Tachycardia**

References

American Heart Association. Part 12: Pediatric Advanced Life Support. *Circulation.* 2005;112:167–187.

Chameides L. Dysrhythmias. In: Barkin RM, ed. *Pediatric Emergency Medicine: Concepts and Clinical Practice.* 2nd ed. St Louis: Mosby-Year Book Inc.; 1997:156–165.

Garson A. Ventricular arrhythmias. In: Gillette PC, Garson A Jr, eds. *Pediatric Arrhythmias: Electrophysiology and Pacing.* Philadelphia: W. B. Saunders Co.; 1990:427–500.

Gewitz M, Vetter V. Cardiac emergencies. In: Fleisher G, Ludwig S, eds. *Textbook of Pediatric Emergency Medicine.* 4th ed. Philadelphia: Lippincott Williams & Wilkins; 2000:676–684.

Gillette P, et al. Preexcitation syndromes. In: Gillette PC, Garson A Jr, eds. *Pediatric Arrhythmias: Electrophysiology and Pacing.* Philadelphia: W. B. Saunders Co.; 1990:360–379.

Kugler JD, Danford DA. Management of infants, children and adolescents with paroxysmal SVT. *J Ped.* 1996;129:324–338.

Ludomirsky A, Garson A. Supraventricular tachycardia. In: Gillette PC, Garson A Jr, eds. *Pediatric Arrhythmias: Electrophysiology and Pacing.* Philadelphia: W. B. Saunders Co.; 1990:380–426.

Perry JC, et al. Pediatric use of intravenous amiodarone: efficacy and safety in critically ill patients from a multicenter protocol. *J Am Coll Cardiol.* 1996;27:1246.

Tinglestad J. Cardiac dysrhythmias. *Pediatr Rev.* 2001;22(3):91–94.

22 ▪ Syncope

Sanjay Mehta

Introduction

- Syncope is defined as temporary loss of consciousness and postural tone due to an abrupt, transient, and diffuse reversible disturbance of cerebral function
- Usually a benign isolated event, fairly common
  - Incidence 0.1–0.5% of children, 1–3% of emergency visits
  - Peaks in adolescents, females > males
- Usually benign, requiring minimal investigation, but may be a result of potentially life-threatening causes

Loss of Consciousness: Differential Diagnosis

- True syncope
  - Transient, acute loss of consciousness caused by a decreased cerebral blood flow secondary to vasodilation or decreased cardiac output
- Neurologic
  - Seizures, migraines
- Hysterical
  - Pseudoloss of consciousness

Common Causes of True Syncope

- Vasovagal
- Orthostatic
- Hyperventilation
- Breath-holding

Vasovagal Syncope ("Simple Faint")

- Common in teenage females
- 50% of childhood syncope
- Altered systemic vascular tone due to exaggerated *Bezold-Jarisch* reflex: responsible for maintaining blood pressure on standing

Table 22.1   Classification

Neural-mediated syncope (NMS)	Vasovagal
	Reflex (breath-holding, cough, micturition)
	Hyperventilation
Orthostatic	Blood or fluid loss
Cardiovascular	Arrhythmias
	Congenital heart disease
	Cardiomyopathy
Metabolic	Hypoglycemia
Hypoxic	Carbon monoxide
Neurologic	Syncopal migraine (rare; basilar artery most common)

- Vasodilation and vagally mediated bradycardia
- Rapid drop in BP and bradycardia, nausea, vomiting, sweating, pallor, numbness, blurred vision, weakness

Triggers

- Prolonged upright posture
- Warm/humid environment (crowds, hot tub, shower)
- Intercurrent illness/over-the-counter medications
- Painful, emotional, fearful, noxious stimuli: coughing paroxysms, hair combing, micturition

Three Phases

1. Prodrome (seconds to minutes)
   - Dizziness or lightheadedness
   - Visual or hearing changes
   - Headache
   - Nausea or abdominal pain
   - Warm, hot, or cold sensation
   - Diaphoresis

2. Loss of consciousness (5–20 seconds)
   * Period generally not recalled by patient
   * Observers describe patients as having a pale or ashen appearance, cold skin, profuse sweating, dilated pupils, and rarely seizure-like activity
3. Recovery period (5–30 minutes)
   * Fatigue, dizziness, weakness, headache, or nausea

Management
Directed at preventing triggers

Cardiac Syncope

▪ Important to rule out cardiac causes of syncope in the emergency department
▪ Often life threatening and can lead to sudden death

Cardiac Causes of Sudden Death

Structurally Abnormal Heart

▪ Cardiomyopathy (hypertrophic, restrictive, dilated)
▪ Postop congenital heart disease
▪ Myocarditis
▪ Congenital coronary abnormality
▪ Aortic stenosis
▪ Pulmonary hypertension

Primary Electrical Disorder

▪ Long QT syndrome
▪ Wolff-Parkinson-White (WPW) syndrome
▪ Atrioventricular fibrillation
▪ Catecholaminergic ventricular tachycardia
▪ Atrioventricular block
▪ Sick sinus syndrome

History

▪ Detailed history of event is critical: precipitating factors such as time of last meal, activities, environmental conditions,

patient position, length of episode, seizure-like activity, details of recovery
■ History of recent medications, past medical history (cardiac conditions, seizures, syncope), metabolic abnormalities, intercurrent illness, pregnancy

History Suggestive of Cardiac Cause

Event History
■ Event occurred during exertion or stress
■ Palpitations; chest pain preceded syncope
■ No premonitory warning symptoms; resulted in bodily injury
■ Seizure-like activity; incontinence
■ Event resulted in cardiopulmonary resuscitation or with neurologic sequelae
■ Event occurred while supine

Prior History
■ Recent fatigue; exercise intolerance
■ Known structural heart disease; arrhythmia

Family History
■ Syncope
■ Premature or unexplained sudden death < 30 years old
■ Unexplained accidents (single motor vehicle accidents, drowning)
■ Known arrhythmia, long QT syndrome, implanted cardiac device
■ Early myocardial infarction
■ Seizure disorder

Life-Threatening Presentations of Syncope
■ Evidence of cardiovascular disease: CHF, abnormal ECG
■ Red-flag cardiac symptoms: chest pain, cyanotic spells, apneic or bradycardic spells requiring vigorous stimulation
■ Abnormal CNS presentation: focal signs, status epilepticus, meningeal irritation
■ Acute toxic ingestions
■ Orthostatic hypotension (resistant to fluid therapy)

Examination

- Vitals (postural), hydration, pallor
- Cardiac and pulmonary exam
- Neurologic exam
- Concurrent injuries

Investigations

- Routine investigations have low yield
- 12-lead ECG for all patients

Consider

- Chest X-ray
- CBC, glucose, carboxyhemoglobin, toxicology screen, βHCG
- Consider neurology referral for EEG, CT, or MRI head as indicated
- Cardiology referral for exercise test, Holter monitoring, echocardiogram if recurrent syncope or history suggestive of cardiac cause

Indications for Referral

- Atypical episodes
- Recurrent or refractory episodes
- Exertional syncope
- Chest pain, arrhythmias, or palpitations
- Abnormal history, exam, or ECG
- Family history of sudden death
- Seizures
- Focal CNS findings

References

Fleisher GR, Ludwig S, eds. *Textbook of Pediatric Emergency Medicine.* 4th ed. Philadelphia: Lippincott Williams & Wilkins; 2000.

Steinberg LA, Knilans TK. Syncope in children: diagnostic tests have a high cost and low yield. *J Pediatr.* 2005;146(3):355–358.

Strieper MJ. Distinguishing benign syncope from life-threatening cardiac causes of syncope. *Semin Pediatr Neurol.* 2005;12(1):32–38.

Wathen JE, et al. Accuracy of ECG interpretation in the pediatric emergency department. *Ann Emerg Med.* 2005;46(6):507–511.

■ PART V

GASTROINTESTINAL EMERGENCIES

23 ▪ Gastroenteritis and Oral Rehydration

LEAH HARRINGTON AND SUZAN SCHNEEWEISS

Introduction

- Gastroenteritis: diarrheal disease of rapid onset
- May be accompanied by nausea, vomiting, fever, or abdominal pain
- Common cause of abdominal pain presenting to the emergency department
- Vomiting alone does not constitute gastroenteritis
- Be cautious in labeling the child with vomiting in the absence of diarrhea as "gastroenteritis"; need thorough assessment to rule out other diagnoses
- Infrequently requires antibiotics

Pathogens

- Viral in up to 80%
- Bacterial etiologies more commonly present with bloody diarrhea

Common Viral Etiologies

- Rotavirus: age 3–15 months; fever, vomiting precedes nonbloody diarrhea; duration 5–7 days
- Norwalk, adenovirus, torovirus

Differential Diagnosis

- Appendicitis
- Intussusception
- Urinary tract infection
- Malrotation with volvulus
- Hemolytic uremic syndrome

Table 23.1 Common Pathogens	
BACTERIAL ETIOLOGIES	ANTIMICROBIAL TREATMENT
Clostridium difficile	Metronidazole, vancomycin
Campylobacter	Erythromycin
Shigella	Amoxicillin, sulfamethoxizole
Yersinia	Trimethoprim-sulfamethoxizole, tetracycline (> 9 yr)
PARASITIC ETIOLOGIES	
Giardia lamblia	Metronidazole

History

- Fluid intake: volume, type (hypertonic, hypotonic, ORS), frequency
- Stool output: frequency, consistency, presence of blood or mucus
- Emesis: frequency, volume, bilious vs nonbilious, hematemesis
- Fever, appetite, weight loss
- Sick contacts including daycare
- Travel
- Underlying illness: cardiac disease, diabetes, renal disease, cystic fibrosis

Examination

- Determine if underlying cause of disease
- First signs of dehydration may not be evident until reach 3–4% dehydration, more signs at 5%, and signs of severe dehydration at 9%
- Difficult to distinguish signs of mild and moderate dehydration on basis of clinical signs; updated recommendations group these patients together (i.e., 3–9%)

Table 23.2   Symptoms and Signs of Dehydration

SYMPTOM/SIGN	MINIMAL OR NO DEHYDRATION (< 3% LOSS BODY WT)	MILD TO MODERATE DEHYDRATION (3–9% LOSS BODY WT)	SEVERE DEHYDRATION (> 9% LOSS BODY WT)
Mental status	Well, alert	Normal, fatigued or restless, irritable	Apathetic, lethargic, obtunded
Fontanel	Normal	Depressed	Sunken
Thirst	Drinks normally; may refuse liquids	Thirsty, eager to drink	Drinks poorly, unable to drink
Mucous membranes	Moist	Dry	Parched
Tears	Present	Decreased	Absent
Eyes	Normal	Slightly sunken	Deeply sunken
Heart rate	Normal	Normal to increased	Tachycardia, bradycardia in severe cases
Blood pressure	Normal	Normal; orthostatic changes	Decreased
Breathing	Normal	Normal; tachypneic	Tachypnea, hyperpnea
Quality of pulses	Normal	Normal to decreased	Weak, thready, or impalpable
Capillary refill	Normal	Prolonged, > 2 sec	Prolonged, > 4 sec
Skin turgor	Instant recoil	Recoil < 2 sec	Recoil > 2 sec
Extremities	Warm	Cool	Cold, mottled, cyanotic
Urine output	Normal to decreased	Decreased	Minimal

Source: Adapted from: Duggan C, Santasham M, Glass RI. *MMWR.* 1992;41(RR–16):1–20, and King CK, Glass R, Bresee JS, Duggan C. *MMWR* 2003;52(RR16):1–16.

Investigations

- Urinalysis for infection and to quantify specific gravity
- Bloodwork:
  - Indicated for moderately dehydrated children when clinical presentation inconsistent with simple diarrheal episode, and in all severely dehydrated children
  - CBC, electrolytes, urea, creatinine, venous gas, glucose
  - Serum bicarbonate best predictor of moderate to severe dehydration

Initial Management

- Based on clinical assessment of dehydration
- Most accurate indicator of magnitude of dehydration is *percentage loss of body weight* during the illness, which represents fluid deficit, but often not available
- Most children present with isonatremic dehydration
- Suspect hypernatremic dehydration if:
  - Oral intake is mostly hypertonic (e.g., salt solutions)
  - Hypotonic fluid loss (e.g., profuse watery diarrhea)
  - Decreased level of consciousness or lethargy beyond expected from apparent mild signs of dehydration

No Dehydration

- Give adequate fluids and continue age-appropriate diet (do not restrict nutrition)
- Increase fluid intake to compensate for losses: can use ORS (oral rehydration solution)
  - 10 mL additional fluid/kg for each episode of vomiting or diarrheal stool
  - *or* give 60–120 mL if < 10 kg, 120–240 mL if > 10 kg

Mild to Moderate Dehydration and Tolerating Fluids

- 50–100 mL ORS/kg over 2–4 hours to replace estimated fluid deficit, plus additional ORS to replace ongoing losses (stool and emesis)

- Give small volume of ORS frequently (i.e., 5 mL aliquots every 1–2 min. (can deliver 150–300 mL/hr)
- As dehydration and electrolyte imbalances correct, may give larger volume at longer intervals
- Solids may be started as early resumption of feeding improves outcome
- Infants: continue breastfeeding, supplement with ORS
- If vomiting, consider NG tube: continuous administration of fluids at low rate
- Observe until signs of dehydration subside; reassess regularly

Severe Dehydration

- Intravenous therapy for severe dehydration (shock/near-shock)
- 20 mL/kg normal saline IV bolus; repeat boluses may be required
- Then 100 mL/kg ORS over 4 hours or D5W 0.45NS IV at 2 times maintenance
- Can continue breastfeeding and age-appropriate diet after initial rehydration
- Replace ongoing losses

Oral Rehydration Therapy (ORT)

- ORT is as effective as IV therapy when rehydrating mild to moderate dehydration: should be the first choice for these patients
- Effective in replacing fluid and electrolyte losses but no effect on duration of diarrhea or stool volume
- May shorten length of hospital stay
- NG tube may be used to administer ORS
- Use of "home-made" ORS strongly discouraged due to risk of serious error in preparation and subsequent metabolic derangement: all commercially prepared ORS acceptable
- Carbohydrate-based drinks (colas, ginger ale, apple juice, sports drinks) can cause osmotic worsening of diarrhea; low sodium content may lead to hyponatremia

Contraindications

- Stupor or coma
- Intestinal ileus, bowel obstruction, acute abdomen

Intravenous Therapy for Dehydration

Indicated for:

- Moderate dehydration and vomiting or worsening diarrhea with inability to keep up with losses
- All severe dehydration and shock or near shock

Antiemetics and Antidiarrheals

Limited/controversial role for antiemetics or antidiarrheals in treatment of pediatric gastroenteritis

Ondansetron

- Selective 5-HT3 receptor antagonist
- Clinically significant effect on cessation of vomiting
- Given as single dose in the emergency department
- Tablets dissolve on tongue
- Dose: 8–15 kg: 2 mg, 15–30 kg: 4 mg, > 30 kg: 8 mg

Metoclopramide

- Not superior to placebo
- High incidence of side effects: somnolence, nervousness, irritability, dystonic reactions

Dimenhydrinate

- Insufficient evidence for use

Loperamide

- Antidiarrheal
- No significant effect on duration of diarrhea
- Not currently recommended

Antibiotics

Antibiotics should not be used unless a bacterial etiology requiring treatment has been identified

Early Refeeding

- Improves fluid and electrolyte uptake and helps to reduce stool losses
- Complex carbohydrates, lean meat, yogurt, fruits and vegetables; avoid foods high in simple sugars
- Start after initial rehydration
- Breastfeeding should continue despite diarrhea
- Early reintroduction of milk (may use lactose-free formula)

Follow-up

- Infants < 3 months must be carefully assessed for hydration; rehydrate under medical observation
- Follow-up within 24–48 hours
- If unable to ensure follow-up, hospital observation or home nurse visit may be required
- Consider admission if:
  - Severe dehydration
  - Hyponatremic or hypernatremic dehydration

References

Borowitz SM. Are antiemetics helpful in young children suffering from acute viral gastroenteritis. *Arch Dis Child.* 2005;50:646–648.

Burkhart DM. Management of acute gastroenteritis in children. *Amer Fam Phys.* 1999;60(9):2555–2563.

Canadian Paediatric Society Statement. Oral rehydration therapy and early refeeding in the management of childhood gastroenteritis. *Can J of Paeds.* 1994;1(5):160–164.

Duggan C, Santosham M, Glass RI. Centers for Disease Control and Prevention. The management of acute diarrhea in children: oral rehydration, maintenance, and nutritional therapy. *MMWR.* 1992;41(RR1–16):1–20.

Fonseca BK, Holdgate A, Craig JC. Enteral vs intravenous rehydration therapy for children with gastroenteritis: a meta-analysis of randomized controlled trials. *Arch Pediatr Adolesc Med.* 2004;158:483–490.

Freedman SB, Adler M, Seshadri R, Powell EC. Oral ondansetron for gastroenteritis in a pediatric emergency department. *NEJM.* 2006;354(16): 1698–1705.

Gorelick MH, Shaw KN, Murphy KO. Validity and reliability of clinical signs in the diagnosis of dehydration in children. *Pediatrics.* 1997:99:5:1–6.

King CK, Glass R, et al. Centers for Disease Control and Prevention. Managing acute gastroenteritis among children: oral rehydration, maintenance, and nutritional therapy. *MMWR Recomm Rep.* 2003;52(RR-16):1–16.

Provisional Committee on Quality Improvement, Subcommittee on Acute Gastroenteritis. Practice parameter: the management of acute gastroenteritis in young children. *Pediatrics.* 1996:97:3:424–435.

24 ▪ Fluid and Electrolyte Disorders

STEPHEN FREEDMAN

Introduction: Fluid Compartments

- Total body water (TBW) = 67% intracellular fluid (ICF) + 33% extracellular fluid (ECF)
- ECF = 25% intravascular + 75% interstitial + transcellular
- As a percentage of body weight, TBW varies inversely with advancing age

Maintenance Fluid and Electrolyte Requirements

- Insensible losses = 400–600 mL/BSA (m^2)/day plus urine and stool output
- Since weight is easily available, used as an adequate alternative to surface area

Electrolyte Requirements

- Sodium: 1–3 mmol/kg/day
- Potassium: 1–3 mmol/kg/day

Table 24.1   Fluid Requirements

WEIGHT (KG)	MAINTENANCE FLUID REQUIREMENT/24 HOURS	MAINTENANCE FLUID REQUIREMENT/HOUR
< 10 kg	100 mL/kg	4 mL/kg
1–20 kg	1,000 mL + 50 mL for each kg > 10 kg	40 mL + 2 mL for each kg > 10 kg
> 20 kg	1,500 mL + 20 mL for each kg > 20 kg	60 mL + 1 mL for each kg > 20 kg

Disorders of Sodium Homeostasis

Hypernatremia (serum sodium > 145 mmol/L)

Etiology

1. Increased total body Na from excess intake or hyperaldosteronism
2. Pure water loss with normal body Na
   - Insensible losses, renal (diabetes insipidus), inadequate access to water
3. Decreased total body water from diarrhea, vomiting, or renal cause
4. Normal total body Na and water with abnormal central regulation
   - Hypothalamic abnormality (essential hypernatremia, hypodipsia)

Clinical Manifestations

- Depend on volume status, degree of hypernatremia, and rate of rise
- Dry mucous membranes, irritability, weakness, lethargy, coma, seizures
- Increased extracellular osmolarity protects perfusion and results in doughy skin

Investigations

- Blood: electrolytes, BUN, creatinine, osmolality
- Urine: urinalysis, specific gravity, Na, osmolality

Approach to Diagnosis

- Urine osmolality > 700 mOsm/kg: normal physiologic response
- Urine osmolality < plasma osmolality: DI (central/nephrogenic)
- Urine osmolality high but < 700 mOsm/kg: loop diuretics, osmotic diuresis, DI

Treatment

- If circulatory compromise, bolus 20 mL/kg normal saline

- Calculate free water deficit:
  - Free water deficit = $0.6 \times$ weight $\times$ [(plasma Na/145) – 1]
  - Simple calculation = 4 mL $\times$ weight (kg) $\times$ desired Δ Na
  - 4 mL/kg water lowers serum Na by 1 mEq/L
- Goal is to reduce serum Na by < 10–12 mmol/L/day to prevent cerebral edema
- Fluid requirement = free water deficit plus ongoing losses plus maintenance
- Give only 75% maintenance fluids due to increased ADH
- Usually reasonable to start with D5W + 0.45 NS solution with frequent monitoring of Na
- Add K after urine output established and if normal renal function
- Monitor Na q 1–4 h initially with glucose, calcium, CNS status
- Admit if symptomatic or Na > 160 mmol/L without an obvious cause
- If severe hypernatremia Na > 170 mmol/L, do not correct serum Na < 150 in first 48–72 hours; consult nephrology and ICU

Hyponatremia (serum sodium < 135 mmol/L)

Etiology

- Pseudohyponatremia (normal total body water and Na) due to hyperosmolar states (hyperglycemia), extreme hyperlipidemia, hyperproteinemia
- Edema and hyponatremia: CHF, hypoalbuminemia, cirrhosis, acute renal failure
- Dehydration and hyponatremia
  - Vomiting, diarrhea, tube drainage, renal losses, third space losses
- Increased total body water with normal total body Na
  - SIADH, primary polydipsia, hypotonic feeds, hypothyroidism

Note: hospitalized patients receiving hypotonic maintenance fluids may have high levels of circulating ADH and are at risk of developing severe hyponatremia

Clinical Manifestations
- Reflect disturbances in volume status, osmolarity, and rate of serum Na fall
- Nausea, lethargy, disorientation, hypothermia, seizures, cerebral edema
- Cerebral edema may present with headache, nausea, vomiting, seizures, respiratory arrest
- Risk of cerebral demyelination if excessively rapid correction of serum sodium:
  - May present with confusion, quadriplegia, pseudobulbar palsy, pseudocoma "locked-in"

Investigations
- Blood: electrolytes, BUN, creatinine, osmolality
- Urine: urinalysis, specific gravity, Na, osmolality

Approach to Diagnosis
- Assess volume status with urine sodium and osmolality to determine diagnosis and treatment

Hypovolemic hyponatremia
- If circulatory compromise, bolus 20 mL/kg normal saline
- If neurologic manifestations, raise plasma Na by 5 mmol/L over 30 min with 6 mL/kg 3% NaCl
- Calculate sodium deficit
  - Na deficit = (desired Na − actual Na) × 0.6 × weight
- Fluid requirements = deficits plus maintenance plus ongoing losses
  - Reduce serum Na by < 12 mmol/L/day to prevent cerebral edema
  - Divide electrolytes by total volume to achieve desired solution
  - Add K only after urine output established and if renal function is normal
  - Rate of correction depends on clinical status, not the absolute Na value

- Monitor plasma Na and CNS status closely
- Admit if symptomatic or Na < 130 mmol/L without an obvious cause

Euvolemic hyponatremia

- Identify underlying etiology; most commonly SIADH
- Acute symptomatic: hypertonic saline to raise plasma Na by 5 mmol/L
- Chronic symptomatic: furosemide to induce water deficit until symptoms resolve, then water restrict
- Asymptomatic: water restriction (consider furosemide if chronic)

Hypervolemic hyponatremia

- Identify underlying etiology
- Water restriction, salt restriction, furosemide

Disorders of Potassium Homeostasis

Hyperkalemia (K > 5.5 mmol/L or > 6.0 mmol/L in newborns)

Etiology

- Pseudohyperkalemia secondary to hemolysis (e.g., tourniquet, heel poke)
- Transcellular shifts (acidosis, drugs, hyperosmolarity, insulin deficiency)
- Increased intake
  - Endogenous (rhabdomyolysis, massive hemolysis)
  - Exogenous
- Decreased excretion
  - Renal failure, hypoaldosteronism, ACE inhibitor, NSAID

Clinical Manifestations

- Paresthesias, weakness, fatigue, ascending paralysis, confusion, dysrhythmias

Investigations

- ECG: peaked T wave, prolonged PR interval, widening of QRS; > 8 mmol/L: P wave disappears and QRS widens and merges into T giving "sine wave"
- Blood: electrolytes, BUN, creatinine, CBC, blood gas, CPK
- Urine: urinalysis, Na, K

Treatment

- ABCs
- Stop K intake
- If K > 8.0 mmol/L or ECG changes other than peaked T waves:

  1. Stabilize cellular membranes
  - Calcium gluconate 10% 0.5–1 mL/kg over 5 minutes

  2. Transfer K into cells
  - Sodium bicarbonate 1–2 mmol/kg over 20 minutes
  - Glucose 1 gm/kg + insulin (regular) 1 unit/3 g glucose over 30 min
  - Nebulized salbutamol (albuterol)

  3. Increase K excretion
  - Sodium polystyrene sulfonate 1 g/kg/dose q 4–6 h PO/PR
  - Dialysis if above measures fail or renal failure present

  4. Recheck plasma K q 1 h until < 6.5 mmol/L
  - If K = 6.5–8.0 mmol/L ± peaked T waves, then perform steps 2 and 3
  - If K < 6.5 mmol/L ± peaked T waves, then perform step 3 and recheck in 4 hrs

Hypokalemia (K < 3.5 mmol/L)

Etiology

- Transcellular shifts: alkalosis, insulin, β_2 catecholamines, periodic paralysis

- Decreased intake: anorexia nervosa, IV fluids without K, low K foods
- Extrarenal loss: vomiting, diarrhea, nasogastric tube losses, laxative abuse
- Urinary loss: diuretics, renal tubular acidosis, diabetic ketoacidosis, excess aldosterone

Clinical Manifestations

- Muscle weakness, ileus, autonomic instability, dysrhythmias, rhabdomyolysis

Investigations

- ECG: premature beats, ST segment depression, U waves
- Serum electrolytes, blood gas, urine K

Treatment

- Search for underlying etiology
- Mild or chronic (K > 3.0 and no ECG changes):
  - Oral supplementation 3 mmol/kg/d plus standard maintenance K
- Severe (K < 3.0 and/or ECG changes):
  - IV KCL 0.2 mmol/kg/hour; maximum concentration of 40 mmol/L via peripheral IV
- Life-threatening: IV KCL via central line 0.2–1 mmol/kg/hour; maximum concentration 80 mmol/L

Disorders of Calcium Homeostasis

Hypercalcemia (Total Ca > 2.75 mmol/L; Ionized Ca > 1.3 mmol/L)

Etiology

- Primary hyperparathyroidism
- Medication related (vitamin A, D, thiazide diuretic, lithium)
- Prolonged immobilization, malignant disease

Clinical Manifestations

- GI: constipation, anorexia, nausea, vomiting, abdominal pain, pancreatitis
- Neurologic: headache, weakness, lethargy, confusion, psychosis, coma
- GU: nephrolithiasis, polydipsia, polyuria, hypokalemia, aminoaciduria

Investigations

- Blood: Ca (ionized, total), phosphorous, alkaline phosphatase, protein, albumin, electrolytes, BUN, creatinine, parathyroid hormone, vitamin D
- Urine: Ca, phosphorus, creatinine
- ECG: short QT, bradycardia, heart block, sinus arrest, dysrhythmias

Treatment

If significant symptoms or cardiac changes, total Ca > 3.5 mmol/L:

ECF expansion

- Rapid rehydration followed by 2 times maintenance

Ca excretion

- Furosemide 1–2 mg/kg q 6–8 h
- Peritoneal or hemodialysis

Hypocalcemia (Total Ca < 2.25 mmol/L; Ionized Ca < 1.1 mmol/L)

Etiology

- True hypoparathyroidism
- Transient neonatal (early, late, maternal hyperparathyroidism)
- Vitamin D deficiency, resistance, or dependence
- Magnesium deficiency
- Massive transfusion of citrated blood
- Hyperphosphatemia

Clinical Manifestations

- ▓ Nonspecific: vomiting, weakness, irritability, fatigue, cramping
- ▓ Neuromuscular: seizures, tetany, laryngospasm, Chvostek and Trousseau signs
- ▓ Rickets, congestive heart failure

Investigations

- ▓ Blood: Ca (ionized, total), phosphorous, alkaline phosphatase, protein, albumin, electrolytes, BUN, creatinine, parathyroid hormone, vitamin D, magnesium
- ▓ Urine: Ca, phosphorus, creatinine
- ▓ ECG: prolonged QT interval, bradycardia, dysrhythmias

Treatment

- ▓ If significant or symptomatic (seizures, arrhythmias):
  - • IV Ca gluconate 10% diluted to 2% solution (10 mL 10% Ca gluconate + 40 mL normal saline = 0.04 mmol/mL Ca); give 0.1 mmol/kg/hr
  - • Adjust infusion q 4 h based on plasma Ca
- ▓ If less severe (muscle cramps, paresthesias):
  - • Give Ca 0.05 mmol/kg/hr

References

Cheng A, Williams BA, Sivarajan BV, eds. *The HSC Handbook of Pediatrics.* 10th ed. Toronto: Elsevier Canada; 2003.

Fleisher GR, Ludwig S, eds. *Textbook of Pediatric Emergency Medicine.* 4th ed. Philadelphia: Lippincott Williams & Wilkins; 2000.

Hoorn EJ, Geary D, et al. Acute hyponatremia related to intravenous fluid administration in hospitalized children: an observational study. *Pediatrics.* 2004;113(5):1279–1284.

Moritz ML, Ayus JC. Disorders of water metabolism in children: hyponatremia and hypernatremia. *Pediatr Rev.* 2002;23(11):371–379.

Moritz ML, Ayus JC. Prevention of hospital-acquired hyponatremia: a case for using isotonic saline. *Pediatrics.* 2003;111(2):227–230.

Strange GR, Ahrens WR, et al, eds. *Pediatric Emergency Medicine: A Comprehensive Study Guide.* 2nd ed. New York: McGraw-Hill; 2002.

25 ▪ Constipation

LEAH HARRINGTON

Introduction

- Constipation: < 3 bowel movements/week, and/or painful passage of hard/large stools
- Functional constipation: not due to organic, anatomic, or pharmaceutical causes
- Fecal soiling: stool deposited on underwear regardless of presence of organic/anatomic lesion
- Encopresis: fecal soiling with functional constipation in the child 4 years of age

Differential Diagnosis

- Gastroenteritis, urinary tract infection, intussusception, appendicitis, chronic recurrent abdominal pain

Acute (1–4 weeks)

- Most common etiologies: viral illness, dietary change

Chronic (> 4 weeks)

- Functional
- Organic/mechanical obstruction (e.g., Hirschsprung's)
- Drug induced (e.g., iron supplementation)
- Endocrine (e.g., hypothyroidism)
- Neuromuscular disorders (e.g., cerebral palsy)

Clinical Presentation

- Affects all age groups
- One of the most common causes of pediatric abdominal pain
- Important questions: passage of meconium within the first 24 hours of life, description of stools, medications taken, recent viral illness

Examination

Acutely Constipated Child

- Well hydrated/nourished
- May have significant pain causing the child to draw the legs into the abdomen

Chronically Constipated Child

- As above if functional etiology
- May present with failure to thrive or unwell/toxic if secondary to organic/obstructive processes

Abdominal Examination

- Stool may be palpated; abdomen is generally soft, diffusely tender with lack of peritoneal signs
- If organic/obstructive process is present, abdomen may appear acutely surgical
- Hard stool may be felt in rectum; overflow loose stool may also be present

Investigations

- Acute functional constipation requires minimal workup (consider urinalysis)
- Radiologic studies not indicated in uncomplicated constipation
- Chronic constipation with suspected organic origin should be investigated as per findings of history and physical examination in a nonemergent setting

Management

- Acute constipation can generally be treated using the oral route, such as stool softeners and dietary adjustments
- Enemas and suppositories can be traumatic for children, so use sparingly

Infants

- Corn syrup: breast-fed: 5–10 mL in 60–120 mL water/fruit juice daily
  bottle-fed: 7.5–30 mL/total formula/day or 5–10 mL every 2nd feed
- Prune juice/infant prunes for infants > 2 months: 30 mL/month of age/day
- Mineral oil *not* recommended for infants < 1 year

Toddlers/Preschoolers/School Age

- Mineral oil/ Lansoyl®: 1–3 mL/kg/day divided into 1–2 doses; double dose every 3 days until results, may take up to 5 days
- Lactulose: 5–10 mL/day; double the dose daily until stool produced
- Senna (Senokot®) syrup: 1–5 yrs 5 mL daily, 5–10 yrs 10 mL daily

Disimpaction of Stool

- For moderate discomfort
- May include manual disimpaction (consider premedication prior to procedure)
- Infant to 2 yrs: glycerin/Dulcolax® suppositories
- Children > 2 yrs: hypertonic phosphate solution (Fleet® enema) ~ 2 mL/kg, and/or normal saline enema 20 mL/kg
- Fleet® enemas and other hyperphospate solutions (e.g., PegLyte®) can be life threatening if used improperly; children < 5 years with congenital/acquired GI/GU abnormalities may be predisposed to metabolic derangement from these solutions
- Picosalax®:
  - Active components are picosulfate sodium and magnesium citrate
  - Combination stimulant cathartic and osmotic laxative
  - 20% or more of magnesium absorbed, therefore contraindicated in renal impairment

- No prospective studies in children
- Orange flavor, pleasant taste
- Dose with 8 oz water: 1–6 yrs: $^1/_4$ packet, 6–12 yrs: $^1/_2$ packet, > 12 yrs: 1 packet
- May repeat × 1 in 8 hrs

Prevention of Reaccumulation

- Infants: see above management recommendations
- Children > 1 yr: mineral oil/Lansoyl® 1–3 mL/kg/day for 3–6 weeks

Fiber Recommendations

- Fiber supplements/purified fiber not suitable for children < 4 years
- Natural food fiber is suitable for infants < 1 yr (pureed fruits, vegetables, and infant cereal)
- Older children may have several servings daily of fiber-rich foods
- Eliminate constipating foods (rice, cheese, bananas)

References

Bulloch B, Tenenbein M. Constipation: diagnosis and management in the pediatric emergency department. *Pediatr Emerg Care.* 2002;18(4):254–258.

Harrington L, Schuh S. Complications of Fleet® enema administration and suggested guidelines for use in the paediatric emergency department. *Pediatr Emerg Care.* 1997; 13(3):225–226.

Loening-Baucke V. Chronic constipation in children. *Gastroenterology.* 1993;105:1557–1564.

Maraffa JM, Hui A, Stork CM. Severe hyperphosphatemia and hypocalcemia following the rectal administration of a phosphate-containing Fleet pediatric enema. *Pediatr Emerg Care.* 2004;20(7):453–456.

Williams CL, Bollella M, Wynder EL. A new recommendation for dietary fiber in childhood. *Pediatrics.* 1995;96(5):985–988.

26 ▪ Abdominal Emergencies

LEAH HARRINGTON

Introduction

- Abdominal pain is a common presenting complaint to the emergency department
- Causes: medical vs surgical
- Etiology varies by age

Principles of Management

- Assess ABCs
- Fluid resuscitation 20 mL/kg normal saline bolus
- NPO
- Surgical consultation
- Pain management

Common Abdominal Emergencies

- Intussusception
- Bowel obstruction: malrotation
- Gastrointestinal bleeding (see Chapter 27)
- Appendicitis (see Chapter 28)

Intussusception

- Telescoping of the bowel at the ileocecal junction leading to ischemia, subsequent necrosis, and death if undiagnosed and untreated
- Triad of intermittent abdominal pain, vomiting, RUQ abdominal mass, plus occult/gross blood per rectum has a positive predictive value of 100%; but only present in 10–20% cases
- Age 2 months to 6 years (peak 5–9 mo), male predominance
- High index of suspicion to avoid missed diagnosis

Table 26.1 Major Diagnosis for Age

	INFANT	CHILD	ADOLESCENT
Medical	UTI	UTI	UTI
	Constipation	Constipation	Constipation
	Gastroenteritis	Gastroenteritis	Gastroenteritis
	Sepsis	Functional	Functional
	Gastroesophageal reflux	HSP	IBD
	Colic	IBD	Pelvic inflammatory disease
		HUS	Sickle cell crisis
		Pneumonia	Diabetic ketoacidosis
		Strep throat	
		Sickle cell crisis	
		Diabetic ketoacidosis	
		Mesenteric adenitis	
Surgical	Malrotation/ volvulus	Intussusception	Appendicitis
	Hirschsprung's disease	Appendicitis	Cholecystitis
	Necrotizing enterocolitis	Testicular torsion	Ectopic pregnancy
	Incarcerated hernia	Pancreatitis	Testicular torsion
	Intussusception		
	Pyloric stenosis		

- May follow an episode of gastroenteritis, with enlarged mesenteric nodes acting as lead points
- Older children may present with intussusception especially if lead points are present (e.g., intestinal lymphosarcoma) or in association with Henoch-Schonlein Purpura
- Differential diagnosis: constipation, gastroenteritis, UTI, appendicitis
- Small bowel intussusception: short segment, no pathological lead point, in otherwise asymptomatic children: conservative observation

Clinical Presentation

- Previously well child or prior gastroenteritis/viral infection
- Intermittent colicky abdominal pain lasting several minutes, inconsolable crying, may draw legs up to the abdomen
- Stops crying with cessation of pain and resumes quiet activity
- ± Vomiting, may be bilious
- ± Lethargy: may be only presenting sign in 10%
- Stools are normal in early stage; rectal blood/currant jelly stools is a late sign
- Abdominal examination
  - May be normal between episodes
  - Diffuse tenderness, distention, RUQ sausage-shaped mass

Investigations

- Abdominal X-ray: low specificity
  - May show signs of obstruction
  - Target sign (pseudokidney sign), crescent sign (intussuscepting lead point protruding into a gas-filled pocket), absent liver edge
- Abdominal ultrasound: negative predictive value 97.4% in one pediatric center
- Air/barium enema:
  - Gold standard for diagnosis and treatment
  - Contraindicated if perforation, complete obstruction, or hemodynamic instability

Bowel Obstruction: Malrotation

- Bilious vomiting in an infant is malrotation with volvulus until proven otherwise
- 1 in 500 live births
- M:F 2:1 (neonatal)
- Age of presentation: 50% in first month, 75% in first year
- May be associated with other gastrointestinal abnormalities such as volvulus, small bowel atresia, Meckel's diverticulum, Hirschprung's disease, intussusception

Differential Diagnosis

- Sepsis: must be considered in infants presenting with vomiting, distress, lethargic/toxic appearance (may precipitate paralytic ileus or may be associated with ischemic/necrotic gut)
- Other congenital/acquired obstructive processes (e.g., duodenal atresia)

Clinical Presentation

- Infancy
  - Sudden onset of abdominal pain and bilious vomiting in previously well infant, or
  - Sudden onset of abdominal pain in infant with transient episodes of bilious vomiting or past "feeding intolerance"
- Older children: symptoms more vague
  - Chronic intermittent vomiting, crampy abdominal pain, failure to thrive, constipation, bloody diarrhea, hematemesis
  - Differential: intussusception, Hirschprung's disease, and necrotizing enterocolitis

Examination

- 50% have normal abdominal exam
- Mild distention, diffuse tenderness, dilated loop of bowel may be palpable
- Rectal exam: gross blood associated with bowel ischemia/necrosis
- Disease progression: intestinal ischemia → gangrene

- Progression of symptoms:
  - Abdominal distention
  - Abdominal pain and peritonitis
  - Tachycardia, hypovolemia
  - May appear lethargic/toxic and progress to shock

Investigations

- Bloodwork
  - CBC and differential, electrolytes, urea, creatinine, venous gas, blood and urine culture, type and cross
- Plain films (supine and upright views)
  - Gastric or proximal duodenal dilatation, ± distal bowel gas
  - Loops of small bowel overriding the liver shadow, dilated loops of bowel with multiple air-fluid levels, markedly dilated stomach and duodenum
- Upper GI series
  - Absent ligament of Treitz and C-loop of duodenum
  - Duodenum lies to the right of the spine
  - Jejunum: coiled spring appearance in right upper quadrant
  - Sensitivity for detecting malrotation: 100%
- Lower GI series
  - Can identify malrotation (false negative 5–20%)
  - Rule out colonic obstruction (e.g., atresia, Hirschsprung's disease, meconium ileus/plug

Initial Management

- ABCs
- NPO, NG tube to suction
- Fluid resuscitation
- Urgent surgical referral
- Intervention is urgent because bowel ischemia can progress rapidly if volvulus is present

References

Barkin RM. *Pediatric Emergency Medicine: Concepts and Clinical Practice.* St. Louis: Mosby-Year Book Inc.; 1992:784–790.

Harrington L, et al. Ultrasonographic and clinical predictors of intussusception. *J Pediatr.* 1998;132:836–839.

Leung A, Sigalet D. Acute abdominal pain in children. *Am Fam Phys.* 2003;67(11):2321–2326.

Schnaufer L, Mahboubi S. Abdominal emergencies. In: Fleisher G, Ludwig S, eds. *Textbook of Pediatric Emergency Medicine.* 4th ed. Philadelphia: Lippincott Williams & Wilkins; 2000:1513–1539.

27 ■ Gastrointestinal Bleeding

LEAH HARRINGTON

Introduction
- Upper gastrointestinal bleeding
  - Hematemesis: bleeding proximal to ligament of Treitz
  - Melena: black, tarry stools, bleeding proximal to ileocecal valve
- Lower gastrointestinal bleeding
  - Hematochezia: bright red blood per rectum

Assessment
- Is the child hemodynamically stable?
- Is this blood?
- For infants: maternal vs infant blood?
- Is this an upper or lower gastrointestinal hemorrhage?
- What are the specific diagnosis and site of the hemorrhage?

Table 27.1   Substances Mistaken for Blood in Emesis and Stool

HEMATEMESIS	HEMATOCHEZIA	MELENA	
Commercial dyes	Menstruation	Iron	Lead
Swallowed maternal blood	Commercial dyes	Licorice	Charcoal
Bleeding from nose, mouth, pharynx	Ampicillin	Blueberries	Dirt
	Hematuria	Spinach	Beets
		Bismuth (Pepto-Bismol®)	

Apt-Downey Test: Maternal vs Infant Blood
■ Mix stool or emesis with water (1:5), centrifuge mixture
■ Add 1 mL 0.25% sodium hydroxide to 5 mL supernatant—
  wait 5 minutes
  • Adult hemoglobin = brown–yellow
  • Fetal hemoglobin = pink

Stool Guaiac (Occult Blood) Test
■ Identifies gross/occult blood in stool

Acute Stabilization
■ Assess for signs of intravascular volume depletion
  • < 15%   No hemodynamic change
  • > 15%   Tachycardia
  • > 30%   Hypotension

Table 27.2	Causes of Upper Gastrointestinal Bleeding	
	COMMON	UNCOMMON
Newborns and infants	Swallowed maternal blood	Gastritis
	Esophagitis	Gastroduodenal ulceration
		Coagulopathy
Toddlers and children	Swallowed blood	Sepsis
	Severe GE reflux	Liver failure
	Mallory-Weiss tear	Vitamin K deficiency
		Mechanical, chemical injury
		Infection
		Esophageal varices
		Duodenal ulcer

- Elevate head of the bed
- Place large-bore IV lines × 2
- Volume replacement with crystalloid 10–40 mL/kg depending on status
- CBC, INR, PTT, consider liver function tests, cross and type for blood
- Vitamin K 5–10 mg IV/IM if elevated INR or known liver disease (keep anaphylaxis kit at bedside for IV dose)

Additional Stabilization for Upper GI Bleed

- Large-bore NG tube: decompression of stomach, confirmation of UGI bleeding, indication of rate of blood loss
- Pantoprazole (Pantoloc®)
  - 5–15 kg: 2 mg/kg IV bolus followed by continuous infusion 0.2 mg/kg/hr
  - 15–40 kg: 1.8 mg/kg IV, then infusion 0.18 mg/kg/hr
  - > 40 kg: 80 mg IV, then infusion 8 mg/hr
- Severe bleeding (especially from variceal source):
  - Octreotide (Sandostatin®) 1 mcg/kg bolus; continuous infusion 1 mcg/kg/hr
- Consider endoscopy with gastroenterology consultation

Transfusion as Required

- PRBCs, fresh frozen plasma, platelets
- FFP to correct coagulation abnormalities, or with every 2–3 units of PRBCs for ongoing loss of coagulation factors
- Platelets reserved for patients with platelet count < 50

UGI Bleeding—Esophageal Varices

- Sudden onset, often life threatening
- Massive hematemesis
- Melena may precede hematemesis

Note: volume overload/excessive transfusion may increase portal pressure and continuance of hemorrhage

Table 27.3   Causes of Lower Intestinal Bleeding

	COMMON	UNCOMMON
Preterm infant	Necrotizing enterocolitis	
Newborn/Infant	Milk protein intolerance	Vascular lesions
	Anal fissure	Hirschsprung's enterocolitis
	Swallowed maternal blood (with rapid transit time)	Meckel's diverticulum
		Intestinal duplication
		Intussusception
		Midgut volvulus
Toddler/ Older child	Anal fissure	Inflammatory bowel disease (< 4 yrs)
	Infectious enterocolitis	Vascular malformations
	Inflammatory bowel disease (> 4 years)	Intestinal duplications
	Intussusception	Solitary rectal ulcer
	Perianal streptococcal cellulitis	Henoch-Schonlein Purpura
	Juvenile/ inflammatory polyp	Colonic or rectal varices
		Sexual abuse
		Rectal trauma
		Meckel's diverticulum
		Typhlitis/cecitis

Lower GI Bleeding—Anal Fissures

- Tear of the squamous epithelial mucosa of the anal canal from passage of hard stool
- Common in infants 6–24 months; most common cause of bright rectal bleeding at any age

Clinical Presentation

- Streaks of bright red blood on surface of hard stool, diaper, or toilet paper after bowel movement

Diagnosis

- Inspection of anal region

Treatment

- Dietary modification, stool softeners, Sitz baths

Juvenile Polyps

- Benign hamartomas with no malignant potential (80% of polyps in children)
- Most commonly seen age 2–8 years (peak 3–4 years)

Clinical Presentation

- Painless rectal bleeding, rectal prolapse (4%), abdominal pain (10%)

Diagnosis

- Sigmoidoscopy, colonoscopy, and/or contrast enema

Treatment

- Observation: may auto-amputate
- Endoscopic resection of distal colonic/rectal polyps if persistent bleeding

Polyp Syndromes

- Juvenile polyposis
- Peutz-Jeghers Syndrome: intestinal hamartomatous polyps with mucocutaneous pigmentation of the mouth, hands, and feet
- Familial adenomatous polyposis:
  - Presents with rectal bleeding, anemia, abdominal pain, or diarrhea
  - Diagnosed by routine screening of children from an affected family

Meckel's Diverticulum

- Most common congenital abnormality of the small intestine
- 45% present in infants < 2 years of age

Clinical Presentation

- < 5 years: acute generally painless lower GI bleeding due to ulceration from heterotopic gastric mucosa

Diagnosis

- Technetium Tc 99m–pertechnetate scintiscan (Meckel's scan)
- 95% accuracy for detection of gastric mucosa

Treatment

- Referral to surgery for excision

Inflammatory Bowel Disease (IBD)

- Idiopathic immune reaction of the body to its own intestinal tract
- Ulcerative colitis (limited to colon) and Crohn's disease (mouth to anus)
- Affects children aged 5–16 years (10% < 18 years)

Clinical Presentation

- Growth failure, weight loss, occult rectal bleeding, bloody diarrhea, abdominal pain
- Less common: fever, arthritis, skin lesions, oral or perianal ulcers
- UC: hallmark is bloody, mucusy diarrhea
- Crohn's: more insidious presentation with abdominal pain, weight loss; diarrhea may not be present if disease confined to small bowel

Diagnosis

- Contrast radiographs and sigmoidoscopy or colonoscopy
- Consult gastroenterologist

Treatment

- 5-Aminosalicylates, followed by corticosteroids if unsuccessful
- Severe disease requires hospitalization for bowel rest, IV steroids ± immunomodulators

Allergic Colitis (cow's milk protein intolerance)

- Hypersensitivity to cow and soy milk, or food allergy induced in breastfed infant by cow's milk proteins ingested by mother
- Immunologic response may vary from classic allergic mast cell activation to immune complex formation
- Affects infants age 2 weeks to 1 year

Clinical Presentation

- Blood and mucus in the stool, vomiting
- Diarrhea after introduction of milk
- Usually a well-appearing infant with normal weight gain

Diagnosis

- Elevated WBC count, low hemoglobin
- ± Eosinophilia, hypoalbuminemia (if protein-losing enteropathy present)

Treatment
- Eliminate offending protein from infant's diet
- Substitute formula containing casein-hydrolysate (Nutramigen®, Pregestimil®, Alimentum®)
- Exclusively breastfed infants: eliminate offending protein (milk) from mother's diet
- Consider proctosigmoidoscopy if gross bleeding continues after 7 days of casein-hydrolysate formula
- Rechallenge with milk at 1 year if treatment successful

Infectious Colitis
- Most common cause of colitis beyond 1 year of age
- Bacterial, viral, parasitic agents
- Viral in > 80% cases
- Most common bacterial causes: *E. coli*, *Shigella*, *Salmonella*, *Campylobacter*, *Yersinia*
- Most common cause of pseudomembranous colitis is *Clostridium difficile* following a course of antibiotics (clindamycin most common antibiotic)

Clinical Presentation
Bacterial Colitis
- More commonly presents with bloody diarrhea compared to viral colitis
- *Salmonella*
  - Outbreaks associated with contaminated eggs, dairy products, meats
  - *Salmonella enteritidis* most common cause of gastroenteritis
  - *Salmonellla typhi* most common cause of typhoid fever (enteric fever)
- *Shigella*
  - Causes intestinal mucosal cell destruction, mucosal ulcerations, bleeding
  - Elaborates exotoxins that produce diarrhea

- *Escherichia coli*
  - Many different pathologic strains including enterohemorrhagic *E. coli* (EHEC), O157:H7, and O26:H11 (risk of HUS post *E. coli* 0157 is 10–15% in children)

Parasitic Colitis
- Watery, foul-smelling stools, cramping; strong secretory component
- *Entamoeba histolytica:*
  - Most common cause of parasitic colitis globally
  - Ingestion of trophozoites
  - Due to water contamination, fecal–oral route transmission
- *Giardia lamblia* frequently isolated from patients with diarrhea

Table 27.4   Management

Organism	Treatment
Campylobacter and Yersinia	Erythromycin, azithromycin
	Antibiotic treatment generally not required; no significant change in course with treatment
E. coli	Antibiotic treatment of enterohemorrhagic *E. coli* infection—no benefit proven in prophylaxis or treatment for HUS; antibiotics may increase risk of HUS
Salmonella	Ampicillin, septra, cefotaxime, ceftriaxone
	Consider treatment for infants, immuno-compromised, systemically unwell patients
Shigella	Ampicillin (80% resistance in some areas), septra (47% resistance), ceftriaxone
	Antibiotic treatment shortens clinical course
Clostridium difficile	Metronidazole, vancomycin
Giardia lamblia	Metronidazole

References

Arain Z, Rossi TM. Gastrointestinal bleeding in children: an overview of conditions requiring non-operative management. *Semin Pediatr Surg.* 1999;8(4):172–180.

Barkin RM. *Pediatric Emergency Medicine: Concepts and Clinical Practice.* St. Louis: Mosby-Year Book Inc.; 1992:784–786.

D'Agostino J. Common abdominal emergencies in children. *Emerg Med Clin North Am.* 2002;20(1):139–153.

Dennehy PH. Acute diarrheal disease in children: epidemiology, prevention, and treatment. *Infect Dis Clin North Am.* 2005;19(3):585–602.

Gibbons TE, Gold BD. The use of proton pump inhibitors in children: a comprehensive review. *Pediatr Drugs.* 2003:5(1):25–40.

28 ▪ Appendicitis

BRUCE MINNES

Introduction

- Most common nontraumatic condition requiring emergency abdominal surgery in children and adolescents
- Missed appendicitis or delays to diagnosis are among the common scenarios resulting in a complaint or lawsuit regarding ED care
- May present at any age, but most common in second and third decades (peak incidence 9–12 years)
- ~1 in 15 lifetime risk of developing appendicitis
- M:F ratio is 2:1
- Incidence of perforation at diagnosis is highest in children < 1 yr (almost 100%), 94% < 2 yrs, and 60–65% < 6 yrs
- Mortality rate 0.1% (nonperforated), 3–5% (perforated)
- Young children can progress to perforation rapidly within 6–12 hrs from symptom onset
- Need a high index of suspicion

Pathophysiology

- Lumen of the appendix vermiformis becomes obstructed
- Less likely in infants due to primitive shape and relative lack of lymphoid tissue in appendix
- Obstruction commonly caused by
  - Hypertrophied lymphatic tissue: seen with viral illnesses
  - Fecaliths, parasites, fruit or vegetable material
- Obstruction leads to venous engorgement, inflammation, and eventual necrosis and perforation
- In adolescents and adults, omentum may help to "wall-off" appendicitis
- Omentum less developed in young children, leading to a higher likelihood of diffuse peritonitis and increased morbidity and mortality

Clinical Presentation

- Classic symptoms: abdominal pain, low-grade fever, and vomiting
- Abdominal pain
  - Typically dull or achy at onset, later colicky, crampy, and finally constant
  - Initially periumbilical or epigastric, later localized to right lower quadrant as parietal peritoneum becomes irritated
- Anorexia and nonbilious emesis
- Some degree of fever is often present
- In many cases, atypical symptoms may occur and lead to misdiagnosis
- Urinary frequency and dysuria if inflamed appendix is close to the ureter and bladder
- Diarrhea (frequent, small volume, and loose stools) and tenesmus (fecal urgency) may occur in retrocecal appendicitis or if appendix is near a segment of colon

Physical Examination

- Resting tachycardia or fever may not be universally present, particularly in nonperforated appendicitis
- May walk with slightly hunched-over gait or prefer to lie still
- Pain increases with movement
- Early, generalized abdominal tenderness with soft abdomen
- Later: pain may localize to RLQ, maximally tender at McBurney's point
- Pain may be increased with palpation or percussion over descending colon (Rovsing's sign)
- Rebound tenderness on light palpation and involuntary guarding of the right lower quadrant may be present
- Positive iliopsoas or obturator signs suggest retrocecal appendicitis:
  - Iliopsoas sign: pain with extension of hip
  - Obturator sign: painful internal rotation of hip
- Digital rectal examination of limited value, may be helpful if equivocal or difficult abdominal examination (i.e., obese

patient) or in female adolescents to help to differentiate appendicitis from pelvic pathology

Investigations

- No laboratory tests are diagnostic
- CBC and differential: may be normal, often WBC: 10,000 with increased neutrophil or band count
- WBC > 15,000 suggests perforation
- Urinalysis usually normal or mildly positive for leukocytes
- If urine highly positive WBC or positive for nitrites, consider UTI
- Pregnancy test in female adolescent (especially preradiographs or CT)

Pediatric Appendicitis Score

- Pediatric Appendicitis Score (PAS) by Samuel: relates different variables to improve diagnostic accuracy and reduce negative laparotomy rate in early suspected appendicitis
- Currently undergoing prospective evaluation for validity (R. Goldman, The Hospital for Sick Children, personal communication):

Table 28.1 Pediatric Appendicitis Score

CLINICALLY SIGNIFICANT VARIABLES	SCORE
Cough/percussion/hopping tenderness	2
Tenderness in RLQ	2
Anorexia	1
Fever	1
Nausea/vomiting	1
WBC > 10×10^9/L	1
Polymorphonuclear neutrophilia	1
Migration of pain from umbilical area to RLQ	1
Maximum score	**10**

- Score ≤ 5 : not compatible with appendicitis
- Score ≥ 6: compatible with appendicitis
- Score 7–10: suggests a high probability of appendicitis
- For low–medium probability patients, the score may help to guide decisions related to serial examination or the use of diagnostic imaging

Diagnostic Imaging

- In presentations of "classic" or high-probability appendicitis, imaging is unlikely to provide more useful information
- Delays to definitive treatment while waiting for CT or ultrasound add to patient discomfort and are associated with higher perforation rates and associated morbidity and increased hospital stay
- Selective strategies of timely radiologic evaluation will provide useful information in equivocal cases, reduce both perforation rates and negative laparotomy rates, and reduce radiation exposure and its associated risks
- Use of selective guidelines can reduce the number of ultrasounds and CT scans with minimal reduction in overall diagnostic accuracy for appendicitis

Ultrasound

- Ultrasound is often considered as a first imaging procedure
- Limited accuracy; equivocal or nondiagnostic tests are common
- In patients with "classic" appendicitis, may further delay treatment as deliberations are made as to whether to proceed with CT

Abdominal CT Scan

- CT scanning is a more accurate imaging tool and focused CT scanning (L3 to tip of acetabulum) with rectal contrast may improve its use

- A nonselective policy of CT scanning will result in excessive use, radiation exposure, and costs without diagnostic value
- Consider a protocol of clinical evaluation, serial reexamination, and selective use of ultrasound or CT scan for equivocal cases

Plain Radiographs

- No role for routine plain abdominal radiography in the evaluation of children with abdominal pain or suspected appendicitis
- Obtain chest X-ray to evaluate for pneumonia if respiratory findings

Differential Diagnosis

- Lower lobe pneumonia
- Mesenteric adenitis: intensity and localization of the pain are more vague
- Gastroenteritis
- Intussusception
- Inflammatory bowel disease
- Urinary tract infections
- Tubo-ovarian or other gynecologic conditions (pregnancy, ectopic pregnancy, ovarian cysts or torsion, pelvic inflammatory disease, or endometriosis)
- Exclude pregnancy prior to any radiation exposure
  - Ultrasound (consider transvaginal scanning) is the imaging modality of choice in this group

Management

- Surgical consultation
- Pain management: use of narcotic analgesia does not reduce diagnostic accuracy
- Intravenous hydration, correct electrolyte imbalance, keep NPO

- In high-probability cases, surgical referral should proceed without imaging
- Serial reexamination or use of imaging may be considered in low- or moderate-risk cases in collaboration with surgeon
- If appendicitis unlikely and the patient is discharged, clear written discharge instructions must be given because the presentation may be atypical or early in the evolution of appendicitis

References

Gore Peña BM, Cook EF, Mani KD. Selective imaging strategies for the diagnosis of appendicitis in children. *Pediatrics.* 2004;113(1):24–28.

Kosloske AM, Love CL, Nohrer JE, Goldthorn JE, Laxy SR. The diagnosis of appendicitis in children: outcome of a strategy based on pediatric surgical evaluation. *Pediatrics.* 2004;113(1):29–34.

Samuel M. Pediatric appendicitis score. *J Pediatr Surg.* 2002;37:877–881.

Thomas SH, et al. Effects of morphine analgesia on diagnostic accuracy in emergency department patients with abdominal pain: a prospective, randomized trial. *J Am Coll Surg.* 2003;196:18–31.

■ PART VI

GENITOURINARY EMERGENCIES

29 ▪ Urinary Tract Infections

DENNIS SCOLNIK

Introduction
- Urinary tract infections (UTIs) occur frequently throughout childhood
- Prevalence in first year of life: 6.5% (girls), 3.3% (boys)
- Prevalence in children: 8.1% (girls), 1.9% (boys)
- Rate of UTIs is 5–20 × higher in uncircumcised boys
- Less common in African American children
- Prevalence in febrile children 2 months to 2 years of age: ~ 5%
- Upper respiratory tract infection or otitis media does not preclude UTI
- Other risk factors: fever > 24 hours, fever > 38.9°C and prior UTIs

Clinical Presentation
Different presentations through childhood:

Infants
- Nonspecific feeding difficulty, anorexia, irritability, vomiting, diarrhea
- $\frac{2}{3}$ have fever, few present with sepsis syndrome or shock
- Late onset jaundice, with elevation of both direct and indirect bilirubin may be the only indication of infantile UTI

Toddlers and Preschool Children
- Nonspecific presentation
- May notice a change in urine smell, color, or pattern of urination

Schoolchildren

- More likely to present with "classic" adult symptoms and signs
- Frequency, dysuria, and urgency are common but not pathognomonic
- May report changed behavior, vomiting, anorexia, fever, abdominal pain, or secondary enuresis
- If untreated, symptoms may subside over 1–3 weeks, although the urine culture remains positive
- In recurrent UTIs, symptoms may be minimal

UTI vs Pyelonephritis

- Not possible to clinically distinguish lower UTIs from pyelonephritis in young children; therefore must maintain a high index of suspicion
- 75% of children < 5 years with febrile UTIs have upper tract involvement
- Costovertebral angle tenderness, rigors, and toxicity suggest upper tract involvement
- Up to 50% of children with febrile UTIs develop renal scarring—may be associated with development of hypertension and end stage renal disease
- Most scars develop in first five years of initial diagnosis

When to Send a Urine Culture?

- Febrile infants < 1 year
- Symptoms/signs suggestive of UTI
- Toxic/septic/shock without obvious cause
- History of recurrent UTI, regular catheterization, or known urinary tract anomaly
- Unexplained fever or symptoms

Obtaining a Urine Sample

- Four methods: midstream/clean catch sample, urine bag, catheterization, and suprapubic aspiration
- Urine must be promptly analyzed and plated

- Refrigerate specimen if > 30-min delay between collection and plating

Midstream/Clean Catch Sample
- Least traumatic method
- Can be used in all children without obvious infection or anomaly of external genitalia
- In infants the parent may prefer to wait with a sterile container and catch urine

Catheterization
- Method of choice for febrile infants, toxic/septic/shock, and in all age groups with an urgent clinical indication to start antibiotic treatment
- Genitalia must be carefully cleansed and strict aseptic technique followed to avoid iatrogenic infection
- Contraindications: gross infection of genital area, labial adhesions, and uncircumcised boys whose urethral opening cannot be visualized
- Foreskin should not be forcibly retracted as predisposes to paraphimosis

Suprapubic Aspiration
- Used in diapered uncircumcised boys whose urethral opening cannot be visualized, and infants/children with urgent indications for initiation of therapy who cannot be catheterized or produce a midstream sample
- Considered gold standard but varied success rates (23–90%) and technical expertise is required
- Bladder is percussed to ensure urine is present
- Sterile technique, 23G 2-cm needle with 5-mL syringe: inserted at right angles to skin in midline of first crease above the pubic bone with constant suction
- Needle is removed from syringe before urine is expelled into a sterile container

Urine Bag

- Discouraged due to high risk of contamination of sample
- Periurethral area should be carefully washed and dried before affixing bag
- May be used for screening of urine to exclude infection if negative, but should *not be used for definitive culture*

How to Interpret Urinalysis and Culture

White Cells and Gram Stain

- Presence of white cells by microscopy or by leukocyte esterase dipstick usually indicates a urine infection
- Controversy regarding number of cells on urine microscopy that indicate infection:

  > 5 cells/mm^3 or positive leukocyte esterase test is usually considered indicative of infection
- Normal urinalysis may not rule out UTI in infants < 8 weeks of age

Table 29.1   Sensitivity and Specificity of Components of Urinalysis

Test	Sensitivity (%)	Specificity (%)
Leukocyte esterase (LE)	83	78
Nitrites	53	98
Positive LE or nitrites	93	72
Microscopy WBCs	73	81
Microscopy bacteria	81	83
LE or nitrites or microscopy positive	99.8	70

Source: Adapted from: American Academy of Pediatrics practice parameter, *Pediatrics.* 1999;103(4):847.

Nitrite Test
- Positive nitrite on dipstick usually indicates infection
- Urine voided shortly after formation does not allow time for bacteria to produce enough nitrites to give a positive result (especially in infants < 3 months)

Culture and Colony-Forming Units
- Negative culture on bag specimen is a reliable indication of absence of UTI (many labs will no longer process bag specimens for culture)
- In midstream/clean catch or bag urine specimens, a mixed growth usually means contamination of specimen
- If vague and nonspecific symptoms, a mixed culture may still be significant
- Reassess and repeat urine culture with meticulous attention to collection and transport technique
- In immunocompetent patients, organisms such as *Lactobacillus,* coagulase negative *staphylococci, Strept viridans,* and *Corynebacterium* species are considered skin contaminants

Treatment

Duration
- Short courses (2–4 days) of oral antibiotics are not currently recommended

Table 29.2   Guidelines for Interpretation of Colony Counts

Specimen	Significant number of colony-forming units ($\times 10^6$/L)
Suprapubic	≥ 1
Midstream, catheter, clean catch	≥ 50

- Short courses may be effective for lower tract disease
- Optimal duration of therapy unknown
- Current guidelines recommend 7–10 days of treatment

Oral vs IV Therapy

- If clinically stable, oral and parenteral therapy in children > 3 months have similar efficacy; consider using oral cefixime
- In young infants IV therapy and admission for closer observation may still be warranted
- In children with symptoms and signs of pyelonephritis a short course of IV antibiotics can be followed by oral treatment
- Single daily dose of aminoglycoside has been shown to be as effective and safe as tid dosing

Antibiotic Choice

- Choice of antibiotics should be based on local resistance patterns
- Organisms: *E. coli* (50%), *Klebsiella pneumoniae, Proteus, Enterococcus, Citrobacter, Pseudomonas, Staph saprophyticus*
- Currently many areas show resistance to amoxicillin and trimethoprim-sulfamethoxazole
- Consider first-generation cephalosporin as first-line agent (e.g., cephalexin)

Admit

- Neonates
- Sepsis or shock
- Complex urologic pathology
- Persistent vomiting or dehydration
- Suspect organism resistant to oral medication
- Psychosocial issues

Follow-up

- All young children with a urinary tract infection require investigation for vesicoureteral reflux or renal anomalies

- Follow-up should include renal ultrasound, voiding cystourethrogram (VCUG)
- If delay to obtaining VCUG, prophylactic antibiotics must be given

References

Chon CH, Lai FC, Shortliffe LM. Pediatric urinary tract infections. *Pediatr Clin North Am.* 2001;48(6):1441–1459.

Crain EF, Gershel JC. Urinary tract infections in febrile infants younger than 8 weeks of age. *Pediatrics.* 1990;86:363–367.

Hoberman A, Wald ER, et al. Oral versus initial intravenous therapy for urinary tract infections in young febrile children. *Pediatrics.* 1999;104(1): 79–86.

Michael M, Hodson EM, Craig JC, Martin S, Moyer VA. Short versus standard duration oral antibiotic therapy for acute urinary tract infection in children. *Coch Data Syst Rev.* 2003;(1):CD003966.

Practice Parameter: the diagnosis, treatment and evaluation of the initial urinary tract infection in febrile infants and young children. American Academy of Pediatrics, Committee on Quality Improvement, Subcommittee on Urinary Tract Infection. *Pediatrics.* 1999;103(4):843–852.

Shaw KN, Gorelick MH. Urinary tract infection in the pediatric patient. *Pediatr Clin North Am.* 1999;46(6):1111–1124.

30 ▪ Renal Emergencies

JENNIFER THULL-FREEDMAN

Introduction

- Most common cause of acute renal failure in children is prerenal
- Common to find varying degrees of functional/transient proteinuria or hematuria

Proteinuria

Common Causes of Isolated Proteinuria

- Functional/transient proteinuria
  - Caused by fever, exercise, dehydration, seizures, exposure to cold, congestive heart failure
  - Urine dip usually < 2+ proteinuria (< 100 mg/dL)
- Benign postural (orthostatic) proteinuria
  - Usually occurs after 7 years of age
  - Urine protein: creatinine ratio in a first morning void is normal
- Glomerulopathy
  - Nephrotic syndrome (see below)
- Tubular
  - Overload proteinuria
  - Tubular dysfunction (reflux nephropathy, ischemic injury, cystinosis)
- Benign persistent proteinuria

Laboratory Evaluation

- Dipstick:
  - False positive with concentrated urine, pH > 8, gross hematuria or pyuria
  - False negative with very dilute, acidic urine (pH < 4.5)
- Urine protein: creatinine ratio (mg/mg)
  - < 0.5 if < 2 years age or < 0.2 for older children considered normal

228

- • > 1 suspicious for nephrotic range proteinuria
- • > 2 suggestive of nephrotic range proteinuria
- ◼ Consider 12–24 hour collection if urine protein:creatine ratio is abnormal
- ◼ Additional evaluation to consider: electrolytes, urea, creatinine, albumin, cholesterol, C3, C4, ANA, CBC, VBG

Nephrotic Syndrome

- ◼ Clinical syndrome of proteinuria due to loss of glomerular membrane selectivity
- ◼ Characterized by proteinuria, hypoproteinemia, edema, hyperlipidemia
- ◼ Secondary disturbances: hypocalcemia (due to hypoalbuminemia), hyperkalemia (due to prerenal azotemia), hyponatremia, hypercoagulability, hypogammaglobulinemia

Epidemiology

- ◼ Primary acquired form (idiopathic minimal-change nephrosis) most common from 18 months to 6 years of age; 80% of cases
- ◼ Secondary acquired form most common > 6 years; causes include infection, drugs, systemic disease (HUS, HSP, SLE, sickle cell, etc.)

Diagnosis

- ◼ Hypoalbuminemia < 3.0 g/dL
- ◼ Urine protein 100–300 mg/dL or > 40 mg/m^2/hour in 24-hour period

Treatment for New-Onset Disease

- ◼ Prednisone 2 mg/kg/day for 4–6 weeks, then taper
  - • Anticipate response in 7–10 days
- ◼ Furosemide may be considered (1–2 mg/kg/day)
- ◼ Albumin infusion if needed to emergently increase oncotic pressure
  - • Indications: symptomatic hypovolemia, peritonitis, clinically significant edema

- 1 g/kg of 25% solution over 4 hours with furosemide midway through transfusion
- Watch for pulmonary edema
■ Optimize dietary protein

Complications

■ Infection: peritonitis, cellulitis, sepsis, meningitis
■ Thrombosis and thromboembolism: caution with femoral venous access
■ Other: ascites, pleural effusion, intravascular hypovolemia (shock, prerenal acute renal failure)

Hematuria

■ > 5–10 RBCs per high-power field from a centrifuged voided urine sample
■ Confirm with microscopy: RBCs, hemoglobin, myoglobin give positive dipstick
■ False positive dipstick can result from drugs (ascorbic acid, sulfonamides, iron sorbitol, metronidazole, nitrofurantoin); beets, dyes, drugs; urate crystals may discolor urine
■ False negative microscopy may occur in setting of low specific gravity causing cell lysis

Common Causes of Persistent Hematuria

■ Without proteinuria: UTI, hypercalciuria, IgA nephropathy, sickle cell trait/disease, renal cystic disease, nephrolithiasis, anatomical abnormalities, trauma, benign familial hematuria
■ With proteinuria: UTI, poststreptococcal glomerulonephritis, IgA nephropathy, HSP, membranoproliferative glomerulonephritis, lupus, HUS, Alport syndrome

Evaluation

■ History: menstruation, vigorous exercise, trauma, dysuria, abdominal pain, medications, recent sore throat or skin rash, viral illness, joint or muscle pain

- Family history: hematuria, renal disease, deafness, stones, sickle cell, coagulopathy
- Exam: edema, hypertension, rash, arthritis, abdominal pain

Laboratory Evaluation

- If microscopic hematuria only, present < 1 month, with normal history and exam, refer to family physician for repeat
- Urine evaluation:
  - Appearance: red color suggests lower urinary source; tea color = glomerular
  - Dipstick: proteinuria suggests glomerulonephritis, intrinsic renal disease
  - Microscopy: casts or dysmorphic RBCs suggest glomerular origin; normal RBC morphology suggests lower tract origin
  - Culture
- If no signs of glomerular disease or urine infection:
  - Consider renal ultrasound (or CT if history of trauma)
  - Urinary calcium, calcium:creatinine ratio
  - Consider hemoglobin electrophoresis, urinalysis of parents
- If signs of glomerular disease (edema, hypertension, proteinuria, or RBC casts):
  - CBC, electrolytes, urea, creatinine, C3, anti-streptolysin O titre (ASOT), streptozyme, albumin
  - Consider ultrasound to rule out polycystic kidney disease, tumor, uretero-pelvic junction obstruction, stones
  - If proteinuria also present, check CBC, C3, C4, ASOT, serum electrolytes, urea, creatinine, serum albumin, ANA

Specific Syndromes Characterized by Hematuria

Acute Poststreptococcal Glomerulonephritis

- Presents with tea-colored urine 7–21 days following pharyngitis or skin infection
- Check urinalysis, microscopy, C3, C4, ASOT, streptozyme or throat culture, electrolytes, urea/creatinine
- Refer to nephrologist if hypertension or signs of acute renal failure

Hemolytic Uremic Syndrome

- Triad of renal failure, microangiopathic hemolytic anemia, thrombocytopenia
- Commonly affects children under 5 years with history of bloody diarrhea
  - *E. coli 0157:H7 implicated in majority of cases*
- Clinical findings:
  - Renal: hypertension, hematuria, proteinuria, acute renal failure
  - Hematologic: anemia, thrombocytopenia, hepatosplenomegaly, bleeding
  - GI: intussusception, GI bleeding, bowel perforation, hepatitis, pancreatitis
  - Cardiac: cardiomyopathy, myocarditis, high-output failure
  - Neurologic: irritability, seizures, encephalopathy, coma
- Evaluation: CBC, reticulocytes, blood smear, PT/PTT, electrolytes, urea/creatinine, LFTs, UA, stool antigen studies for *E. coli 0157:H7*
- Antibiotics contraindicated due to risk of bacterial lysis and toxin release
- Treatment involves management of hypertension, renal failure, electrolyte disturbances, bleeding, anemia, and other complications

Henoch-Schonlein Purpura

- Characterized by palpable nonthrombocytopenic purpura predominantly over buttocks and lower extremities, abdominal pain, arthralgia or arthritis, and glomerulonephritis
- Check urinalysis for hematuria and microscopy
- Serum electrolytes, urea/creatinine, CBC, coagulation studies
- Renal manifestations in approximately 50%, chronic impairment in 2%
  - May include hematuria, proteinuria, glomerulonephritis, renal failure
  - Refer to nephrologist if hypertension or signs of acute renal failure

Renal Failure
Acute Renal Failure

- Sudden inability of the kidneys to regulate water and electrolyte homeostasis
- Usually characterized by oliguria (urine output < 300 mL/m2/day or < 0.5 mL/kg/hour), decreased glomerular filtration rate, decreased creatinine clearance
- Classified as prerenal, intrarenal, postrenal
  - Prerenal due to decreased perfusion (dehydration, DKA, shock, ischemia)
  - Intrarenal due to renal parenchymal disease (glomerulonephritis, HUS, toxins)
  - Postrenal due to obstruction (posterior urethral valves, stones)
- Often reversible, but may progress to chronic renal failure

Management

- If prerenal, challenge with isotonic fluid (10–20 mL/kg, repeat if needed)
- If postrenal, identify and treat obstruction (catheter, urology consultation)
- Consider furosemide 1 mg/kg if intrarenal
- Treat electrolyte imbalances: hyperkalemia, hypocalcemia, hyperphosphatemia

Table 30.1	Laboratory Findings	
PRERENAL	INTRARENAL	POSTRENAL
Osmolality > 500	Osmolality < 300	Osmolality 300–400
Urine/plasma osm > 1.3	Urine/plasma osm < 1.3	
Urine Na+ < 15 mEq/L	Urine Na+ > 20 mEq/L	
Urine:plasma Cr > 40:1	Urine:plasma Cr < 20:1	
↑ BUN/Cr ratio		

- Treat hypertension: if hypertensive crisis, consider nitroprusside or nifedipine to decrease systolic blood pressure by 15–25%
- Fluid administration should equal insensible losses (400 mL/m^2/day) plus urine losses
- Consider dialysis for hypertension, electrolyte imbalances, volume overload, or acidosis that does not respond to medical therapy
- Consider central venous pressure monitoring

Chronic Renal Failure

- Defined as an irreversible and progressive decline in GFR for more than 3 months
- Priority in emergency setting is identification and management of complications

Clinical Manifestations

- Uremia: anorexia, fatigue, vomiting, encephalopathy, seizures, paresthesias
- Electrolyte abnormalities: acidosis, hyperkalemia, hyponatremia, hypocalcemia
- Cardiovascular: hypertension, pericarditis, heart failure, stroke
- Musculoskeletal: renal osteodystrophy, osteomalacia, rickets
- Anemia
- Growth retardation, delayed puberty

Management

- See management of acute renal failure (above)
- Fluid restriction if edema, hypertension, or CHF
- Controlled protein, low phosphate, low potassium, low salt, vitamin replacement
- Calcium carbonate for hyperphosphatemia; Na bicarbonate or citrate for acidosis
- Iron supplement and erythropoietin for anemia, growth hormone for short stature
- Dialysis if medical management ineffective

References

Cronan K, Norman ME. Renal and electrolyte emergencies. In: Fleisher G, Ludwig S, eds. *Textbook of Pediatric Emergency Medicine.* 4th ed. Philadelphia: Lippincott Williams & Wilkins; 2000:811–859.

Lowe A. Nephrology. In: Cheng A, Williams BA, Sivarajan BV, eds. *The HSC Handbook of Pediatrics.* 10th ed. Toronto: Elsevier; 2003:530–564.

Meyers KEC. Evaluation of hematuria in children. *Urol Clin North Am.* 2004;31:559–573.

Roth KS, Amaker BH, Chan JCM. Nephrotic syndrome: pathogenesis and management. *Pediatrics Rev.* 2002;23:237–247.

Weinberg JA, Castillo J, Combest FE, et al. Urinary and renal disorders. In: Barkin RM, ed. *Pediatric Emergency Medicine: Concepts and Clinical Practice.* 2nd ed. St. Louis: Mosby-Year Book Inc.; 1997:1127–1174.

31 ■ Urologic Emergencies

LEAH HARRINGTON

Introduction

- Need to distinguish true emergencies from benign complaints
- Testicular torsion: 6-hour window to treat to achieve salvage rate > 80%

Phimosis

- Inability to retract neonatal/infantile foreskin is a normal condition secondary to congenital adhesions between the glans and foreskin
- Congenital phimosis rates: 1–3 months: 91%; 3 years: 35%; 8–13 years: 3–6%; 17 years: 1%
- Numbers quoted in the literature vary widely
- Phimosis should be treated if accompanied by symptoms of urinary obstruction or infection/balanitis or balanoposthitis
- Foreskin ballooning during voiding is a benign occurrence and does not require treatment
- Controversy in the literature as to definition of true phimosis requiring treatment
- Some authors consider nonretractable foreskin with a whitish ring of hardened sclerotic skin at the tip of the prepuce to be a true phimosis (balanitis xerotica obliterans): extremely rare in pre-school boys
- Normal developmental foreskin tightness is commonly misdiagnosed as phimosis requiring treatment
- Medical management: 65–90% of cases can be treated with topical steroids (i.e., betamethasone 0.05% cream or triamcinolone 0.1% applied to tip of foreskin 2–3 times daily, 85–90% response)
- Surgical management includes dorsal or ventral slit, circumcision

Paraphimosis

- Fixation of foreskin behind glans
- Occurs when foreskin is retracted and not replaced immediately
- Fibrous ring of foreskin causes venous congestion; results in extreme pain and swelling of glans
- If untreated may lead to ischemia, necrosis; can present as a surgical emergency

Treatment

- No prospective, randomized, controlled studies comparing efficacy of treatment options
- Preparation: sedation, analgesia, and/or penile block may facilitate reduction process
- Topical anesthetic 2% lidocaine gel, 2.5% lidocaine (EMLA cream) applied to skin for 45–60 minutes prior to reduction may be effective
- Ice application or manual compression of the foreskin glans and penis helps decrease edema
- Coban tape may be used to apply pressure to glans and prepuce to reduce edema: apply from distal tip of glans to proximal shaft of penis. Manual pressure may also be used following application of tape
- Manual reduction: "inverting the sock": place both index fingers on dorsal aspect of penis proximal to retracted prepuce. Place both thumbs on tip of glans. Apply pressure to tip of glans while using index fingers to pull prepuce back into position over glans
- Puncture technique requires a 21G needle to puncture one or more openings into edematous foreskin: release of edema facilitates manual reduction of foreskin
- Dorsal slit procedure: vertical incision along dorsal aspect of preputial ring will loosen constricting ring of tissue and facilitate reduction of foreskin

Balanitis

- Inflammation of glans; may be associated with inflammation of inner surface of foreskin (balanoposthitis)
- 3% of male children
- Etiology: infectious origin (case reports of group A beta hemolytic *streptococcus*), contact irritation, trauma, and allergy

Treatment

- Treat underlying cause
- Gentle cleaning, antibiotic ointment, oral antibiotics (i.e., cephalosporin providing staphylococcal coverage) if more extensive involvement of foreskin
- Consider circumcision in recurrent cases

Priapism

- Painful erection unaccompanied by sexual excitation
- > 60% pediatric patients also have sickle cell disease, more typical in older adolescents
- Two types:
  - *Low-flow, ischemic*: painful, although pain may disappear with prolonged priapism. Associated with thromboembolic/hypercoagulable states, sickle cell disease, polycythemia, thalassemia, vasculitis
  - *High-flow, nonischemic*: generally painless, may be episodic. Associated with blunt, penetrating injury to the perineum, straddle injury

Treatment

- Sickle-cell-related priapism: oxygenation, IV morphine, hydration, alkalinization, exchange transfusion to maintain hematocrit value > 30%, hemoglobin-S < 30%
- Surgical decompression if conservative management fails; consider early urological consultation
- Complications: fibrosis and impotence result from prolonged persistent erection; urinary retention

Table 31.1 Scrotal Swelling: Approach

CONDITION	ONSET OF SYMPTOMS	AGE	TENDERNESS	URINALYSIS	CREMASTERIC REFLEX	TREATMENT
Testicular torsion	Acute	Early puberty	Diffuse	Negative	Negative	Surgical exploration
Appendiceal torsion	Subacute	Prepubertal	Localized to upper pole	Negative	Positive	Bed rest and scrotal elevation
Epididymitis	Insidious	Adolescence	Epididymal	Positive or negative	Positive	Antibiotics

Source: Adapted from: Galejs LE, Kass EJ. Diagnosis and treatment of the acute scrotum. *Am Fam Physician*. 1999;59:817–824.

Hydrocele

■ Collection of fluid between layers of tunica vaginalis surrounding testis

Classification

■ *Communicating (congenital) hydrocele*: patent processus vaginalis permits flow of peritoneal fluid into the scrotum, changes in size with crying or exertion
  • Associated with indirect inguinal hernias
■ *Noncommunicating hydrocele*: processus vaginalis not patent thus no communication with the peritoneal cavity, fluid reabsorbed in first 12–18 months of life

Incidence

■ > 80% of newborn boys have a patent processus vaginalis
■ Majority close spontaneously within 18 months of age
■ Incidence increasing due to improving survival rate of premature infants

Presentation

■ Located superior and anterior to testis
■ Bilateral in 7–10%
■ Frequently associated with hernia, especially on right side

- If hydrocele collapses with gentle pressure, a hernia component is likely
- Size and consistency varies with position: smaller and softer when supine, larger and more tense following prolonged standing
- Bluish hue to overlying scrotal skin often detected
- Transillumination is positive but not adequate to discount acute scrotum

Treatment

- < 1 year of age: spontaneous resolution common (even large noncommunicating hydroceles)
- > 1 year of age: elective repair recommended, spontaneous resolution unlikely
- Hernia: surgical intervention recommended because of risk of incarceration

Varicocele

- Collection of venous varicosities within scrotum

Incidence

- Age 10–20 years: 12–18%
- Rare in preadolescents

Presentation

- 95% left side; 22% bilateral
- Generally asymptomatic, nontender, not associated with inflammation of overlying skin
- Ipsilateral testis may be smaller than contralateral testis due to interference with testicular development
- Varicoceles may be missed if patient examined in supine position (varicocele collapses); in standing position, varicocele distends within the scrotum "bag of worms"

Treatment

- Varicoceles associated with pain or testicular atrophy should be repaired surgically

- Presence of varicocele < 5 years age may be presentation of neoplasm (Wilm's tumor)

Testicular Torsion

Newborn

- Testis twists about its blood supply outside of the tunica vaginalis leading to infarction
- Related to loose attachment between tunica vaginalis and scrotal wall
- Occurs from birth to 6 weeks

Presentation

- Typically infants demonstrate no distress
- Scrotum is slightly swollen with occasional bluish cast to affected side
- Does not transilluminate and is firm with absence of tenderness to palpation

Treatment

- Urgent exploration generally not helpful
- Salvage rate minimal for testis with neonatal torsion, secondary to torsion occurring in utero/intrapartum
- Elective exploration: rule out presence of tumor (indistinguishable from torsion on clinical or ultrasound)
- Contralateral testis: suture to scrotal wall to prevent torsion

Older Child

- Torsion due to deficient attachments between epididymis and tunica vaginalis
- Testis twists on vascular pedicle
- Majority of torsions occur in late childhood or early adolescence

Presentation

- Age 13–17 years
- Acute onset of intense testicular pain, swelling, and redness
- Elevated, horizontal lie of affected testis

- Bell-clapper deformity: lack of anchoring of testis to tunica vaginalis, leaves testis free to swing and rotate; mimics clapper inside bell
- No pain relief with scrotal elevation (Prehn sign): not reliable in children
- Cremasteric reflex usually absent
- Pain may not be localized to scrotum; may be referred to lower quadrant of abdomen or flank

Treatment
- Surgical emergency: need to treat within 6 hours
- Repair salvage rates:

6 hours	80–100%
> 6–8 hours	55–85%
24 hours	0%

- Scrotal ultrasound with color flow Doppler or radionuclide scrotal scanning establishes presence of blood flow to testis (specificity 77–100%, sensitivity 86–100%)
- Imaging studies should be obtained only if relatively sure that torsion does not exist and seeking supportive evidence to rule out diagnosis
- Treatment should not be delayed for imaging if obvious clinical evidence of torsion
- 5–10% spontaneously detorse; risk of retorsion remains high

Manual Detorsion: "opening the book"
- Majority of torsions twist inward and toward midline
- Manual detorsion of testicle involves twisting outward and laterally, as if opening a book
- May be used as temporizing measure prior to surgical management
  - Place patient in supine or standing position
  - Grasp affected testicle between thumb and forefinger
  - Rotate the affected testicle from the medial to lateral position 180°

- Maneuver may need to be repeated 2–3 times for resolution of pain and complete detorsion
- Successful in 30–70%

Torsion of Testicular Appendage

- 5 appendages of testis (all vestigial and functionless)
- May infarct or twist
- Appendix testis, located at superior pole of testicle, is most commonly affected appendage

Presentation

- Scrotal pain, swelling, erythema (not as intense as with testicular torsion)
- Cremasteric reflex generally present
- Twisted appendage may be palpated directly or identified through skin as a "blue dot" at superior pole of testis

Treatment

- Ultrasound, color flow Doppler exam assists in diagnosis
- Surgery generally not required
- No clinical trials published to evaluate conservative measures
- Bed rest, scrotal elevation to minimize inflammation
- NSAIDs and analgesics not routinely used
- Inflammation usually resolves within a week

Inguinal Hernia

- Abdominal or pelvic viscera enter the patent processus vaginalis and travel through internal ring into inguinal canal

Presentation

- Symptomatic or asymptomatic bulges in the lower abdomen, scrotum, or labia, commonly seen with straining, crying
- Most common in infants 1–3%, especially premature infants 3–5%
- Boys 3 to 10 × more likely than girls

- Indirect hernia: 99% of cases
- Incarceration occurs most commonly in first 6 months of life
- Silk glove sign: gently passing fingers over pubic tubercle may reveal patent processus vaginalis; thickened cord of hernia sac within spermatic cord provides feel of fingers of a silk glove rubbing together

Treatment

Reduction of inguinal hernia:

- Administration of narcotic and/or sedative may be helpful (e.g., intranasal midazolam)
- Place patient in mild Trendelenberg position
- Gently squeeze most dependent portion of the hernia in the direction of the inguinal canal with one hand, while providing gentle pressure on the external ring with the thumb and forefinger of the other hand. Apply traction to the hernia mass, as this aligns hernia with inguinal canal. Maintain continuous pressure for 10+ minutes
- If reduction fails, hernia is considered incarcerated and requires emergent surgical repair
- Strangulation or compromise of blood supply to bowel in hernia sac can occur within 2 hours, leading to perforation and peritonitis

Epididymitis

- Inflammation/infection of epididymis, a convoluted duct that lies on posterior surface of testicle
- Extension to adjacent testicle: epididymoorchitis

Etiology

- Generally idiopathic
- Postpubertal males: consider sexually transmitted disease: *C. trachomatis* (50–60%), *N. gonorrhea*
- Prepubertal boys: postinfectious inflammatory reaction; elevated titers for *M. pneumoniae*, enteroviruses, adenoviruses in affected population vs controls

- Chemical /inflammatory reaction due to reflux of sterile urine
- Coliform bacteria (*E. coli*) predominates in bacterial cases
- Rarely due to hematogenous spread

Presentation

- May develop in association with urinary tract infection in prepubertal boys
- Epididymis enlarged, tender; testis normal
- Pain may be alleviated with elevation of scrotum (Prehn's sign): not reliable to rule out torsion
- Urine is positive for leukocytes in most cases

Treatment

- Antibiotics until results of urine culture available; if negative, treat as viral/chemical epididymitis with NSAIDs/analgesia
- If urine infection present, consider renal ultrasound, VCUG to rule out genitourinary anomaly
- Scrotal elevation
- Ultrasound of testis to rule out torsion if diagnosis uncertain

References

Choe JM. Paraphimosis: current treatment options. *Am Fam Physician.* 2000;62(12):2623–2628.

Galejs LE, Kass EJ. Diagnosis and treatment of the acute scrotum. *Am Fam Physician.* 1999;59(4):817–829.

Kapur P, Caty M, et al. Pediatric hernias and hydroceles. *Pediatr Clin North Am.* 1998;45(4):773–790.

Katz D. Evaluation and management of inguinal and umbilical hernias. *Pediatr Ann.* 2001;30(12):729.

Langer J, Coplen D. Circumcision and pediatric disorders of the penis. *Pediatr Clin North Am.* 1998;45(4):801–812.

Lee-Kim SJ, Fadavi S, et al. Nasal versus oral midazolam sedation for pediatric dental patients. *J Dent Child.* 2004;71(2):126–130.

Weinberg JA, Castillo J, Combest FE, et al. Urinary and renal disorders. In: Barkin RM, ed. *Pediatric Emergency Medicine: Concepts and Clinical Practice.* 2nd ed. St. Louis: Mosby-Year Book Inc.; 1997:1127–1174.

32 ▪ Hypertensive Emergencies

SAVITHIRI RATNAPALAN

Introduction
- High–normal blood pressure (BP): 90–95th percentile
- Moderate hypertension: 95–99th percentile
- Severe hypertension: persistently at or above 99%
- Hypertensive urgency: elevated BP without end-organ damage
- Hypertensive emergency: elevated BP with evidence of end-organ damage

Risk Factors for Hypertension
- Prematurity, low birth weight, or other neonatal complications
- Congenital heart disease
- Certain urinary or kidney problems
- Organ or bone marrow transplant
- Treatment with medications known to raise blood pressure
- Illnesses associated with high blood pressure, such as neurofibromatosis

Table 32.1	Causes of Hypertension
Newborns	Renal artery thrombosis, renal artery stenosis, congenital renal malformation, coarctation of the aorta, bronchopulmonary dysplasia
Infancy to 6 years	Renal parenchymal disease, coarctation of the aorta, renal artery stenosis
6–10 years	Essential hypertension (including obesity), renal artery stenosis, and renal parenchymal diseases
Adolescence	Essential hypertension (including obesity), renal parenchymal diseases

History

- Neurologic symptoms: headaches, vomiting, irritability, seizures, features of encephalopathy
- Renal symptoms: decreased urine output, edema
- Endocrine symptoms: sweating, flushing, palpitations, fever, weight loss
- Past history: UTI, fever, hematuria, dysuria, edema, umbilical artery catheterization
- Medications including birth control pill, toxins, illicit drugs
- Family history: renal disease, hypertension, stroke

Physical Exam

- Growth
- Evidence of congestive heart failure (tachypnea, hepatomegaly)
- Femoral pulses, four limb blood pressures
- Thyroid
- Neurologic exam and fundoscopy (papilledema, hemorrhage, edema, infarcts)
- Abdominal bruit, abdominal masses

Investigations

Basic: CBC, urea, creatinine, ESR, electrolytes, calcium, uric acid, lipid profile
          Urinalysis, microscopy, culture
          ECG, CXR

Consider: Renal ultrasound, echocardiogram
          Urinary catecholamines and toxicology screen

Management

Emergency pharmacologic treatment depends on:

- Acuteness of rise in blood pressure
- Presence of symptoms
- Preexisting conditions
- Extent of end-organ damage

If life-threatening:
- ABCs, vascular access
- Rapid but cautious reduction of BP to stabilize patient
- Frequent BP monitoring
- Slow reduction of BP if due to increased intracranial pressure
- Reduce BP gradually (30–40% in first 6 hours; 30% over next 12–36 hours; 30% over next 48–96 hours)
- Identify and correct underlying cause

Table 32.2	Anti-hypertensives with Rapid Onset of Action		
DRUG	ROUTE	DOSE	ONSET
Nifedipine	Bite and swallow	0.15 mg/kg/dose q4h	5–10 minutes
Hydralazine	IV	0.1–0.8 mg/kg q4–6 h	10–20 minutes
Nitroprusside	IV infusion	0.5–10 mcg/kg/min	Immediate
Labetalol	IV IV infusion	1–3 mg/kg over 1 hour 1mg/kg/hour	5–10 minutes
Captopril	PO	0.01–0.05 mg/kg/dose q8 h	15–30 minutes

Nifedipine
- Calcium channel blocker: short-acting preparation can be used initially
- Can be given by sublingual route and orally as bite and swallow
- Dose 0.15 mg/kg/dose bite and swallow q 4 h as needed, maximum 10 mg/dose
- Frequent BP monitoring necessary to avoid rebound hypertension once effect wears off
- Used in: angina, hypertension, migraine, cardiomyopathy, Raynaud's phenomenon

Adverse Effects
- Sudden drop in BP, tachycardia, dizziness, flushing, nausea, constipation, dependent edema

Hydralazine

- Arteriolar vasodilator
- IV or oral; IV used in moderate to severe hypertension
- Dose 0.1–0.8 mg/kg IV q 4–6 h, maximum 20 mg/dose OR infusion 1.5 mcg/kg/min IV
- Adverse effects: tachycardia, myocardial stimulation, sodium and water retention, nausea, drug-induced lupus

ACE Inhibitors

- Captopril used to treat hypertension in neonates
- Dose: 0.01–0.05 mg/kg/dose
- Provides after-load reduction
- Captopril q 8 h, Enalapril q 12 h, Lisinopril q d
- Caution with compromised renal function
- Contraindicated in renal artery stenosis, risk of ARF
- Adverse effects: more common with captopril (neutropenia, skin rashes, taste problems), decreases BP with first dose, dry cough, headache, dizziness, fatigue

Table 32.3   Antihypertensive Infusions

Nitroprusside	• Drug of choice in hypertensive emergency
	• Reduces BP rapidly, easily titratable, well tolerated, easily reversed by discontinuing infusion
	• Vasodilator (arterioles and venules)
	• Dose: 0.5–10 mcg/kg/min IV continuous infusion
	• Maximum cumulative dose 2.5 mg/kg/day
	• Reconstituted solution has to be wrapped in aluminum foil to prevent deterioration with light exposure
	• Ideal for accurate blood pressure control
	• Requires ICU monitoring
	• Side effects: nausea, vomiting, muscle twitching, cyanide toxicity
	• Renal insufficiency worsens cyanide toxicity

(continues)

Table 32.3 Antihypertensive Infusions (continued)
Labetalol • Alpha + beta effects
• Ideal for treatment of pheochromocytoma
• Dose: Acute hypertension 1–3 mg/kg over 1 hour
• IV infusion 1 mg/kg/hour
• Requires careful monitoring as BP may drop suddenly
• Adverse effects: β-blocker effects cause hyperkalemia (ARF), bronchospasm, orthostasis, dizziness

References

Dillon M. The diagnosis of renovascular diseases. *Pediatr Nephrol.* 1997;11(3):366–372.

Elkasabany A. Prediction of adult hypertension by K4 and K5 in children. *J Pediatr.* 1998;132(4):687–692.

Gutgesell H. Common cardiovascular problems in the young. *Am Fam Physician.* 1997;56(8):1993–1998.

Moss AJ, Adams FH. Heart disease in infants, children and adolescents. In: Fleisher G, Ludwig S, eds. *Synopsis of Pediatric Emergency Medicine.* Philadelphia: Lippincott Williams & Wilkins; 1996.

Sadowski R. Hypertension in pediatric patients. *Am J Kidney Dis.* 1996;27(3):305–315.

■ PART VII

INFECTIOUS EMERGENCIES

33 ▪ Fever

JONATHAN PIRIE

Introduction

- Optimal management of febrile children < 3 years without infectious focus is controversial
- Management variables: age, temperature at presentation, and low vs high risk for serious bacterial infection

Definitions

- Fever: rectal temp > 38°C (100.4°F)
  - Temperature documentation essential
  - Core temperature (rectal) more reliable than other methods in children < 1 yr
- Fever without source (FWS): acute febrile illness, etiology not apparent
- Serious bacterial infection (SBI): meningitis, sepsis, bone and joint infections, urinary tract infections, pneumonia, and enteritis
- Occult bacteremia (OB): pathogenic bacteria in the blood without appearance of toxicity
- Toxic: clinical picture consistent with sepsis syndrome (lethargy with signs of poor perfusion, marked hypoventilation or hyperventilation, or cyanosis)
- Lethargy: level of unconsciousness characterized by poor or absent eye contact, or failure of a child to recognize parents or to interact with persons or objects in the environment

General Principle

- All clinically septic or toxic patients should undergo a full septic workup, admission, and initial empiric intravenous antibiotics according to age

■ The remainder of the guidelines will pertain to those infants and children who appear nontoxic and without a focus of infection at presentation

Management of Febrile Neonates 0–1 month

■ High risk for SBI, incidence of SBI 12–13%
■ Cannot use same risk stratification protocols used in infants 1–3 months in < 1 month age group: 2–3% risk of missing SBI

Recommendations

■ Full-septic workup and hospitalization
  • Blood, catheter urine, and CSF cultures; CXR if indicated
■ Treatment: broad-spectrum parenteral antibiotics pending culture results
  • Ampicillin and cefotaxime (may vary depending on local resistance patterns)

Management of Nontoxic Febrile Infants 1–3 months

■ Risk stratification criteria have been developed to identify nontoxic patients at lower risk of SBI
■ Over the last 10–15 years, different criteria have been proposed by various authors to identify infants at low risk for SBI (< 1%)
■ Two examples include the Rochester and Baker criteria
■ Criteria may be difficult to compare at different age groups; some studies included lumbar puncture and/or stool examination

Rochester Criteria

Age group:
■ 60 days

Past health:
- Born at 37 weeks gestation
- Home with or before mother
- No subsequent hospitalizations
- No perinatal, postnatal, or current antibiotics
- No treatment for unexplained hyperbilirubinemia
- No chronic disease

Physical examination:
- Rectal temperature 38.0°C
- Appears generally well with no evidence of skin, soft tissue, bone, joint, or ear infection

Laboratory:
- Total WBC $5.0–15.0 \times 10^9$/L
- Bands $< 1.5 \times 10^9$/L
- Urine   10 WBC/HPF
- Stool (if diarrhea)   5 WBC/HPF

Baker Criteria

Age group:
- 29–56 days

Past health:
- No known immune deficiency

Physical examination:
- Rectal temperature 38.2°C
- Infant observation score > 10

Laboratory:
- WBC $< 15.0 \times 10^9$/L
- Band/mature PMN ratio   < 0.2
- Urine   10 WBC/HPF
- CSF non-bloody $< 8 \times 10^6$ WBC/L; Neg. Gram stain
- CXR   No evidence of discrete infiltrate

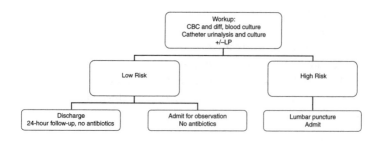

■ **Figure 33.1   Management of Febrile Infants 1 to 3 Months**

Management of Nontoxic, Febrile Infants 3–36 months

- Previous studies: high occult bacteremia and SBI rates 3–11% in highly febrile children; therefore recommended blood cultures and empiric antibiotics
- Recent data suggest rate of occult bacteremia is 1.6%
- Bacterial organisms:
  - > 90% pneumococcus
  - 10% *N. meningitidis, nontyphoidal Salmonella,* group A and B *Streptococcus, E. coli, S. aureus,* others
- Relationship of height of fever and WBC on bacteremia rates:
  - Rate of bacteremia is 0.9% if temperature 39–39.4°C (102–103°F) vs 2.8% if ≥ 41.0°C (106°F)
  - Rate of bacteremia is 0.5% if WBC 10–15 and increases to 18.3% if WBC > 30
- However, positive predictive value for WBC > 15,000 is 5.1% while WBC > 20,000 is 8.1%
- Decreasing rates of SBI with introduction of conjugated pneumococcal vaccine

Recommendations

■ Fever alone should not be the main criteria for obtaining CBC and blood cultures

■ Consider urinalysis for all infants < 1 year, uncircumcised males < 2 yrs, and all females < 2 years. Obtain catheter urine culture whenever possible if not toilet trained

■ CBC and blood cultures should be considered at the discretion of the physician; depend on a number of factors including age, duration of fever, clinical appearance, previous medical history, immunization status, and reliability of parents

■ Little evidence to support routine administration of empiric antibiotics for patients with high WBC counts

■ May be reasonable to judiciously use empiric antibiotics in selected circumstances (e.g., poor clinical appearance, previous medical history, lack of immunization, unreliable parents)

References

Avner JR, Baker MD. Management of fever in infants and children. *Emerg Med Clin North Am.* 2002;20(1):49–67.

Baker M, Bell L, Avner J. Outpatient management without antibiotics of fever in selected infants. *N Engl J Med.* 1993;329:1437–1441.

Baker MD, Bell LM. Unpredictability of serious bacterial illness in febrile infants from birth to 1 month of age. *Arch Pediatr Adolesc Med.* 1999;153(5):508–511.

Baraff L, Bass J, Fleisher G. Practice guidelines for the management of infants and children 0 to 36 months of age with a fever without a source. *Pediatrics.* 1993;92:1–12.

CPS Statement. Management of the febrile one- to 36-month-old child with no focus of infection. *Pediatr Child Health.* 1996;1(Summer):41–45.

Girodias JB, Bailey B. Approach to the febrile child: a challenge bridging the gap between the literature and clinical practice. *Paediatr Child Health.* 2003;8(2):76–82.

Jaskiewicz J, McCarthy C, Richardson A. Febrile infants at low risk for serious bacterial infection: an appraisal of the Rochester criteria and implications for management. *Pediatrics.* 1994;94:390–396.

Kadish HA, Loveridge B, Tobey J, et al. Applying outpatient protocols in febrile infants 1–28 days of age: can the threshold be lowered? *Clin Pediatr.* 2000;39(2):81–88.

Lee GM, Harper MB. Risk of bacteremia for febrile young children in the post-*Haemophilus influenzae* type b era. *Arch Pediatr Adolesc Med.* 1998;152(7):624–628.

34 ▪ Meningitis and Encephalitis

SUZAN SCHNEEWEISS

Introduction
- Important and serious infection of childhood
- Marked decline in incidence of bacterial meningitis since introduction of *Haemophilus influenzae b* vaccine
- Clinical presentation of meningitis or encephalitis often nonspecific

Bacterial Meningitis
- *Neisseria meningitidis* and *Streptococcus pneumoniae* continue to be important pathogens
- Increasing concerns with penicillin-resistant *S. pneumoniae*:
  - Varies according to region (up to 20% in some regions)
  - May have cross resistance to cephalosporins; add vancomycin therapy if suspect *S. pneumoniae*
  - Higher doses of third-generation cephalosporin and vancomycin synergistic against penicillin-resistant *S. pneumoniae*

Clinical Presentation
- Often nonspecific: fever, poor feeding, lethargy, irritability, and vomiting
- Clinical signs: bulging fontanelle, apnea, seizures, purpuric rash
- Older children more classic symptoms: headache, neck stiffness, photophobia
- Kernig and Brudzinksi signs lack sensitivity

Investigations
- CBC and differential
- Electrolytes, urea, creatinine, blood glucose, INR, PTT

- Blood culture:
  - Positive in 40–50% meningococcal disease, 80–90% pneumococcal and *H. influenzae* meningitis if no prior antibiotics
  - Neonatal meningitis: blood cultures positive in only 50%

CSF Examination

Newborn

- $> 30 \times 10^6$/L WBC, with $> 60\%$ polymorphonuclear cells
- CSF protein > 1.7 g/L
- CSF/ blood glucose ratio < 0.5–0.6
- Presence of microorganisms on Gram stain
- Latex agglutination for group B *Streptococcus*
  Note: Coliforms found in CSF 2–3 days after antibiotic treatment; however, group B *streptococcus* clears from CSF within 8 hours of treatment

Infants and Children

- WBC: 10×10^6/L in very young infants; $> 5 \times 10^6$/L older infants and children, mainly polymorphonuclear cells (generally WBC $> 500 \times 10^6$/L)
- CSF protein > 0.6 g/L
- CSF glucose/blood glucose ratio < 0.4 obtained simultaneously
- Cellular and biochemical changes remain in CSF fluid for 44–68 hrs after start of antibiotic treatment
- CSF culture may be negative 2 hours post parenteral antibiotics with meningococcal meningitis and 6 hours post antibiotics with pneumococcal meningitis
- PCR for *N. meningitidis* and *S. pneumoniae*

CT head

- Limited use
- Obtain if uncertain diagnosis and to rule out other causes (e.g., posterior fossa tumor)

- Rule out complications of meningitis (e.g., cerebral abscess)
- Decision to perform CT scan should not delay use of antibiotics

Contraindications to Lumbar Puncture

■ Focal neurologic signs
■ Cardiorespiratory compromise
■ Signs of cerebral herniation:
  - GCS < 8
  - Abnormal pupil size and reaction (unilateral or bilateral)
  - Absent dolls eye movements
  - Abnormal tone (decerebrate/decorticate posturing, flaccidity)
  - Tonic posturing
  - Respiratory abnormalities (hyperventilation, Cheyne-Stokes breathing, apnea, respiratory arrest)
  - Papilledema
    Note: CT scan may be normal in a child with signs of cerebral herniation

Treatment

General Principles

■ Immediate treatment of shock and increased intracranial pressure
■ Control of seizures
■ Restoration of normal hydration and electrolyte imbalance

Empiric Therapy

Dexamethasone—controversial
■ 0.15 mg/kg q 6 h × 4 days or 0.4 mg/kg q 12 h × 2 days
■ Indications: infants and children with *H. influenzae type b* meningitis; consider for pneumococcal meningitis in infants and children > 6 wks
■ Relative contraindications: aseptic or "partially treated" meningitis, infants < 6 weeks of age

Table 34.1 Etiologic Agents by Age and Initial Empiric Antibiotics

AGE GROUP	COMMON BACTERIAL PATHOGENS	INITIAL ANTIBIOTIC REGIMEN
Newborn	Group B *streptococcus* *E. coli* *Klebsiella pneumoniae* *Listeria monocytogenes* *Enterococcus sp.* *Salmonella sp.*	*< 0– 7 days, > 2 kg:* Ampicillin 150 mg/kg/day IV ÷ q 8 h +cefotaxime 100–150 mg/kg/day IV ÷ q 8–12 h *> 7 days, > 2 kg:* Ampicillin 200 mg/kg/day IV ÷ q 6 h + cefotaxime 150–200 mg/kg/day IV ÷ q 6–8 h
4–12 weeks	Group B *streptococcus* *E. coli* *Listeria monocytogenes* *Haemophilus influenzae* *Streptococcus pneumoniae* *Neisseria meningitidis*	Ampicillin 200–400 mg/kg/d IV ÷ q 6 h (maximum 12 g/day) + cefotaxime 200 mg/kg/day ÷ q 6 h (max 8 g/day) ± vancomycin
12 weeks and older	*Haemophilus influenzae* *Streptococcus pneumoniae* *Neisseria meningitidis*	Vancomycin 60 mg/kd/day IV ÷ q 6 h + ceftriaxone 100 mg/kg/dose: at 0, 12, and 24 h followed by 100 mg/kg/dose IV q 24 h (max 2 g/dose, 4 g/day)

Source: Adapted from: Griffiths K, ed. *The 2006–2007 Formulary of Drugs, The Hospital for Sick Children.* 25th ed. Toronto: The Graphic Centre, HSC; 2006.

- May have some benefit for *H. influenzae type b* meningitis; greatest benefit if given 10–20 minutes before first dose of antibiotics
- In vitro studies: decreases penetration of vancomycin and ceftriaxone in blood–brain barrier although no clinical failures documented
- Risk of gastrointestinal bleeding

Aseptic Meningitis

- Fever, headache, vomiting, irritability
- Signs of meningeal irritability: Kernig and Brudzinski signs
- CSF:
  - $20–2,000$ WBC $\times 10^6$/L; $< 30\%$ polymorphonuclear cells
  - Gram stain negative; cultures negative
  - Glucose normal or slightly decreased
  - CSF protein slightly elevated ($0.3–0.8$ g/L)

Encephalitis

- Primary encephalitis: direct infection-related encephalitis
- Post infectious: CNS neurologic effects from host immune response to infection
  - Usually presents days to weeks following infection
  - Demyelination causes focal or global CNS dysfunction
  - Often called acute disseminating encephalomyelitis (ADEM)
  - Distinctive findings on MRI
  - Treated with high dose steroids
  - Consider IVIG and plasma exchange

Etiology

- Often no etiologic agent identified
- Herpes group: HSV 1 and 2 (see Chapter 11, Newborn Emergencies), EBV, CMV, varicella, human herpes types 6 and 7
- Measles, mumps, rubella group
- Arboviruses:
  - Mosquito borne: Western equine, Eastern equine, Venezuelan equine, St. Louis, California, La Crosse, West Nile virus
  - Tick borne: Colorado tick fever, Powassan virus
- Respiratory group: adenovirus, influenza A and B, parainfluenza, RSV
- Enteroviruses: coxsackie, echo virus
- Rotavirus

- Parvovirus
- Rabies
- Bacterial: *Mycoplasma pneumoniae*, *Bartonella henselae* (cat-scratch disease), *Rickettsia* sp

Clinical Presentation

- History: travel, camping, mosquito exposures, contact with animals (horses, cats, mice, hamsters), rash, varicella, mononucleosis-like syndrome, recent immunizations
- Fever, headache, vomiting, irritability, poor appetite, and restlessness may precede neurologic symptoms
- Altered level of consciousness: disorientation, confusion, somnolence, coma
- Altered mental status, aggressiveness, or apathy
- Ataxia
- Focal neurologic signs
- Seizures

Specific Investigations

- CBC and differential
- Acute and convalescent serum (2–4 weeks):
  - Adenovirus, arboviruses, enteroviruses, HSV, mycoplasma, influenza, parainfluenza, bartonella, varicella, measles, EBV, CMV, parvovirus, HHV-6
- CSF: may be normal
  - WBC often elevated, predominance of lymphocytes
  - Protein mildly elevated
  - Glucose varies
  - CSF culture and PCR
- NP swab (influenza, parainfluenza)
- Viral throat swab (adenovirus, enterovirus, HSV)
- Bacterial throat swab (mycoplasma PCR)
- Viral stool cultures (adenovirus, enterovirus)
- CT head: may be normal in early disease

- MRI: more sensitive than CT for acute changes associated with encephalitis
- EEG: seizure activity; may be helpful for localizing encephalitic involvement
- Consider blood cultures, PPD skin test

Treatment

- If infectious encephalitis, consider empiric acyclovir for HSV and antibacterials for meningitis pending test results
- Consult neurology or infectious disease for specific treatment recommendations

References

Canadian Paediatric Society Infectious Diseases and Immunization Committee. Therapy of suspected bacterial meningitis in Canadian children six weeks of age and older. *Paediatr Child Health.* 2001;6:147–152.

Griffiths K, ed. *The 2006–2007 Formulary of Drugs, The Hospital for Sick Children.* 25th ed. Toronto: The Graphic Centre, HSC; 2006.

Lewis P, Glaser CA. Encephalitis. *Pediatr Review.* 2005;26:10:353–362.

Pickering LK, ed. *Red Book: 2003 Report of the Committee on Infectious Diseases.* 26th ed. Elk Grove Village, Il: American Academy of Pediatrics; 2003:293,493.

Riordan FAI, Cant AJ. When to do a lumbar puncture. *Arch Dis Child.* 2002;87:235–237.

35 ▪ Fever and Tropical Infections

AMINA LALANI

Introduction

- Immigrant children most likely to visit country of origin
- Unaware of travel risks, lack of parental knowledge of immunity
- May not seek travel advice or malaria prophylaxis prior to visits
- Multiple tropical infectious agents can cause fever
- Important to consider key infections in emergency department

The Travel History: Key Elements

- Place of travel, urban/rural
- Exposures: water, uncooked foods, animals, insects, activities
- Onset of symptoms and fever, duration of fever
- Pre-travel advice, travel immunizations
- Malaria prophylaxis and compliance

Tropical Infections

Malaria

- Fever from the tropics is malaria until proven otherwise
- Most deaths occur in children
- Severe malaria < age 4; mortality decreases over age 5
- Protozoan infection with one of four species: *Plasmodium falciparum, vivax, ovale,* and *malariae*
- Transmitted by female *Anopheles* mosquito
- Infected mosquito transmits the parasite to human → matures in liver → infects red blood cells and produces clinical findings of malaria

Clinical Presentation
- Incubation period 10–20 days before symptoms
- Short prodrome of headache, myalgias, joint pains, low fever
- Intermittent paroxysms of high fever, chills, and sweats as parasite released from RBCs
- Nausea, vomiting, abdominal pain, headache
- Anemia, mild jaundice, hepatosplenomegaly

Fever Pattern
- Classic fever spike has three stages:
  - Initial cold stage with chills
  - Hot stage with high fever
  - Profuse sweating
- Pronounced fatigue after defervescence
- Parasite often released in 48–72-hour cycles
- May see characteristic fever spikes every 48–72 hours but usually persistent irregular pattern
  Note: Fever pattern cannot be used as a reliable diagnostic tool

Species
P. falciparum
- Most severe form, especially in naïve hosts
- Mortality rates up to 25%
- 98% present within 2 months of return
- Most prevalent in sub-Saharan Africa

P. vivax
- Less severe, relapses common if dormant form not treated
- Most prevalent on Indian subcontinent

Complications
- Cerebral malaria
  - Most serious complication, clinical diagnosis
  - Progressive lethargy, seizures, confusion, coma
- Acute respiratory distress syndrome, liver failure, shock
- Hemolysis and severe anemia, hypoglycemia

Diagnosis

- Minimum of three thick and thin blood films, separated by 12 hours
- One negative film does not rule out diagnosis
- Thrombocytopenia
- ± Anemia, increased bilirubin, and LDH
- Severe malaria: defined as parasitemia > 5% or presence of complications
- Reportable disease

Treatment

- Chloroquine-sensitive area: Chloroquine
- Chloroquine-resistant: Quinine plus clindamycin/doxycycline, OR atovaquone-proguanil, OR mefloquine
- Primaquine for radical cure of liver phase

Severe malaria:

Quinine/quinidine **plus** clindamycin/doxycycline/atovaquone-proguanil

Chemoprophylaxis

- Chloroquine: weekly
- Mefloquine (Lariam®): weekly
  - Neuropsychiatric side effects: insomnia, anxiety, dizziness, hallucinations in 1/250
- Doxycycline: daily, > age 8, risk of photosensitivity
- Atovaquone-proguanil (Malarone®): newest antimalarial
  - More expensive but fewer side effects, daily, 95% effective
  - Used if history of depression, anxiety, psychiatric problems, seizures
- Primaquine
  - Kills liver (dormant) phase of *vivax* and *ovale*
  - 90% effective

Chemoprophylaxis: Regimen

- Chloroquine-sensitive area: Chloroquine weekly
  - Start 1–2 weeks pre travel to 4 weeks post travel

- Chloroquine-resistant area: Mefloquine weekly (Lariam®)
  - Start 1–2 weeks pre travel to 4 weeks post travel
- Chloroquine-resistant area and mefloquine contraindicated:
  - Doxycycline daily if > 8 yrs, or Malarone® daily

Malaria Testing
- Rapid antigen detection tests available but miss low parasitemia and cannot quantitate parasitemia

Dengue
- Arbovirus, transmitted by mosquito *Aedes aegypti*
- Consider if fever and travel to tropics in last 2 weeks
- Found in Africa, Indian subcontinent, Asia, South and Central America
- Urban disease
- Sudden onset of high fever, frontal headache, retro-orbital pain, myalgia
- Erythroderma, thrombocytopenia, leukopenia
- Diagnosis: acute and convalescent serology
- Treatment: none
- Prevention: avoid daytime mosquitoes

Dengue Hemorrhagic Fever
- Uncommon, more severe form of dengue
- Reinfection with a different subgroup
- Fever lasts 2–7 days, nausea, vomiting, abdominal pain
- Later develop hemorrhagic manifestations: purpura, mucosal bleeding, thrombocytopenia, DIC

Enteric (typhoid) Fever
- Infection with *Salmonella typhi* or *paratyphi*
- Found in Indian subcontinent, Asia, Africa, Latin America
- Usually rural areas, transmitted by contaminated food and water
- Death in up to 30% of untreated patients
- Most common in children > age 5 in endemic areas
- Incubation period: 2–4 weeks, up to 3 months

- Insidious onset: prolonged fever, headache, malaise, anorexia, cough, colon, abdominal pain
- Diarrhea or constipation
- Hepatosplenomegaly, rose spots, relative bradycardia for fever
- Complications: small bowel ulcers, perforation or hemorrhage; septicemia
- Relapsing infection in 10%
- Diagnosis: blood, stool, urine, bone marrow culture
- Treatment: ceftriaxone, fluoroquinolones
- Prevention: vaccine, only 75% effective

Gastrointestinal Illness: Travelers' Diarrhea

- Affects one-third of tropical travelers
- Food or water borne pathogens transmitted by fecal-oral route
- Younger children at higher risk and more serious consequences
- Relative lack of gut immunity in children
- Bacterial pathogens cause over 80% of travelers' diarrhea
- Common causes: *enterotoxigenic E. coli, Salmonella, Shigella, Campylobacter*
- Increasing worldwide resistance to antibiotics
- Diagnosis: stool cultures
- Treatment: 3-day course of fluoroquinolones in older children, macrolide in young children

Hepatitis A

- RNA virus
- Often asymptomatic in young children
- Severity of illness increases with age
- Infection usually causes clinical hepatitis in adults and teens
- Fever, malaise, anorexia, nausea, abdominal pain, followed by jaundice
- Recovery often takes 4–6 weeks but may take months
- Oral-fecal transmission, direct contact with infected persons, or ingestion of contaminated food or water
- Virus can persist for weeks in environment

- Shedding in feces peaks 2 weeks before clinical illness
- Incubation period 2–6 weeks
- Combined hepatitis A/B vaccines also available: Twinrix®
- Vaccines have 90% efficacy

Fever in the Returning Traveler—Investigations

Consider:
- Thick and thin smears for malaria × 3
- Cultures of blood, stool, urine
- CBC, liver function tests
- Chest X-ray
- Specific serology as indicated
- TB skin test

References

Batres LA, Marino R. Index of suspicion. *Pediatr Rev.* 1999;20(2):53–55.

Ellerin T, et al. Fever in a returned traveler: an "off the cuff" diagnosis. *Clin Infect Dis.* 2003;36:1074–1075.

Health Information for International Travel 2001–2002. Atlanta: US Department of Health and Human Services, Public Health Service; 2001.

Plourde PJ. Travellers' diarrhea in children. *Paediatr Child Health.* 2003;8(2):99–103.

Schwartz MD. Fever in the returning traveler, part one: a methodological approach to initial evaluation. *Wilderness and Environ Med J.* 2003;14(1): 24–32.

Silvie O, Danis M, Mazier D. Malaria—the disease and vaccine development. *Vaccines: Children and Practice.* 2002;5:9–13.

PART VIII

HEMATOLOGIC/
ONCOLOGIC
EMERGENCIES

36 ▪ Sickle Cell Disease

D. ANNA JARVIS AND MELANIE KIRBY

Introduction

- A group of genetic disorders in which a single point mutation results in substitution of valine for glutamic acid at the sixth position on the β-hemoglobin chain
- Common sickle cell syndromes include hemoglobin SS disease, hemoglobin S-hemoglobin C disease, hemoglobin S-β thalassemia disease
- High risk of infection due to splenic dysfunction: overactive reservoir function and ineffective filtration
- Splenomegaly may be present by 4–5 months of age
- Spleen is palpable in 50% by 12 months of age

Sickle Cell Emergencies

1. Vaso-occlusive crisis
2. Aplastic crisis
3. Splenic sequestration crisis
4. Acute chest syndrome
5. Fever/sepsis syndrome
6. Stroke/cerebrovascular accident
7. Priapism
8. Gallstones

Vaso-occlusive Crisis (VOC)

- Painful VOC is the most common sickle cell complication

Cause

- Ischemic tissue injury results from obstructed blood flow by sickled RBCs
- Precipitants: infection, fever, acidosis, hypoxia, dehydration, extremes of heat and cold

Clinical Presentation

- Individual patients often have a recurrent pattern of pain
- Pain can be symmetrical, asymmetrical, or migratory
- Any area of the body may be affected:
  - Infants: dactylitis (hand/foot syndrome)
  - Others: limb pain, abdominal pain, back pain
- Bone pain is the most frequent VOC and may be accompanied by low-grade fever, redness, and warmth
- History should include:
  - Nature, duration, and severity of pain
  - Comparison to previous painful crises
  - Analgesics already taken for current episode
  - Previous experience with analgesics/side effects
  - Associated symptoms (e.g., fever/dyspnea)
  - Consider other etiologies (e.g., osteomyelitis)

Management

- ± Oxygen
- Maintain hydration and adequate pain control
- Hydration: 1.5 × maintenance normal saline
- Rule out other pathologies and concurrent sickle crises
- Measure pain intensity with age and developmentally appropriate tools (see Ch. 64, Pain Management)
- Check with caregivers for child's usual response to pain
- Children with chronic pain syndromes develop coping mechanisms and may not appear as distressed
  - Mild to moderate pain: acetaminophen (15 mg/kg) with codeine (1 mg/kg) q 4 h
  - Moderate to severe pain: morphine 0.1 mg/kg IV
- May require morphine infusion 10–40 mcg/kg/h
  $1/2$ child's weight in kg = morphine in mg added to 50 mL D5W, 1 mL/hr = 10 mcg/kg/hr
- Transfuse if hemoglobin 15 g/L or more below baseline

Aplastic Crisis

Cause

- Parvovirus B19, other viruses
  - Parvovirus B19 is a common cause of aplastic crisis, highly contagious
  - Infected pregnant healthcare providers have risk of fetal complications
  - Family contacts with SCD at high risk of developing aplastic crises

Clinical Presentation

- Rapid fall in hemoglobin to 30–50 g/L
- Reticulocytes < 0.1%
- Usually lasts 7–10 days
- Marrow recovery is heralded by the presence of many nucleated RBCs in the peripheral blood smear
- Less severe in SC or sickle β-thalassemia
- Presentation may be subtle: "fatigue, less active"

Management

- Transfuse to Hb 80–90 g/L:
  - Caution as transfusion may precipitate congestive cardiac failure
- Partial exchange transfusion may be needed
- Monitor cardiovascular status closely
- Monitor family members with SCD

Splenic Sequestration Crisis

- Sequestration of half or more of a child's blood volume may occur over hours
- Results in sharp fall in hemoglobin ± platelets
- Can occur in older children with HbSC disease, sickle β-thalassemia, or SS patients with persistent splenomegaly

Cause
- Pooling of blood in spleen associated with viral infections

Clinical Presentation
- 6 months to 5 years age
- Fever (60%)
- Grossly enlarged spleen
- May present with pallor and shock
- 14% mortality during first episode
- Hb > 20–30 g/L below baseline
- WBC normal/elevated, reticulocytes elevated
- Platelets < 50,000

Management
- PRBC transfusion
- Splenectomy for patients > 2 years age
- Chronic transfusion program if < 2 years age
- Monitor closely for congestive cardiac failure during PRBC transfusion
- Platelet infusions may be indicated
- Although a viral etiology is most likely in young febrile patients, cover for bacterial infections (see Fever Sepsis Syndrome below)

Acute Chest Syndrome (ACS)
- Second most common reason for hospitalization
- Causes 25% of sickle cell patient deaths
- May result in restrictive chronic lung disease

Cause
- Infectious and noninfectious causes
  - Infectious: bacteria, viruses
  - Noninfectious: pulmonary infarction
- Infections are more common in younger children

Clinical Presentation

- Young children—fever and cough
- Older children—severe pain, dyspnea, chills

Management

- Chest X-ray, blood culture, arterial gas
- IV normal saline at maintenance rate (do not overhydrate)
- Oxygen to maintain saturation ≥ 94%
- Consider intensive care unit admission
- Pain control
- Antibiotics:
  - Ceftriaxone 100 mg/kg IV, max 2 g/dose
  - Add erythromycin IV/PO if suspect atypical pneumonia > 5 yrs age
- Exchange transfusion:
  - Extensive infiltrates
  - Oxygen requirement > 40%
  - Deteriorating ABGs
- Moderately severe disease and Hb 15 g/L < baseline: PRBC 10 mL/kg to maximum Hb 100 g/L (Hct 30%)

Fever Sepsis Syndrome

Cause

- Impaired splenic function develops by 3–4 months age in SCD and sickle β-thalassemia
- Risk of overwhelming sepsis and death due to encapsulated organisms
- < 6 years age: *Streptococcus pneumoniae* (66% cases) and other encapsulated organisms (e.g., *Haemophilus influenzae*, *Salmonella*)
- > 6 years age: Gram-negative organisms (> 50%)
- History should include previous febrile events and compliance with prophylactic medications/vaccines

Clinical Presentation

- Sepsis responsible for 20–25% of deaths
- Pneumococcus is predominant pathogen
- Temperature > 38°C

Management

- Blood culture
- ± Other cultures ± chest X-rays as clinically indicated

Antibiotics:

- Ceftriaxone 100 mg/kg IV (max 2 g/dose) as soon as possible after blood culture drawn
  - Aim to administer within 30 minutes of patient's arrival
  - Do not delay antibiotics to complete investigations
  - Use of other antibiotics depends on clinical status, allergies, and past history
- Vancomycin 60 mg/kg/d IV ÷ q 6 h (max 4 g/d)
  - Suspected meningitis, multilobar pneumonia, shock, altered sensorium, coagulopathy, previous severe pneumococcal sepsis
- Erythromycin 40 mg/kg/d IV ÷ q 6 h (max 4 g/d) for respiratory symptoms in children > 5 years or if < 5 years with suspected mycoplasma
  - Older children may receive erythromycin 40 mg/kg/d PO ÷ q 6–12 h (max 2 g/day) or clarithromycin 15 mg/kg/d PO ÷ bid

Outpatient Management

- For outpatient treatment, patients may receive oral antibiotics (see below), or return within 24 hours for a second dose of IV ceftriaxone
- Duration of treatment depends on findings at reassessment, including the focus of infection

Give 3-day supply of an oral antibiotic:

- Cefixime 8 mg/kg/day, given once daily (max 400 mg/day) OR

Table 36.1   Admission/Outpatient Criteria

ADMISSION CRITERIA	OUTPATIENT CRITERIA
• Age < 1 year	• Age > 1 yr
• Temperature > 40°C	• Temperature < 40°C
• Hb < 60 g/L, WBC < 5 or > 30, Plt < 150	• WBC 5–20, platelets > 100
• Pulmonary infiltrate/respiratory distress	• Not missed recent doses of penicillin VK
• Previous sepsis	• Fully immunized including Prevnar®
• Follow-up uncertain	• No systemic toxicity
• Two or more emergency visits for same episode	• No respiratory distress
	• First dose IV ceftriaxone given
	• Follow-up can be ensured within 24 hours
	• Family able to pay for medication

Source: Adapted from: Kowalczyk A, ed. *The 2005–2006 Formulary of Drugs, The Hospital for Sick Children.* 24th ed. Toronto: The Graphic Centre, HSC; 2005.

- Cefuroxime axetil 30 mg/kg/day PO ÷ bid (max 1 g/day) as suspension, or 250 mg PO bid as tablets, OR
- Cefprozil (6 months to 12 years of age): 30 mg/kg/day ÷ bid (max 1 g/day); > 12 yrs: 250–500 mg bid, OR
- Clarithromycin 15 mg/kg/day ÷ bid (max 1 g/day), OR
- Clindamycin 30 mg/kg/day PO ÷ q 6–8 h (max 1.8 g/day)

Stroke/Cerebrovascular Accident

Frequency

- Much higher incidence in SCD than in general population
- 11% risk of stroke in sickle cell patients by 20 years of age
- Less common in sickle β-thalassemia and HbSC disease
- Age risk: highest 1–9 years of age—usually ischemic stroke; ages 20–29—usually hemorrhagic stroke

Ischemic Stroke: Risk Factors
- Prior transient ischemic attack
- Low steady-state hemoglobin
- Rate of and recent acute chest syndrome
- Elevated systolic blood pressure
- Abnormal transcranial doppler velocities

Clinical Presentation/Investigations
- May be subtle: visual field defects, aphasia, acute changes in behavior, headache, seizure
- Consider other diagnoses: e.g., meningitis (if fever), poisoning, metabolic substance
- CT may be normal in early stage
- MRI is investigation of choice

Treatment
- For children > 2 yrs, screen for stroke with transcranial Doppler; screen with intermittent MRI if Doppler unavailable
- For ischemic stroke, treat with IV hydration and exchange transfusion to reduce Hb S levels to < 30% total hemoglobin
- After initial exchange transfusion consider long-term transfusion program

Recurrence Risk
- 50% SCD:SS will have a second stroke within 3 years
- 10% SCD:SS on transfusion treatment have a second stroke
- Increased risk with low protein C and S levels
- Untreated: two-thirds of CVA patients will have recurrent strokes

Cognitive, Behavioral, Educational Issues
- SCD:SS patients 16% experience "silent strokes"
- MRI and detailed psychoeducational testing essential
- Skills most likely to be affected: attention span, visual-spatial skills, ability to decode/process concepts

Priapism

- Occurs at least once in 75% of males with SCD < age 21
- Peak occurrence ages 5–13 and 21–29
- Precipitating events: majority occur during early morning sleep, 20% sexual activity, 40% no precipitating event identified

Cause

- Local stasis and sickling in the corporal cavernosa of the penis

Clinical Presentation/Investigation

- Stuttering priapism lasts < 3 hours
- Major priapism lasts ≥ 24 hours and results in impotence
- Obtain CBC, retics, blood type, and cross match

Management

- Oxygen, IV morphine
- Bolus 10 mL/kg normal saline followed by 1.5 × maintenance
- Give 1 dose of oral pseudoephedrine (30 mg < 12 yrs, 60 mg > 12 yrs)
- Avoid ice or cold packs, sitting in warm bath may be helpful
- If priapism continues > 2 hours, consult urology urgently: may require penile aspiration and irrigation with epinephrine
- After 12 hours, exchange transfusion to maintain hematocrit > 30%, hemoglobin S < 30%
- Complications: fibrosis and impotence result from prolonged persistent erection; urinary retention
- Positive outcome if prepubertal, early presentation, and treatment with resolution within 2 hours

Gallstones

Differential diagnosis of abdominal pain in SCD:
- Vaso-occlusive episode
- Cholecystitis
- Acute hepatic vaso-occlusive episode
- Splenic sequestration

- Liver sequestration
- Appendicitis
- Pancreatitis
- Acute chest syndrome
- Urinary tract infection
- Pelvic inflammatory disease

Cause

- Increased hemolysis results in an elevated serum bilirubin, cholelithiasis, and cholestasis
- Occurs in 14% children < 10 years age, 30% adolescents
- Lower incidence in HbSC disease or sickle β-thalassemia

Clinical Presentation/Investigations

- Early satiety, nausea, vomiting, RUQ pain, ± change in color of sclera/skin/stool +/or urine
- Obtain CBC, retics, blood culture, liver function tests, GGT, alk phos, bilirubin, amylase
- Gallstones are usually radiopaque: may see on plain X-ray
- Ultrasound abdomen

Management

- Antibiotics if febrile (fever protocol)
- IV hydration 1.5 × maintenance
- Pain management: see Vaso-occlusive Crisis (VOC)

Complications

Acute cholecystitis, cholangitis, pancreatitis, common bile duct obstruction

Cholangitis

Fever, jaundice, RUQ pain

Treatment

- Ampicillin 100 mg/kg/d ÷ q 6 h IV (max 10 g/day)
- Gentamicin 7.5 mg/kg/d ÷ q 8 h IV/IM (max 120 mg/dose prior to TDM)
- Metronidazole 30 mg/kg/d ÷ q 6–8 h IV (max 4 g/day)
- Penicillin allergy: vancomycin 60 mg/kg/day ÷ q 6–8 h (max 4 g/day)

References

Dampier C, Yamaja Setty BN, et al. Vaso-occlusion in children with sickle cell disease, clinical characteristics and biologic correlates. *J Pediatr Hematol Oncol.* 2004;26(12):785–790.

Golden C, Styles L, Vichinsky E. Acute chest syndrome and sickle cell disease. *Curr Opin Hematol.* 1998;5:89–92.

Kirby M, Carcao MD, Cook D, et al. Guidelines for the inpatient management of children with sickle cell disease. Haemoglobinopathy program, The Hospital for Sick Children. Revised February 2006 by Kirby MA, Williams S, Friedman J, Lau W, Farhat W, Jarvis DA. http://www.sickkids.ca/HaematologyOncology/custom/SickleCellguidelines2004.pdf.

Kowalczyk A, ed. *The 2005–2006 Formulary of Drugs, The Hospital for Sick Children.* 24th ed. Toronto: The Graphic Centre, HSC; 2005.

Miller ST, Macklin EA, et al. Silent infarction as a risk factor for overt stroke in children with sickle cell anemia: a report from the Cooperative Study of Sickle Cell Disease. *J Pediatr.* 2001:385–390.

Saad STO, Lajolo C, et al. Follow-up of sickle cell disease patients with priapism treated by hydroxyurea. *Am J Hematol.* 2004;77:45–49.

Steinberg MH. Management of sickle cell disease. *NEJM.* 1999;340(13): 1021–1030.

37 ▪ Oncologic Emergencies

ZAID AL-HARBASH

Introduction

- Incidence of childhood malignancy 1:100,000
- Most common: leukemia, followed by solid tumors of the brain and spinal cord

Fever and Neutropenia

- Infections remain the major cause of morbidity and mortality among cancer patients
- Most common bacterial organisms found in febrile neutropenia: *Staphylococcus, Streptococcus, Enterococcus, Corynebacterium, E. coli, Klebsiella, Pseudomonas*
- Neutropenia is defined as absolute neutrophil count (ANC) $< 0.5 \times 10^9$/L, or $0.5-1 \times 10^9$/L and expected to fall
- Absolute neutrophil count is the sum of all mature and band forms of polymorphonuclear cells

Risk of Infection

- Bacteremia or sepsis   12–32%
- Pneumonia   3–13%
- Urinary tract infection   1–5%
- No documented infection   67%

Clinical Assessment

- Obtain thorough history and examine for sites of infection
- Pay special attention to:
  - Mucosa and perioral areas, skin, and perianal areas for ulcerations or lesions
  - Central line for cellulitis

- Abdomen for typhlitis or neutropenic colitis
■ Signs of inflammation may be minimal in neutropenia:
  - Abscess may manifest as pain without erythema or swelling
  - Pneumonia may manifest as tachypnea alone

Investigations
■ CBC and blood cultures should be taken peripherally and from the central line
■ Obtain peripheral cultures immediately on arrival in the emergency department
■ Urinalysis and culture: avoid catheterization in neutropenic patients
■ Chest X-ray in patients with respiratory symptoms

Treatment
■ Initiate antibiotic therapy immediately if febrile and neutropenic
■ Involves IV dual therapy with a β-lactam and aminoglycoside
■ Add vancomycin if suspect central line infection
■ If signs of perirectal involvement, consider anaerobic coverage
■ If signs of herpes simplex virus or varicella zoster virus infection, add acyclovir
■ Admit and monitor with hourly vital signs for first 4 hours and then q 4 h as indicated

Tumor Lysis Syndrome
■ Due to breakdown of cells of a rapidly growing tumor (e.g., Burkitt's lymphoma, T-cell leukemia)
■ Can occur at onset of therapy
■ Intracellular contents are released leading to:
  - Hyperkalemia → cardiac arrhythmias
  - Hyperuricemia → uric acid nephropathy
  - Hypocalcemia → weakness, tetany, seizures, and arrhythmias
  - Hyperphosphatemia → binds with calcium to form calcium phosphate crystals that precipitate in renal tubules

Table 37.1   Empiric Antibiotic Therapy

Stable patient, no beta-lactam allergy	**Tazocin®** (Tazobactam-piperacillin) 80 mg/kg/dose piperacillin IV q 8 h max single dose 4 g *AND* **Gentamicin** 1 mo to 9 yrs: 10 mg/kg/dose IV q 24 h 9 to 12 yrs: 8 mg/kg/dose IV q 24 h ≥ 12 yrs: 6 mg/kg/dose IV q 24 h
Stable patient and beta-lactam allergy	**Ciprofloxacin** 10 mg/kg/dose IV q12h (max single dose 400 mg) *AND* **Gentamicin** as above *AND* **Clindamycin** 10 mg/kg/dose IV q 8 h (max 600 mg/dose)
Unstable patient including sepsis	**Meropenem** 20 mg/kg/dose IV q 8 h (max single dose 1 g) *AND* **Gentamicin** as above *AND* **Vancomycin** 15 mg/kg/dose IV q 6 h (max single dose 1 g)
Unstable patient and beta-lactam allergy	**Ciprofloxacin** 10 mg/kg/dose IV q 12 h (max single dose 400 mg) *AND* **Amikacin** 20 mg/kg/dose IV q 24 h *AND* **Vancomycin** 15 mg/kg/dose IV q 6 h (max single dose 1 g)

Source: Adapted from: Griffiths K, ed. *The 2006–2007 Formulary of Drugs, The Hospital for Sick Children.* 25th ed. Toronto: The Graphic Centre, HSC; 2006.

Management

- Hydration: maintain good urine output with 1.5–2 × fluid maintenance, monitor accurate intake/output
- Alkalinize: keep urinary pH 6.5–7.5

- Alkalinization of urine ionizes uric acid and increases solubility and excretion
- Overalkalinization leads to precipitation of hypoxanthine and calcium phosphate crystals
- Use 50 mEq $NaHCO_3$ per liter of fluid
- Test urinary pH of each void
- Adjust rate of bicarbonate infusion according to urinary pH
- Do not add KCL to fluids due to risk of hyperkalemia
- Allopurinol 400 mg/m^2/day divided tid: xanthine oxidase inhibitor, inhibits formation of uric acid. Recombinant urate oxidase at 0.2 mg/kg IV is a more effective agent
- Cardiac monitoring
- Monitor blood work every 6 hours initially: electrolytes, calcium, phosphate, urate, CBC

Mediastinal Mass

Anterior Mediastinal Mass

- Hodgkin's and non-Hodgkin's lymphoma (NHL) most common
- Others: thymoma, teratoma, thyroid carcinoma, thymic hyperplasia or cysts, sarcoid
- All large tumors cause compromise

Middle Mediastinal Mass

- Hodgkin's and NHL most common
- Others: neuroblastoma (rare), sarcoma (rare)

Posterior Mediastinal Mass

- Neuroblastoma, neurofibrosarcoma, other tumors of neuronal origin

Management

- May cause airway compromise: elevate head of bed, continuous cardiac monitoring, avoid sedation

- Risk of cardiovascular compromise especially if large and compressing superior vena cava
- Superior vena cava (SVC) syndrome:
  - May present with cough, orthopnea, dyspnea, and/or edema of head and neck
  - Present in 6% of patients with anterior mediastinal tumors
  - Do not start IV in upper limbs if evidence of SVC
- Upper thoracic tumors may cause Horner's syndrome: miosis, ptosis, anhydrosis, enophthalmos
- May need treatment with steroids and/or radiation prior to biopsy if tumors are large and cause compromise
- Thoracentesis may provide diagnosis if pleural effusion present, thus avoiding sedation and biopsy of mass
- Consult anesthesia and oncology early

Spinal Cord Compression

- Radicular pain, back pain, difficulty walking, paralysis, or urinary/stool incontinence
- Exam may be unremarkable or show percussion tenderness over spinous processes, weakness, absent deep tendon reflexes, inability to walk on heels or toes
- MRI is the best imaging modality
- Therapy: dexamethasone—1–2 mg/kg IV bolus
- Urgent neurosurgical consultation

Hyperleukocytosis

- WBC > 100,000/mm^3
- Risk of renal, cerebral thrombosis, or pulmonary embolism due to blood hyperviscosity
- Treat with hyperhydration (1.5–2 × maintenance) and follow tumor lysis protocol
- Transfuse if platelets < 20,000/mm^3
- May need leukophoresis to reduce WBC load and risk of metabolic derangements

References

Diamond S, Doyle J. Management of hematology/oncology & BMT patients with fever: antimicrobial guidelines. In: Griffiths K, ed. *The 2006–2007 Formulary of Drugs, The Hospital for Sick Children.* 25th ed. Toronto: The Graphic Centre, HSC; 2006:180–185.

Hogarty MD, Lange B. Oncologic emergencies. In: Fleisher G, Ludwig S, eds. *Textbook of Pediatric Emergency Medicine.* 4th ed. Philadelphia: Lippincott Williams & Wilkins; 2000:1157–1190.

Kennebeck SS. Tumors of the mediastinum. *CPEM.* 2005;6(3):156–164.

Ruddy RM. Emergency presentations of cancer in childhood. *CPEM.* 2005;6(3):184–191.

Shah SS. Device-related infections in children. *Pediatr Clin North Am.* 2005;52:1189–1208.

38 ▪ Hematologic Emergencies

AMINA LALANI AND RAHIM VALANI

Introduction

- Immune thrombocytopenic purpura
- Hemolytic uremic syndrome
- Henoch-Schonlein purpura
- Anemia
- Hemophilia

Immune Thrombocytopenic Purpura (ITP)

- Most common platelet disorder in children ages 1–4 yrs
- Presents classically in preschool age, M = F
- Autoimmune disorder: autoantibodies to platelets
- Develop low platelet count and mucocutaneous bleeding
- May be primary or secondary to underlying disorder
- Two forms: acute < 6 months, chronic > 6 months
- Sudden onset of petechiae or purpura in otherwise healthy child
- Usually recent viral or bacterial illness
- Resolves within 6 months in majority
- Risk of bleeding decreases after first week of illness
- Compensatory increase in platelet production

Clinical Manifestations

- Petechiae, ecchymoses, conjunctival hemorrhage, epistaxis, gum bleeds, hematuria, menorrhagia
- Spleen tip palpable in 10%
- Major complication: intracranial hemorrhage (ICH), often without trauma: may have only mild symptoms such as headache

Diagnosis

- Diagnosis of exclusion
- Thrombocytopenia in absence of underlying disease
- May be secondary to SLE, immunodeficiencies, infections, drugs
- Infants < 3 months: exclude passively acquired antibodies from mother

Investigations

- Bloodwork: decreased platelets, normal WBC and Hg
- Peripheral smear
- Bone marrow aspirate: controversial, must be performed if atypical features

Treatment

- Controversial because favorable outcome in majority without treatment
- Based on risk of ICH and activity restrictions
- Incidence of ICH 0.2–1%
  - Risk increases if plt < 20,000 and highest if < 10,000
  - Risk factors: head trauma, antiplatelet drugs
  - Most ICH occurs within 4 weeks of presentation, usually in first week
- Consult hematology if atypical features

Treatment Options

Observation

- Most children with typical ITP recover completely within few weeks without treatment
- No proof that treatment prevents ICH
- Need to follow as outpatient

IVIG

- Shortens duration of severe thrombocytopenia (< 20,000)
- Blocks uptake of antibody-coated platelets by macrophages in spleen

■ Dose 0.8–1 g/kg, second dose 24 hrs later if platelets < 40,000–50,000
■ Adverse reactions: headache, fever, aseptic meningitis (rare)

Anti-D Immune Globulin (Rhogam®)
■ Antibody vs D antigen of red blood cells
■ Effective in Rh+ patients
■ Dose 50–75 mcg/kg
■ Adverse reactions: headache (rare), hemolytic anemia
■ Preferred over IVIG if Rh positive due to ease of administration and cost
■ Response rate 70%, lasts ~ 3 weeks

Oral Steroids
■ May need high-dose steroids: significant side effects
■ Controversial for newly diagnosed patient with no serious bleeding
■ Consult hematology prior to starting steroids: may require BMA

Emergency Management—Intracranial Hemorrhage

■ Rare if platelets > 50,000
■ For mild head trauma and no signs of bleeding:
  • Observe
  • Give IVIG or antiD IG if platelets < 20, signs of easy bruising, within 1 week of diagnosis or uncertain follow-up
■ For severe head trauma:
  • Consult hematology
  • Methylprednisolone 30 mg/kg/d IV over 20–30 mins, max 1 g/d × 2–3 days
  • IVIG 1 g/kg/d × 2–3 days
  • Platelet infusion
  • Consider splenectomy
■ For mucosal bleeding, consider antifibrinolytic therapy (aminocaproic acid)
■ For persistent epistaxis, use nasal packing

Hemolytic Uremic Syndrome

- Microangiopathic hemolytic anemia, thrombocytopenia and renal dysfunction
- Mainly affects infants and young children < 5 yrs
- Multisystem disorder; most common cause of renal failure in young children
- Vascular endothelial injury results in thrombi that cause clinical manifestations
- Platelets are consumed at sites of vascular injury
- Caused by bacterial and viral infections
- Occurs sporadically and in epidemics
- Two forms: with diarrhea (D+ HUS) and without diarrhea (D– HUS)

Diarrhea Form (75%)

- Usually healthy children < age 5 yrs
- Prodrome of diarrhea, develop hemorrhagic colitis
- Usual cause is enterohemorrhagic *E. coli* 0157:H7: produces verotoxins or Shiga toxins
- Risk of HUS with *E. coli* 0157:H7 infection is 15%
- Incidence highest in summer and fall
- Infected via ingestion of poorly cooked meats and unpasteurized milk
- Toxin causes glomerular injury

Nondiarrhea Form (25%)

- Sporadic form, not associated with toxin
- Rare in children, may relapse, worse prognosis
- May be caused by pneumococcus, OCP, malignancy, pregnancy, medications

Clinical Presentation

- Usually abrupt onset
- History of abdominal pain, diarrhea, vomiting, bloody stools

- Rarely fever in *E. coli* 0157 infections
- Pallor, listless, irritable, dehydrated, oliguria
- May have edema, hypertension, petechiae, hepatosplenomegaly, encephalopathy, neurologic abnormalities

Diagnosis

- Mainly clinical diagnosis: combination of hemolytic anemia, thrombocytopenia, and renal failure
- Obtain blood: CBC, reticulocytes, coagulation profile, electrolytes, urea, creatinine, liver function tests
- Anemia often severe: Hg 50–90
- Increased urea, metabolic acidosis, hyperbilirubinemia, increased LDH
- Peripheral smear: helmet cells, burr cells, schistocytes
- Urinalysis: hematuria, proteinuria, casts
- Stool culture including 0157 antigen

Treatment

- Supportive, admit
- Dialysis necessary if severe uremia, congestive heart failure, encephalopathy, hyperkalemia
- Consider dialysis if urea > 35 mmol/L
- Blood transfusions as needed if symptomatic anemia
- Platelet transfusions only if active bleeding
- Treat hypertension to prevent congestive heart failure and encephalopathy
- Survival rate > 90%
- 25% have long-term renal dysfunction, hypertension, or proteinuria
- No role for antibiotics—may worsen disease

Henoch-Schonlein Purpura

- Small blood vessel hypersensitivity vasculitis
- Most common vasculitic disease of childhood

- Affects skin, joints, gastrointestinal tract, and kidneys
- Triad of abdominal pain, arthritis, and nonthrombocytopenic purpura
- Often renal involvement with glomerulonephritis
- Cause unknown, peak age 3–7 yrs, M > F

Clinical Presentation

- Often follows an upper respiratory illness
- Purpuric rash over buttocks and lower extremities followed by arthralgias, angioedema, colicky abdominal pain
- Gastrointestinal symptoms may precede rash: abdominal pain, bleeding, intussusception, edema of intestinal wall
- GI involvement occurs in 80%
- Migratory arthritis of larger joints
- Renal involvement may develop within 3 months of onset of rash

Investigations

- CBC, electrolytes, albumin, and total protein
- Stool occult blood test
- Urinalysis: asymptomatic microhematuria in 80%
- Blood pressure

Treatment

- No specific treatment
- Usually benign and self-limited course
- Manage as outpatient if limited to skin and joints: NSAIDs for arthralgias
- May have fluctuating course for several months, up to 50% recur within 6 weeks
- Admit if severe abdominal pain or hemorrhage
- Use of steroids is controversial, only weak evidence to date:
  - May decrease abdominal pain
  - Risks of masking intussusception/bowel perforation, side effects

Prognosis

- Primary long-term complication is renal disease in 5% of patients
- Nephritic-nephrotic syndrome carries 50% risk of end-stage renal disease
- If renal disease on presentation, consult pediatric nephrology
- Need 6-month follow-up: check urinalysis even if initial urinalysis is normal
- Follow-up can be discontinued at 6 months if urinalysis remains normal

Anemia

- Decrease in hemoglobin concentration
- Hemoglobin is highest in the neonatal and adolescent periods
- Physiologic anemia from 2–6 months of age due to decreased erythropoietin production
- MCV formula: age 1 month to 9 years: 70 + age in years
- Important to review blood smear

History

- Neonatal anemia: complications during labor or delivery, infections during pregnancy (consider TORCH infections), maternal medications, and diet
- Patient history:
  - Bleeding, jaundice, prematurity (poor iron stores, increased susceptibility to infection)
  - Diet: exclusive milk diet in children
  - Medications
  - Infection
  - Growth history: increased iron demand during growth spurts
  - Exercise tolerance
- Family history of hematologic disorders, thalassemia, or sickle cell disease

Exam
- Tachycardia: compensatory increased cardiac output
- Jaundice: suggestive of hemolysis
- Splenomegaly or hepatomegaly, adenopathy, petechiae, bruising

Approach

Microcytic Anemia (usually a disturbance in Hg synthesis)

Causes:
- Iron deficiency
  - Leading cause of anemia in early childhood
  - Full-term infants have sufficient stores for the first 4–6 months
  - May be due to inadequate intake of iron, ingestion of cow's milk leading to milk protein intolerance, and poor dietary sources of iron
  - Children > 3 years with iron deficiency anemia require GI evaluation to rule out occult blood loss
  - Improved Hg with iron supplementation is evidence of iron deficiency
  - Reticulocyte count increases by 1 week, Hg improves over 4 weeks
- Thalassemia
- Chronic inflammation
- Sideroblastic anemia
- Lead poisoning
- Drugs: isoniazid

Normocytic Anemia
- Hemolytic: autoimmune, enzyme deficiency (2,3-DPG deficiency), membrane defects, microangiopathic (DIC, HUS, TTP)
- Nonhemolytic: anemia of chronic inflammation, acute blood loss, chronic renal failure

Macrocytic Anemia

- Megaloblastic: B_{12} deficiency, folate deficiency, drugs (methotrexate)
- Nonmegaloblastic
  - Aplastic anemia, Diamond-Blackfan syndrome

Management

- ABCs: may require transfusion with severe anemia of acute onset
- Management is based on etiology
  - Consider marrow infiltration, cancer, infection, autoimmune diseases if other cell lines affected
  - Assess morphology or abnormalities of RBCs, WBCs, and platelets on peripheral smear
- Trial of iron supplementation if suspect iron-deficiency anemia: 3–6 mg/kg/day of elemental iron as ferrous sulfate
- Restrict cow's milk if this is major source of dietary intake; increase solid food in diet

Hemophilia

- One of the most common severe inherited bleeding disorders, sex linked
- Hemophilia A: Factor VIII deficiency (85%)
- Hemophilia B, Christmas disease: Factor IX deficiency (10–15%)
- Other factor disorders less common
- Prolonged PTT seen with all forms of hemophilia
- The severity of deficiency is defined by amount of factor present
- Hemostasis levels for FVIII: 30–40%, FIX: 25–30%
- Avoid antiplatelet agents or NSAIDs because of risk of bleeding

Clinical Presentation

- Hallmark presentation: hemarthrosis
- Easy bruising, prolonged bleeding during surgery or circumcision
- Family history of bleeding disorders
- Common sites of bleeding: deep muscle, joints, urinary tract

Table 38.1   Subtypes of Hemophilia

Severity	% Functioning Factor	Bleeding risk
Mild	> 5	Minimal
Moderate	1–5	Minor trauma can precipitate bleeding
Severe	< 1	Spontaneous bleeding is common

- Inguinal or flank pain or trauma: risk of iliopsoas muscle bleed
- Even minor trauma may be significant especially in severe hemophiliacs
- Risk of intracranial bleeding: obtain CT head if history of head injury or neurologic symptoms

Management

- Management depends on severity of deficiency, risk of injury, expected delayed or continued bleeding, and presence of antibodies
- Known hemophiliac: use care plan for management of bleeds

Treatment for Hemophilia A

- Mild: DDAVP (most respond), Factor VIII concentrate, tranexamic acid
- Moderate: DDAVP (if responder), Factor VIII concentrate, tranexamic acid
- Severe: Factor VIII concentrate, tranexamic acid
- 1 U/kg of Factor VIII increases levels by 2%
- 1 U/kg of Factor IX increases levels by 1%
- Always treat prior to CNS imaging if suspect ICH
- Antifibrinolytic therapy (tranexamic acid) also needed for oral bleeds
- May require prophylaxis to prevent spontaneous bleeding, especially if severe or develop target joints

Table 38.2 Factor Dosing

Type of bleed	Hemophilia A	Hemophilia B	Von Willebrand's disease
Treatment	Recombinant FVIII	Recombinant FIX	Humate P
Joint	30 U/kg	50 U/kg	60 RICOF U/kg
Muscle	30 U/kg	50 U/kg	60 RICOF U/kg
Oral mucosa	30 U/kg	50 U/kg	40 RICOF U/kg
Epistaxis	30 U/kg	50 U/kg	40 RICOF U/kg
GI bleed	50 U/kg	75 U/kg	60 RICOF U/kg
GU bleed	50 U/kg	75 U/kg	60 RICOF U/kg
CNS bleed	75 U/kg	125 U/kg	80 RICOF U/kg
Trauma or surgery	75 U/kg	125 U/kg	80 RICOF U/kg

DDAVP (Desmopressin)

■ Useful in mild hemophilia A: releases stored Factor VIII; not suitable for severe hemophilia A because limited or no stores
■ Useful for von Willebrand's disease (known responders)
■ Intranasal DDAVP: 150 mcg for < 50 kg, 300 mcg for > 50 kg/adults
■ IV dose: 0.3 mcg/kg, maximum 20 mcg
■ Not effective for Factor IX deficiency

Inhibitors: **consult hematologist**

Treatment options for patients with inhibitors:
■ FEIBA: Factor VIII inhibitor bypassing agent
■ rVIIa: short half-life, dose 90 mcg/kg
■ Hyate-C: porcine factor, not licensed

Complications

Immediate: increased bleeding
Chronic:
- Chronic joint destruction
- Transfusion-related infectious diseases
- Production of inhibitors to Factor VIII or IX
- Factor IX immune tolerance and nephritic syndrome

References

Blackall DP, Marques MB. Hemolytic uremic syndrome revisited. *Am J Clin Path.* 2004;121(suppl 1):S81–S88.

Cines DB, Blanchette VS. Immune thrombocytopenic purpura. *NEJM.* 2002;346(13):995–1008.

Cohen AR, Manno CS. Hematologic emergencies. In: Fleisher G, Ludwig S, Henretig F, eds. *Textbook of Pediatric Emergency Medicine.* 5th ed. Philadelphia: Lippincott Williams & Wilkins; 2005:921–949.

Glader B. The anemias. In: Behrman RE, Kliegman RM, Jenson HB, eds. *Nelson Textbook of Pediatrics.* 17th ed. Philadelphia: W. B. Saunders; 2004.

Hamilton GC, Janz TG. Anemia, polycythemia, and white blood cell disorders. In: Marx JA, Hockberger RS, Walls RM, eds. *Rosen's Emergency Medicine: Concepts and Clinical Practice.* 5th ed. Chapel Hill, NC: Mosby Inc; 2002.

Haroon M. Should children with Henoch-Schonlein purpura and abdominal pain be treated with steroids? *Arch Dis Child.* 2005;90:1196–1198.

Hermiston ML, Mentzer WC. A practical approach to the evaluation of the anemic child. *Pediatr Clin North Am.* 2002;49(5):877–891.

Janz TG, Hamilton GC. Disorders of hemostasis. In: Marx JA, Hockberger RS, Walls RM, eds. *Rosen's Emergency Medicine: Concepts and Clinical Practice.* 5th ed. Chapel Hill, NC: Mosby Inc; 2002.

Montgomery R, Scott JP. Hereditary clotting deficiencies and von Willebrands disease. In: Behrman RE, Kliegman RM, Jenson HB, eds. *Nelson Textbook of Pediatrics.* 17th ed. Philadelphia: W. B. Saunders; 2004.

Narchi H. Risk of long term renal impairment and duration of follow-up recommended for Henoch-Schonlein purpura with normal or minimal urinary findings: a systematic review. *Arch Dis Child.* 2005;90:916–920.

Narula N, Gupta S, Narula J. The primary vasculitides: a clinicopathologic correlation. *Am J Clin Pathol.* 2005;124(suppl 1):S84–S95.

Sadowitz PD, Amanullah S, Souid A-K. Hematological emergencies in the pediatric emergency room. *Emerg Med Clin North Am.* 2002;20(1):177–198.

Tarr PI, Gordon CA, Chandler WL. Shiga-toxin-producing *Escherichia coli* and hemolytic uraemic syndrome. *Lancet.* 2005;365:1073–1086.

■ PART IX
RHEUMATOLOGIC EMERGENCIES

39 ▪ Rheumatologic Emergencies

SUSA BENSELER

Introduction
▪ Juvenile idiopathic arthritis (JIA)
▪ Pediatric systemic lupus erythematosus (pSLE)
▪ Juvenile dermatomyositis (JDM)
▪ Vasculitis
▪ Macrophage activation syndrome (MAS)

Juvenile Idiopathic Arthritis (JIA)
▪ Arthritis (inflammation of the synovium) with onset < 16 years of age
▪ Previously called juvenile rheumatoid arthritis
▪ Name changed to reflect difference between juvenile and adult forms of arthritis
▪ Likely due to genetic, infectious, and environmental factors
▪ Arthritis in children may resemble joint pain associated with infections, cancer, bone disorders, and other inflammatory disorders: must exclude before giving diagnosis of JIA

Types of JIA
▪ Five main types based on number of joints involved during first 6 months of disease and involvement of other organs:
1. Oligoarthritis: < 5 joints, 50% of JIA
   • Children with anti-nuclear antibodies (ANA) often also have uveitis
2. Polyarthritis: ≥ 5 joints
3. Systemic arthritis: 10–20% of JIA
   • High fevers, rash, and inflammation of other organs, in addition to arthritis

4. Enthesitis-related arthritis: often affects spine, hips, and entheses; mainly boys > 8 years
5. Psoriatic arthritis: arthritis and psoriasis

Clinical Presentation

■ Active arthritis: evidence of swelling, effusion, or two of the following: heat, limited or tender range of movement
■ Additional symptoms:
  • Fevers, weight loss, fatigue (sJIA), rash (sJIA, psoriasis), organomegaly, lymphadenopathy (sJIA)
  • Enthesitis, tendonitis
  • Uveitis, red eye, synechiae, impaired vision

Investigations

■ Inflammatory markers: ESR, CRP, CBC
■ ANA, RF, HLA B27
■ LDH to rule out malignancy
■ Consider PPD to rule out TB
■ X-rays to rule out tumors, fractures, lytic lesions, osteomyelitis
  • Look for osteopenia, effusions, joint damage

Differential Diagnosis

■ Septic arthritis: *If in doubt, tap the joint*
■ Reactive arthritis, transient synovitis
■ Leukemia
■ Tumors (osteoid osteoma, malignant bone or cartilage tumors)
■ Trauma
■ Inflammatory/allergic diseases: serum sickness, HSP, drug reactions
■ Rare joint diseases

Management

■ Rule out important differential diagnoses: septic joint, malignancy, trauma

- Symptoms < 6 weeks: physician reassessment in 2 weeks, consider ophthalmology or optometry assessment for uveitis
- NSAIDs:
  - Naproxen 20 mg/kg/d divided bid or indomethacin 2 mg/kg/d divided tid for at least 2 weeks (give repeats)
  - Potential adverse effects: headaches, stomach pain, nausea
- Consult rheumatology if:
  - Persistent arthritis (> 6 weeks)
  - Severe (poly) or systemic arthritis

Pediatric Systemic Lupus Erythematosus (pSLE)

- Multisystem autoimmune disease with substantial variability in presentation and course

Clinical Features

- New rashes, facial redness, mouth ulcers, nosebleeds, joint pain, chest pain
- CNS symptoms including hallucinations, headaches, seizures, other neurologic deficits
- Constitutional symptoms: fever, fatigue, weight loss, hair loss

Classification Criteria

- Diagnosis requires presence of 4 of 11 criteria
- Remember criteria with mnemonic: "MD SOAP BRAIN"

Investigations

- Inflammatory markers: ESR, CRP, CBC/diff
- C3 and C4 complement, IgG
- Creatinine, urea, albumin, protein, LFTs
- Urinalysis including dipstick, microscopy, and protein:creatinine ratio
- Autoantibodies: ANA, ds-DNA (IF and ELISA), anti-SM, anti-Ro, anti-LA, anti-cardiolipin, RF
- Lupus anticoagulans (anti-phopholipid screen)
- Chest X-ray, ECG

Table 39.1   Classification Criteria for SLE

Malar rash	Fixed erythema over malar eminences, sparing nasolabial folds
Discoid rash	Erythematous raised patches
Serositis	Pleuritis: pleuritic pain or audible rub or pleural effusion *OR*
	Pericarditis: documented by ECG or rub or evidence of pericardial effusion
Oral ulcers	Visible oral or nasopharyngeal ulceration, usually painless
Arthritis	Nonerosive arthritis involving ≥ 2 joints with tenderness, swelling, or effusion
Photosensitivity	Skin rash due to unusual reaction to sunlight
Blood (hematologic disorder)	Hemolytic anemia OR
	Leukopenia—WBC $< 4,000/mm^3$ OR
	Lymphopenia $< 1,500/mm^3$ OR
	Thrombocytopenia—platelets $< 100,000/mm^3$
Renal (Nephritis)	Persistent proteinuria > 0.5 grams per day or $> 3+$ *OR* cellular casts
ANA	Abnormal titer of antinuclear antibody
Immunologic disorder	Anti-DNA: antibody to native DNA in abnormal titer *OR*
	Anti-Sm: presence of antibody to Sm nuclear antigen
Neurologic disorder	Seizures *OR* psychosis

Differential Diagnosis

■ Infections
■ Malignancies
■ Other autoimmune diseases

Complications
- Infections
- Macrophage activation syndrome (see Macrophage Activation Syndrome [MAS])

Common Emergency Presentations
- Infections: immunodeficient, therefore risk of severe infections (e.g., pneumococcus)
  - Others: systemic viral infections (CMV), atypical infections, and focal infections (i.e., septic arthritis)
  - Clinical presentation may be modified due to immunosuppression
  - *If in doubt: treat a suspected infection*
  Note: pSLE patients with infections often require stress steroid dosing and a transient increase of daily steroid dose if patient is taking an adrenal-suppressive dose of prednisone
- Disease flares: worsening constitutional symptoms or new or worsening organ manifestations; commonly requires increased immunosuppressive therapy
- MAS: macrophage activation syndrome can occur at any point during disease course, most commonly seen at or in close proximity to initial presentation; may be life threatening

Juvenile Dermatomyositis (JDM)
- Relatively rare
- Clinical features:
  - Symmetrical proximal muscle weakness
  - Typical cutaneous findings: heliotrope rash (lilac periorbital rash often with swelling), Gottrons papules
  - Nail fold abnormalities: dropouts, decreased density of capillaries, tortuosity of vessels
- Elevated inflammatory markers (ESR, CRP) and muscle enzymes (LDH, AST, ALT aldolase)

Complications

- Laryngeal muscle weakness: risk of aspiration
- Chest wall weakness: respiratory distress
- Cardiac involvement
- Consider rheumatology consultation

Common Emergency Presentations

- Infections: clinical presentation may be modified due to ongoing immunosuppressive treatment. *If in doubt: treat*
- Disease flares: worsening muscle weakness requires increased immunosuppressive therapy after consultation with rheumatology
  Note: JDM patients with infections may require steroid stress dosing

Vasculitis

- Common in children: see Henoch-Schonlein Purpura (Ch. 30, Renal Emergencies, and Ch. 40, Kawasaki Disease)
- *Systemic vasculitides:*
  - Anticytoplasmic neutrophil antibodies (ANCA) are a hallmark of a group of systemic vasculitides that are rare in childhood: may present with acute life-threatening symptoms such as pulmonary bleeds or acute renal failure
  - Includes Wegener's granulomatosis and microscopic polyarteritis nodosa
- *Organ limited vasculitides* of skin, CNS, or kidney are often difficult to diagnose
  - Organ function commonly altered
  - Cutaneous polyarteritis nodosa (cPAN): limited to skin/cutaneous fat tissue, frequently associated with streptococcal infections
  - CNS vasculitis: idiopathic or associated with varicella infections within previous 12 months. May present with newly acquired focal or diffuse neurologic deficit (stroke, seizures, decreased level of consciousness, headaches)

- Pauci-immune glomerulonephritis: presents with proteinuria, hematuria, constitutional symptoms, and hypertension

Investigations
- Inflammatory markers
- Organ function assessment
- Auto-antibodies
- Infection workup
- Imaging

Management
- Treatment of acutely impaired organ function
- Anti-inflammatory therapy after consultation with appropriate service

Macrophage Activation Syndrome (MAS)
- Rare and serious complication of childhood systemic inflammatory disorders
- Also called secondary HLH (hemophagocytic lymphohistiocytosis)
- Occurs in a variety of diseases: infections, neoplastic conditions, hematological conditions, and rheumatic disorders, typically systemic JIA
- May also occur with therapeutic regimens, modifications of immunosuppressive therapy, nonhistiocytic malignancies, SLE, and Kawasaki

Clinical Presentation
- Sepsis-like presentation with high fever, volume refractory hypotension, organomegaly, features of multi-organ involvement/failure: i.e., seizures
  Note: Often rapidly progressive

Laboratory Features

- Low ESR, but elevated CRP
- Pancytopenia
- High ferritin (sometimes delayed)
- Coagulopathy/DIC-like picture: ↓ fibrinogen, prolonged PTT
- High cholesterol and triglycerides
- High LFTs and LDH
- Elevated creatinine, but normal renal output

Differential Diagnosis

- Sepsis and multi-organ failure
- Disease flare of underlying rheumatic disease (i.e., sJIA, pSLE)
- Malignancy
- Primary HLH

Management

- Close monitoring, consider ICU admission
- Volume-resuscitation 40–60 mL/kg, early inotropic support
- Infection workup and empiric broad-spectrum antibiotic coverage

Treatment

- IVIG 2 g/kg
- IV methylprednisolone pulse therapy 30 mg/kg, max 1 g
- Hematology and rheumatology consult to consider cyclosporine A, VP16

References

Benseler SM, Silverman ED, Aviv RI, et al. Primary CNS vasculitis in children. *Arthritis Rheum.* 2006; in press.

Daoud MS, Hutton KP, Gibson LE. Cutaneous periarteritis nodosa: a clinicopathological study of 79 cases. *Br J Dermatol.* 1997;136:706–713.

Frosch M, Foell D. Wegener granulomatosis in childhood and adolescence. *Eur J Pediatr.* 2004;163:425–434.

Hashkes PJ, Laxer RM. Medical treatment of juvenile idiopathic arthritis. *JAMA*. 2005;294:1671–1684.

Muise A, Tallett S, Silverman E. Are children with Kawasaki disease and prolonged fever at risk for macrophage activation syndrome? *Pediatrics*. 2003;112:495–497.

Peco-Antic A, Bonaci-Nikolic B, Basta-Jovanovic G, et al. Childhood microscopic polyangiitis associated with MPO-ANCA. *Pediatr Nephrol*. 2005;21(1):46–53.

Petty RE, Southwood TR, et al. International League of Associations for Rheumatology classification of juvenile idiopathic arthritis, 2nd rev. Edmonton, 2001. *J Rheumatol*. 2004;31:390–392.

Sawhney S, Woo T, Murray KJ. Macrophage activation syndrome: a potentially fatal complication of rheumatic disorders. *Arch Dis Child*. 2001;85:421–426.

40 ▪ Kawasaki Disease

SUSA BENSELER

Introduction

- Kawasaki disease (KD) is an inflammatory syndrome that causes a systemic vasculitis with predilection of the coronary arteries
- Etiology unclear; however, a wide variety of infections is associated with development of KD in children
- Primarily affects young children, 80% < 5 years
- Japan has highest incidence
- Most common cause of acquired heart disease in Western countries
- Kawasaki's is a potential complication/common pathway of multiple triggers/infections; *should be considered in all children with prolonged fever*

Diagnostic Criteria

Clinical diagnosis based on presence of fever for at least 5 days plus 4/5 criteria

Fever ≥ 5 days plus:

- Conjunctival injection/nonpurulent conjunctivitis (red eyes)
- Oral changes: red, cracked lips/oral erythema, prominent follicles of lip (strawberry tongue), diffuse redness of oral cavity
- Cervical lymphadenopathy (> 1.5 cm in diameter)
- Polymorphous rash
- Swelling/redness of hands and feet

Infants < 1 year and older children > 9 years often do not meet all criteria

Clinical Presentation

Frequency of clinical features:

- Fever in all patients, mean duration 6.5 days

Table 40.1 Definitions

Typical KD	Fever for at least 5 days plus 4/5 criteria
Atypical KD	Not fully meeting KD criteria (i.e., fever + 3/5 KD criteria), but evidence of coronary artery lesions on echocardiogram
Incomplete KD	Does not fully meet KD criteria
	No echocardiogram data are implicated in this term

- < 5 days of fever: 11.8%
- Oral changes in 94%
- Conjunctivitis in 92%
- Rash in 90%
- Extremity changes in 77%
- Cervical lymphadenopathy in 64%

May also present with:
- Cardiac: hypotension, tachycardia, myocarditis, pericarditis, pericardial effusion, arrhythmia, valvulitis (< 1%), mitral regurgitation
- CNS: headaches, aseptic meningitis, acute encephalitis
- LN: lymph node abscess/severe adenitis, generalized lymphadenopathy
- Lungs: pneumonitis, pleuritis
- Abdominal symptoms: gallbladder hydrops, noninfectious hepatitis, mesenteric vasculitis, ischemic strictures, pseudo-obstruction
- MSK: arthritis, myositis
- Systemic vasculitis (1%)

Associated features may be presenting symptom: risk of missing diagnosis

Consider Kawasaki disease in every child with ≥ 5 days of fever

Investigations

Bloodwork

Inflammatory Markers

- ESR, CRP
- CBC: high WBC, low hemoglobin, high platelets
- Vasculitis markers: low albumin, elevated IgG
- Hepatic inflammation: elevated AST, ALT

Additional Blood Tests

- Venous gas, creatinine, urea, electrolytes, IgA, IgM
- If indicated: CPK, troponin

Microbiology

- Blood and urine cultures
- Nasopharyngeal swab for respiratory viruses
- Other swab/cultures/serology according to clinical presentation
- CSF analysis if indicated

Ancillary Tests

- ECG: tachycardia/bradycardia, other arrhythmias (block, other), ST changes, low voltage
- Chest X-ray: pneumonia, cardiomegaly, pleural effusions
- Echocardiogram: coronary artery lesions including dilatations and aneurysms; myocardial dysfunction/collapse, decreased ejection fraction, myocarditis/myocardial edema, valvulitis, pericarditis, ischemia

Additional Tests, If Indicated

- Ultrasound: gallbladder hydrops
- Abdominal X-ray: obstruction

Differential Diagnosis

- Group A *Strept.* tonsillitis/scarlet fever, other bacterial infections
- Viral infections: adenovirus, EBV, other
- Drug reactions
- Toxin-mediated diseases
- Leukemia
- Macrophage activation syndrome (MAS)
- Systemic juvenile idiopathic arthritis (JIA)
  Note: Infections do not exclude or override diagnosis of KD

Management

IVIG

- 2 g/kg IVIG, max dose 60 g total given by slow infusion
- Informed consent required as IVIG is a blood product
- Potential adverse effects: allergic reactions and transient post infusion headache—occurs after 24 hrs and responds to acetaminophen

Aspirin

- 100 mg/kg/d divided in 4 doses (25 mg/kg/dose)
- Dose reduction may be required if elevated LFTs
- May cause transient sensorineural hearing loss

Antibiotics

- Treat all suspected bacterial infections

Additional Therapy

- Anticoagulation, abciximab, or other treatment (i.e., steroids may be required)
- Therapy is directed and monitored by cardiologist and/or rheumatologist

Risk Assessment

Coronary Artery Lesions (CAL)

Risk of developing CAL is associated with a number of factors:

Duration of Fever

- The longer the duration of fever, the higher the risk for CAL
- > 10 days of fever: significantly higher CAL risk than patients with 5 days of fever

Age

- Higher risk for development of CAL < 1 yr
- Disease features often incomplete; recognition more difficult
- Young children more likely to develop CAL after same duration of fever compared to older children; cause unknown

Gender

- Higher risk for adverse coronary outcome in males

Treatment

- Untreated: 25% risk of aneurysms
- Treated with IVIG and aspirin: 5–8% risk for aneurysms when treated within 10 days of illness
- CAL common even with treatment, but most resolve spontaneously

Myocardial Dysfunction

- High risk of myocardial dysfunction/collapse if:
  - Hypotension/borderline low blood pressure
  - Tachycardia
  - Hepatomegaly
  - Significantly elevated inflammatory markers with significant anemia
- May rapidly deteriorate with volume challenge: *avoid fluid bolus*

- Echocardiogram will demonstrate myocardial edema and borderline low ejection fraction
- Consult cardiologist if suspect myocardial dysfunction

Arrhythmia

- May present with various arrhythmias: check ECG
- May reflect serious underlying heart problems including myocardial ischemia
- Therapy can lead to transient arrhythmia (i.e., steroid-related bradycardia)
- Consult cardiology if arrhythmia present

Infections

- Need to work up for infections
- Often concurrent infections: need to diagnose and treat
- IVIG does not treat infection (infection can smolder along and cause serious problems)

References

Akikusa JD, Laxer RM, Friedman JN. Intestinal pseudo-obstruction in Kawasaki disease. *Pediatrics.* 2004;113:e504–e506.

Benseler S, McCrindle BW, Silverman ED, Tyrrell PN, Wong J, Yeung RSM. Infections and Kawasaki disease: implications for coronary artery outcome. *Pediatrics.* 2005;116(6):e760–e766.

Burns JC, Glode MP. Kawasaki syndrome. *Lancet.* 2004;364:533–544.

Han RK, Sinclair B, Newman A, et al. Recognition and management of Kawasaki disease. *CMAJ.* 2000;162:807–812.

Newburger JW, Takahashi M, Gerber MA, et al. Diagnosis, treatment, and long-term management of Kawasaki disease: a statement for health professionals from the Committee on Rheumatic Fever, Endocarditis, and Kawasaki Disease, Council on Cardiovascular Disease in the Young, American Heart Association. *Pediatrics.* 2004;114:1708–1733.

41 ▪ Limp

LEAH HARRINGTON

Introduction

- Common presentation to emergency department
- May be difficult to localize source of pain (e.g., hip pain may be referred to knee)
- Young children often not able to localize pain

Table 41.1	Motor Development Milestones
10–12 mo	Cruising: walks holding onto stationary objects for support
12–18 mo	Walks independently
36 mo	Mature walking pattern

Table 41.2	Common Abnormal Gaits
Antalgic	Shortened stance phase gait associated with pain (e.g., septic hip, transient synovitis, fracture)
Trendelenburg	Side lurching gait, trunk shifts toward and pelvis tilts away from painful or weak extremity, decreasing force transmitted through extremity (e.g., congenital hip dislocation, Legg-Calvé-Perthes disease, slipped capital femoral epiphysis)

History

- Age: diagnosis by age groups—see Table 41.3
- Onset of pain: sudden vs insidious
- Duration of pain: intermittent vs constant
- Quality of pain: severe vs mild
- Location of pain: reproducible/localizable, referred pain common

- History of trauma: accidental vs nonaccidental
  - Often not witnessed
  - Does trauma mechanism match development abilities?
- Constitutional symptoms: fever, weight loss, night sweats, malaise (neoplasms and rheumatologic infections)

Physical Examination

- General: vital signs, adenopathy, organomegaly, skin changes
- Stance: pelvic tilt, scoliosis, knee flexion, leg asymmetry, rotation of foot
- Gait: shortened stance phase, antalgic, Trendelenburg, slap foot
- Muscle strength: Trendelenburg test children > 3 yrs, school age heel-toe walk
- Passive/active limitation of range of motion or pain
- Measure leg length discrepancy, calf and thigh diameter
- Neurovascular exam: reflexes, sensation, tone, power

Table 41.3   Differential Diagnoses by Age

BIRTH–2 YEARS	2–10 YEARS	10–18 YEARS
Septic arthritis	Septic arthritis	Fractures
Toddler's fracture (spiral fracture of tibia in ambulating child)	Transient synovitis	Slipped capital femoral Epiphysis (SCFE)
Osteomyelitis	Osteomyelitis	Osteomyelitis
Congenital hip dislocation	Legg-Calvé-Perthes	Patellofemoral problems
Nonaccidental trauma	Juvenile idiopathic arthritis	Tumors
	Leukemia	Sickle cell crisis
	Fractures	
	Sickle cell crisis	

Table 41.4   Differential Diagnoses: Systems Approach

INFECTIOUS	MUSCULOSKELETAL	INFLAMMATORY	HEMATOLOGICAL	NEUROMUSCULAR
Osteomyelitis	Child abuse	JRA	Sickle cell crisis	Guillain-Barré
Septic arthritis	SCFE	Myositis	Hemophilia	Tick paralysis
Cellulitis	CHD	Transient synovitis	Leukemia	
Discitis	Fractures			
Abscess	Neoplasms			
CNS infections				
Appendicitis				
Epididymitis				

Specific Conditions

Transient Synovitis

- Acute self-limiting aseptic inflammation of synovial lining
- Idiopathic; often history of preceding viral infection
- Peak incidence 3–8 years
- Male predominance 2:1
- Diagnosis of exclusion

Note: Most common cause of hip pain/limp in children

Clinical Presentation

- Antalgic gait, may refuse to walk
- Afebrile or low-grade fever
- Hip held in flexion/external rotation

Investigations

- CBC, ESR generally normal
- Radiographs usually noncontributory
- Ultrasound may show effusion but cannot differentiate infectious vs noninfectious

Management

- Rest, NSAIDs, reevaluation in 24–48 hours
- Recurrence within 6 months 4–17%

Septic Arthritis

■ See Ch. 42, Osteomyelitis and Septic Arthritis
■ Fluid/pus accumulates in synovial space raising intra-articular pressure and injuring vessels/articular cartilage
■ Pathogen enters synovial space via hematogenous spread, locally from contiguous infection, or via traumatic/surgical intervention
■ Organisms: *S. aureus, group A Strept, pneumococcus*
  Neonates: *N. gonorrheae, group B Strept*
  Sexually active adolescents: *N. gonorrheae*
  Sickle cell disease: *Salmonella*

Clinical Presentation

■ Fever, antalgic gait, refusal to weight bear
■ Severely limited internal rotation, adduction/extension
■ Affected hip rests in abduction/external rotation
■ If fever, difficulty bearing weight, ESR > 40 mm/h, peripheral WBC > 12,000 cells/mm^3:
  Probability of SA: 99.6% if all four factors present
              93.1% if three factors present

Investigations

■ Joint aspiration—Synovial fluid:
  • WBC count > 100,000/mL suggests SA
  • WBC count consistently demonstrates 90% PMN cells
  • Culture has poor sensitivity (60–70%)
  • Glucose concentration averages 30% of serum in SA
■ Positive blood cultures in 33%
■ Hip X-ray: widened joint space rarely present; asymmetry of hip joint spaces of > 2 mm using the teardrop distance suggestive of SA
■ Hip ultrasound highly sensitive (90–100%) for effusion, cannot be used to assess cause; absence of fluid excludes septic arthritis

Treatment

- Orthopedic consult for joint aspiration/washout
- Admit for intravenous antibiotics
  - \> 4 years: penicillinase-resistant penicillin
  - \< 4 years or unimmunized for *H. influenzae* type b: add coverage for ampicillin-resistant strains of *H. influenzae*
  - Neonates, immunocompromised, IV drug use: Aminoglycoside + penicillinase-resistant penicillin to cover enteric Gram-negative bacilli and *Pseudomonas* species

Osteomyelitis

- See Ch. 42, Osteomyelitis and Septic Arthritis
- Acute or chronic bone infection due to pyogenic organisms
  - Neonates: *S. aureus, Enterobacter, groups A and B Strept*
  - Children/adolescents: *S. aureus (80%), group A Strept, H. infl., Enterobacter*
  - Sickle cell disease: *S. aureus, Salmonella*
  - Puncture wound in running shoe: *S. aureus, Pseudomonas*
- Most commonly hematogenous bacterial seeding in children
- Distal metaphysis predisposed to bacterial seeding due to slowing/sludging of blood flow in sharp angled vessels in this area
- Direct inoculation: spread from a contiguous focus of infection, or sepsis after a surgical procedure; more predominant in adolescents, adults
- Male-to-female 2:1

Clinical Presentation

- Hematogenous osteomyelitis: slow, insidious progression of symptoms
- Neonates: fever present in 50%, pseudoparalysis of limb
- Restriction of movement, local edema, erythema, point tenderness

Investigations

- WBC elevated or normal, left shift is common

- CRP elevated, nonspecific, earlier elevation (6 hrs) vs ESR (24 hrs)
- ESR elevated (90%)
- Radiographic evidence:

  Days 3–5   Soft-tissue edema

  Days 14–21   Periosteal elevation, later bone lucencies

  Day 28   90% have radiographic abnormality
- Culture/aspiration of infected site: negative in 25% of cases
- Blood cultures: positive in 50% of hematogenous osteomyelitis
- Skeletal scintigraphy: sensitivity 94%, specificity 95% (technetium Tc-99m methylene diphosphonate, radiopharmaceutical agent of choice)
- MRI valuable in delineating axial skeleton, pelvic involvement, localized (Brodie's) abscess
- MRI vs bone scan: equivalent/greater sensitivity, specificity, and accuracy for detection of osteomyelitis

Management

Admit for parenteral antibiotics

Slipped Capital Femoral Epiphysis (SCFE)

- Displacement of proximal femoral metaphysis anterolaterally and superiorly
- Often history of minor trauma
- Peak incidence at start of adolescent growth spurt
- Risk factors: male sex, obesity

Clinical Presentation

- Nonradiating, dull aching pain in thigh, groin, hip, or occasionally knee
- Pain worsens with activity
- Antalgic or Trendelenburg gait from pain/weakened hip abductors
- Hip tender to palpation, decreased internal rotation and flexion
- Mild atrophy of thigh in longstanding pathology

Investigations

- CBC/ESR normal
- Hip X-ray: slip more obvious on frog-leg lateral view
- Klein's line:
  - Drawn along superior border of proximal femoral metaphysis: normally transects femoral epiphysis by 20%
  - Line touching lateral margin of epiphysis indicates slippage of femoral epiphysis inferiorly and medially
- Subtle cases of SCFE: physis may be widened or irregular

Management

- Orthopedic consult, bed rest, traction, surgical fixation
- Failure to diagnose increases risk of avascular necrosis

Osgood-Schlatter Disease

- Chronic microtrauma to tibial tuberosity secondary to overuse of quadriceps
- Heterotopic bone formation occurs at tendon insertion site, visible lump present
- Bone growth velocity > soft-tissue growth, results in muscle tendon tightness across the joint, loss of flexibility
- Exacerbated by exercise
- 50% describe precipitating trauma
- 25% have bilateral lesions
- Risk factors:
  - Age 11–18 years, male
  - Rapid skeletal growth
  - Repetitive jumping sports

Clinical Presentation

- Pain exacerbated by running, jumping, kneeling, stairs; relieved by rest, restriction of exercise
- Present for several months on intermittent basis
- Reproducible by extending knee against resistance, stressing quadriceps, or squatting with knee in full flexion

- Tenderness, soft-tissue edema over proximal tibial tuberosity at patellar tendon insertion
- Firm mass may be palpable
- Erythema of tibial tuberosity may be present

Investigations
- Clinical diagnosis; lab evaluation not indicated unless considering other etiologies
- Plain film findings best seen on lateral view, with knee in slight internal rotation
- Irregular ossification of proximal tibial tuberosity
- Calcification and thickening within patellar tendon

Management
- Benign, self-limited condition
- No prospective studies evaluating treatment, including conservative approach (ice, analgesics, activity restriction, stretching, strengthening, or anti-inflammatory medications)
- Corticosteroid injections not recommended; case reports of subcutaneous atrophy
- Avoidance of pain-producing activities

Legg-Calvé-Perthes Disease
- Avascular necrosis of femoral head, followed by collapse and subsequent repair
- Etiology: idiopathic, interruption of blood supply to femoral head via trauma, steroid use, hip dislocation, septic arthritis
- Peak incidence 4–9 years
- Risk factors: male, low birth weight, shorter than average stature

Clinical Presentation
- Painful or painless limp
- Pain usually mild, intermittent, referred to thigh/knee

- Limp related to pain, limb-length discrepancy, or limited internal rotation and abduction of hip
- Muscle atrophy may be present

Investigations

Hip X-ray:
- Initial phase: small radiodense femoral head, widened medial joint space
- Few months: crescent-shaped subchondral radiolucent line
- Fragmentation phase: areas of radiodensity and radiolucency
- Reossification phase: abnormal femoral head shape and size

Management
- Orthopedic clinic follow-up, conservative treatment

References

Eich GF, Superti-Furga AS, Unbricht FS, Willi UV. The painful hip: evaluation of criteria for clinical decision-making. *Eur J Pediatr.* 1999;158:923–928.

Kocher MS, Zurakowski D, Kasser JR. Differentiating between septic arthritis and transient synovitis of the hip in children: an evidence-based clinical prediction algorithm. *J Bone Joint Surg Am.* 1999;81(12):1662–1670.

Lawrence LL. The limping child. *Emerg Med Clin North Am.* 1998;16(4): 911–929.

Lazzarini L. Antibiotic treatment of osteomyelitis: what have we learned from 30 years of clinical trials? *Int J Infect Dis.* 2005;9(3):127–138.

Loder RT. Slipped capital femoral epiphysis. *Am Fam Physician.* 1998; 57(9):2135–2148.

42 ▪ Osteomyelitis and Septic Arthritis

KELLY KEOGH AND ANDREW MASON

Osteomyelitis

- Osteomyelitis results from hematogenous dissemination of an organism into the metaphysis of a long bone
- Occasionally direct inoculation into bone from trauma
- Bacterial proliferation evokes an inflammatory exudate leading to destruction of bone, necrosis of cortex, and elevation, then rupture of periosteum
- Causes pain in affected limb
- Lower limbs most often affected

Pathophysiology

- Often associated with septic arthritis in children < 1 year and in joints with intracapsular metaphyses (proximal radius, humerus, and femur)

Children < 1 year:

- Called septic osteomyelitis of infancy
- Epiphysis contains capillaries that facilitate spread of osteomyelitis to contiguous joint space

Children > 1 year:

- Hematogenously spread infection starts in metaphyseal sinusoidal veins
- Infection contained within metaphysis and diaphysis by avascular epiphysis, which acts as a barrier
- Infection spreads laterally to break through cortex and lifts the loose periosteum, creating a subperiosteal abscess

Clinical Presentation

■ Very similar to septic arthritis; clinical differentiation may be difficult
■ Sudden onset of bone pain, often with high fever
■ Bone pain is manifested according to age:
  • Infants: pseudoparalysis (voluntary immobilization of affected limb), crying with movement of limb
  • Child: pseudoparalysis, refusal to weight bear, limp
■ Examination: look unwell, may hold affected limb immobile, point tenderness at site of infection: difficult to assess in struggling toddler
  • Local erythema and edema if purulent material has ruptured through the cortex
■ Often an effusion is detectable

Investigations

■ CBC (WBC normal in > 50%)
■ Blood culture (causative organism 50–70%)
■ ESR (acute phase reactant; insensitive, nonspecific), CRP
  • Elevated in 90% and 98% of cases, respectively
  • Useful for monitoring effectiveness of therapy
  • ESR peaks 3–5 days after initiation of therapy and normalizes in ~ 3 weeks
  • CRP peaks at day 2 and normalizes within 1 week in uncomplicated cases
■ X-ray: to exclude fracture
  • Initially, films will be normal
  • At 10–12 days: osseous destruction visible, reflecting 40% bone loss
■ Ultrasound: to rule out joint effusion if necessary to differentiate osteomyelitis from septic arthritis and to exclude concomitant septic arthritis
■ Bone radionuclide scan:
  Technetium scan-tracer = Tc99m bound to phosphorus

- Accumulates in areas of increased osteoblast activity with increased blood flow and new bone formation
  - Test of choice; sensitivity and specificity 95%
  - Usually positive within 2–3 days of onset of infection
- Gallium citrate scan:
  - Radioactive gallium citrate acts as an analog of calcium and iron and attaches to transferrin to accumulate at sites of inflammation
  - Most sensitive and specific for *vertebral* osteomyelitis
- Bone biopsy: definitive diagnosis based on positive bone or blood cultures or histopathologic changes consistent with osteomyelitis
  - If cultures are negative, needle biopsy may be necessary to provide tissue for histopathologic analysis
- CT scan/MRI useful in select cases (sequestra, abscess)

Treatment

Medical Management

- Antibiotics: empiric parenteral antibiotics based on most likely organism (see Table 42.1)
- Directed antibiotics according to culture and sensitivities
- If child not vaccinated for *H. influenzae* b, add coverage for ampicillin-resistant strains
- Acute osteomyelitis in infants and children usually responds to medical therapy alone
- Duration of treatment 4–6 weeks
- Treat for 7–14 days with IV antibiotics
- If adequate clinical response, may switch to oral antibiotics if child is afebrile, oral antibiotic tolerated, strict compliance assured, adequate blood levels demonstrated, and resolving signs of inflammation (ESR)

334 ■ Chapter 42: Osteomyelitis and Septic Arthritis

Surgical Treatment
- If initial medical management fails, open medullary or soft-tissue surgical debridement may be necessary

Complications
- High risk of developing chronic osteomyelitis if acute form not treated promptly and optimally

Septic Arthritis
- Septic arthritis results from hematogenous dissemination of an organism into a joint
- Bacteria in the joint space evoke an inflammatory response and an accumulation of purulent material distends the joint capsule
- Causes pain and limited motion
- Septic arthritis often associated with osteomyelitis in children < 1 year and in joints with intracapsular metaphyses

Clinical Presentation
- Very similar to osteomyelitis; clinical differentiation may be difficult
- Look unwell
- Sudden onset of joint pain and swelling with low-grade fever
- Joint pain is manifested according to age: see osteomyelitis section
- Position of comfort protects joint from movement
- In a septic hip, leg will be held flexed, **ab**ducted, and **e**xternally **r**otated to minimize distension of hip capsule (FABER)
- Exquisite tenderness with minimal movement of joint

Investigations
- CBC, ESR, CRP, blood culture (causative organism in 70%)
- X-ray: to exclude fracture, films will be normal initially; periosteal changes seen at 7 days

- Ultrasound: to delineate joint effusion
- Joint aspiration: send joint fluid analysis for:
  - WBC, differential (WBC > 100,000 mm^3)
  - Gram stain, culture
  - Latex agglutination
- Septic joint: WBC > 100,000 mm^3 and decreased glucose

Treatment

- Treat as an "abscess" with both medical and surgical management
- Prognosis is time dependent

Medical Management

- Empiric parenteral antibiotics based on most likely organisms
- Depends on age and directed according to culture and sensitivities (see Table 42.1)
- Supportive measures: analgesia, immobilization
- Duration of treatment:
  - Adequate blood levels of culture-specific antibiotics required for at least 21 days
  - ESR and CRP are valuable indictors of clinical response
  - Generally IV antibiotics are continued until clinical condition and ESR or CRP normalize
- Delivery of antibiotic: IV vs PO
  - Adequate clinical response can be discharged on home IV therapy
  - Switch to oral antibiotics is acceptable provided that the child has defervesced, antibiotic is tolerated, strict compliance assured, adequate blood levels

Surgical Management

- Drainage: percutaneous aspiration in easily accessible peripheral joints
- Open drainage and aggressive irrigation in the operating room is the most effective treatment

Table 42.1 Empiric Antibiotic Treatment for Septic Arthritis and Osteomyelitis

AGE	SUSPECTED MICROBIAL AGENT	ANTIMICROBIAL OF CHOICE	ALTERNATIVE THERAPY OR COMMENTS
Septic arthritis			
Neonate	Gr B streptococci, *S. aureus,* Gm neg enteric bacilli (e.g., *E. coli*)	Cloxacillin + tobramycin	Therapeutic and diagnostic aspirate are essential.
Infant 1–3 mos	*H. influenzae, Streptococcus spp., Staphylococcus spp.* Also pathogens as for neonate	Cefuroxime; cefotaxime	Drain any abscess first. Consider late-onset Group B streptococci.
Child	Gr A streptococci, *S. aureus, S. pneumoniae*	Cefazolin	Cloxacillin; clindamycin.
Osteomyelitis (acute)			
Neonate	*S. aureus,* Gr B streptococci, Gm neg enteric bacilli (e.g., *E. coli*)	Cloxacillin + tobramycin	Cloxacillin + cefotaxime. Drain any abscess first. Consider late-onset Group B streptococci.

Table 42.1 Empiric Antibiotic Treatment for Septic Arthritis and Osteomyelitis (continued)

Osteomyelitis (acute)

Infant 1–3 mos	H. influenzae, Streptococcus spp., Staphylococcus spp. Also pathogens as for neonate.	Cefuroxime; cefotaxime	Cloxacillin; clindamycin.
Child	S. aureus, S. pneumoniae	Cefazolin	Clindamycin + gentamicin.

Sickle cell disease

	S. aureus, Salmonella spp., S. pneumoniae	Cefotaxime	

Puncture wound of foot

Sneakers	P. aeruginosa	Piperacillin + gentamicin	Significant β-lactam allergy: ciprofloxacin + gentamicin.
No sneakers	S. aureus	Oral: cephalexin; IV: cefazolin	Culture and sensitivity desirable.

Source: With permission from: Kowalczyk A, ed. *The 2005–2006 Formulary of Drugs, The Hospital for Sick Children,* 24th ed. Toronto: The Graphic Centre, HSC; 2005.

References

Asensi V, Alvarez V, Valle E, et al. IL-1alpha (- 889) promoter polymorphism is a risk factor for osteomyelitis. *Am J Med Genet.* 2003;119A(2):132–136.

Bradley JS, Kaplan SL, Tan TQ, et al. Pediatric pneumococcal bone and joint infections. The Pediatric Multicenter Pneumococcal Surveillance Study Group (PMPSSG). *Pediatrics.* 1998;102(6):1376–1382.

Kowalczyk A, ed. *The 2005–2006 Formulary of Drugs, The Hospital for Sick Children.* 24th ed. Toronto: The Graphic Centre, HSC; 2005.

Lew DP, Waldvogel FA. Osteomyelitis. *N Engl J Med.* 1997;336(14):999–1007.

Morrissy RT. Bone and joint sepsis. In: Lovell WW, et al, eds. *Lovell and Winter's Pediatric Orthopaedics.* 4th ed. Philadelphia: Lippincott Williams & Wilkins; 1996:579–624.

Peltola H, Kallio MJ, Unkila-Kallio L. Reduced incidence of septic arthritis in children by *Haemophilus influenzae* type-b vaccination: implications for treatment. *J Bone Joint Surg Br.* 1998;80(3):471–473.

Schwentker EP. Septic arthritis. In: Hoekelman RA, ed. *Primary Pediatric Care.* 4th ed. St. Louis: Mosby-Year Book Inc.; 2001:1806–1808.

■ PART X
ENDOCRINE EMERGENCIES

43 ▪ Diabetic Emergencies

AMINA LALANI

Introduction

- Type 1 diabetes accounts for 5–10% of all diabetes
- 50% of type 1 DM present in childhood
- Trend toward lower age at presentation
- Pancreatic β-cell destruction results in insulin deficiency
- Often associated with other autoimmune diseases: thyroid disorders, Addison's disease, celiac disease, vitiligo
- Major emergencies
  - Diabetic ketoacidosis
  - Intercurrent illness
  - Hypoglycemia
- Complications:
  - Microvascular: retinopathy, nephropathy, neuropathy
  - Macrovascular: cardiovascular, cerebrovascular, peripheral vascular
- Hemoglobin A_1c: Measure of glycemic control over last 90–120 days

Canadian Diabetes Association Clinical Practice Guidelines

- Insulin is given as multiple daily injections: NPH or ultralente given once or twice daily with boluses of regular insulin before meals
- Recently fast-acting (insulin aspart and insulin lispro) and very long acting insulin analogs (insulin glargine or detemir) available
- Use of insulin pumps is increasing: fast-acting insulin provided at a continuous rate, with boluses before meals

Table 43.1 Targets for Plasma Glucose and HbA$_1$c		
AGE (YRS)	PLASMA GLUCOSE (mmol^L)	HBA$_1$C (%)
< 5	6–12	≤ 9
5–12	4–10	≤ 8
13–18	4–7	≤ 7

Diabetic Ketoacidosis (DKA)

- Most frequent cause of death due to diabetes in children
- Risk of mortality < 0.5%
- Rate of presentation in DKA ~ 25%; more likely to present in DKA at younger age
- Causes of DKA in known diabetics:
  - Omitting insulin dose (most frequent cause)
  - Infection or illness
  - Malfunction of insulin pump: catheter displacement
- Most deaths are due to cerebral edema

Clinical Presentation

- Polyuria, polydipsia, nocturia, weight loss, polyphagia, abdominal pain, vomiting
- May appear as an acute abdomen
- Signs of dehydration: tachycardia, decreased capillary refill, cool extremities, dry mucous membranes, poor skin turgor
- Metabolic acidosis stimulates tachypnea with classic Kussmaul respirations (deep sighing respirations)
- Acetone production produces fruity breath odor
- Usually normal or minimal decrease in level of consciousness

Investigations

- Immediate capillary glucose
- Serum glucose, electrolytes, venous gas, urea, creatinine
- Intravenous access
- Urine for ketones and glucose

Diagnosis

■ Hyperglycemia: glucose > 11 mmol/L
■ Acidosis: pH < 7.30
■ Serum bicarbonate < 18 mmol/L
■ Ketonuria

Electrolyte Changes

Glucose:
  • Variable serum glucose may be due to degree of hydration
  • Severe dehydration results in higher glucose concentrations

Metabolic acidosis:
  • Increased anion gap metabolic acidosis due to ketones and lactate

Serum sodium:
  • Decreased due to fluid movement into intravascular space as a result of hyperglycemia

Serum potassium:
  • Potassium moves from intracellular to extracellular space due to acidosis, therefore serum measurements are normal
  • Total body potassium concentration is decreased due to urine losses
  • Serum potassium drops rapidly with insulin therapy

Serum phosphate:
  • Concentrations are normal initially but fall with treatment

Treatment

Fluids

■ Start with intravenous normal saline to restore perfusion
■ May require initial bolus of 10–20 mL/kg if dehydrated
■ If blood pressure stable, give fluids cautiously:
  7 mL/kg NS × 1 hour then 3.5–5 mL/kg/hr
■ Serum glucose usually falls significantly with fluid treatment alone

Insulin and Glucose
- Insulin treats acidosis and hyperglycemia
- Start insulin infusion 0.1 U/kg/hr IV (1 mL/kg/hr of 25 U regular insulin in 250 mL NS)
- Do NOT give bolus of insulin
- Serum glucose often normalizes before acidosis has resolved: add dextrose to IV fluids when glucose < 15 mmol/L or glucose falls > 5 mmol/L/hr, and decrease insulin infusion to 0.05 U/kg/hr

Electrolytes
- Potassium moves from extracellular to intracellular space with insulin treatment
- Add potassium 40 mEq/L to IV fluids once urine output present and K < 5.5
- Use potassium chloride +/− potassium phosphate

Bicarbonate
- Routine administration *not* recommended
- Acidosis can usually be corrected with insulin and fluids
- Possible detrimental effects of bicarbonate:
  - May increase hepatic ketone production
  - Increased risk of hypokalemia during treatment
  - May lead to paradoxical acidosis of CSF due to decreased respiratory drive and rise in partial pressure of CO_2
  - May increase risk of cerebral edema
- Consider if pH < 7.0 in consultation with endocrinologist

Monitoring
- Admit to PICU
- Measure capillary blood glucose every hour
- Measure serum glucose, electrolytes, and venous blood gas every 2–4 hours
- Monitor vital signs and neurovitals every hour

■ Monitor fluid intake/output every hour
■ Follow osmolality

Complications

■ Most frequent complications are hypoglycemia and hypokalemia

Life-threatening complications:
■ Cerebral edema
■ Pulmonary edema
■ CNS hemorrhage or thrombosis due to prothrombotic state
■ Cardiac arrhythmias due to abnormal electrolytes
■ Pancreatitis
■ Renal failure

Cerebral Edema
■ Most frequent life-threatening complication of DKA
■ 0.3–1% of pediatric DKA episodes
■ Present with headache, altered LOC, irritability, vomiting, hypertension, bradycardia, signs of increased ICP
■ Up to 24% mortality rate, 25% have permanent neurologic deficits
■ May be mild asymptomatic cerebral edema in most children with DKA
■ Cause is controversial—various theories:
  • Due to rapid changes in serum osmolality and aggressive fluid resuscitation during treatment: not supported by clinical studies and cerebral edema may occur prior to treatment
  • Vasogenic cause with abnormal blood-brain barrier function
■ Risk factors: high urea concentration at presentation, worsening hypocapnia, only small rise in serum sodium with treatment

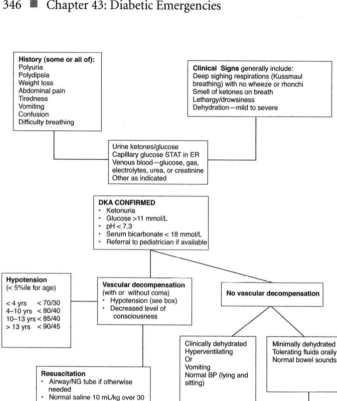

Figure 43.1 Emergency Guidelines for Management of Diabetic Ketoacidosis

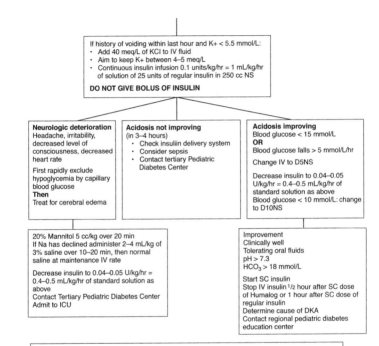

If history of voiding within last hour and K+ < 5.5 mmol/L:
- Add 40 meq/L of KCl to IV fluid
- Aim to keep K+ between 4–5 meq/L
- Continuous insulin infusion 0.1 units/kg/hr = 1 mL/kg/hr of solution of 25 units of regular insulin in 250 cc NS

DO NOT GIVE BOLUS OF INSULIN

Neurologic deterioration
Headache, irritability, decreased level of consciousness, decreased heart rate

First rapidly exclude hypoglycemia by capillary blood glucose
Then
Treat for cerebral edema

Acidosis not improving
(in 3–4 hours)
- Check insuliin delivery system
- Consider sepsis
- Contact tertiary Pediatric Diabetes Center

Acidosis improving
Blood glucose < 15 mmol/L
OR
Blood glucose falls > 5 mmol/L/hr

Change IV to D5NS

Decrease insulin to 0.04–0.05 U/kg/hr = 0.4–0.5 mL/kg/hr of standard solution as above
Blood glucose < 10 mmol/L: change to D10NS

20% Mannitol 5 cc/kg over 20 min
If Na has declined administer 2–4 mL/kg of 3% saline over 10–20 min, then normal saline at maintenance IV rate

Decrease insulin to 0.04–0.05 U/kg/hr = 0.4–0.5 mL/kg/hr of standard solution as above
Contact Tertiary Pediatric Diabetes Center
Admit to ICU

Improvement
Clinically well
Tolerating oral fluids
pH > 7.3
HCO_3 > 18 mmol/L

Start SC insulin
Stop IV insulin 1/2 hour after SC dose of Humalog or 1 hour after SC dose of regular insulin
Determine cause of DKA
Contact regional pediatric diabetes education center

Observation and Monitoring
- Hourly blood glucose (capillary)
- Aim for a decrease in blood glucose of 5 mmol/L/hr
- Hourly documentation of fluid input/output
- Hourly, at least, assessment of neurological status
- 2–4 hours after start of IV: electrolytes, venous gases—then q 2–4 h
- Follow effective osmolality = (2 × measured Na+ measured blood glucose)
- Avoid a decrease of > 2–3 mmol/L/hr in effective osmolality by increasing IV sodium concentration

■ **Figure 43.1   Emergency Guidelines for Management of Diabetic Ketoacidosis (continued)**

Treatment of Cerebral Edema
- Mannitol 20% 5 cc/kg over 20 minutes
- If sodium has fallen, give 3% saline 2–4 mL/kg over 10–20 minutes
- Do not hyperventilate intubated patients
- Decrease insulin to 0.05 U/kg/hr
- CT head to rule out other CNS pathology such as thrombosis
- Admit to ICU

Intercurrent Illness
- Patient presents with vomiting
- For all patients:
  - Obtain capillary glucose, electrolytes, glucose, urea, creatinine, venous gas
  - Check urine for ketones

Management
See Figure 43.2, emergency guidelines for intercurrent illness
- Do not omit insulin
- Adjust insulin dosing as per guidelines and give oral or intravenous fluids

Hypoglycemia
- Most common acute complication associated with treatment of type 1 DM
- Causes:
  - Inadequate caloric intake
  - Excess insulin dose
  - Inadequate preparation for exercise
- Severe hypoglycemia episodes predispose patient to further episodes
- Need to balance food intake, insulin dose, and physical activity
- May lead to seizures, loss of consciousness, permanent brain damage

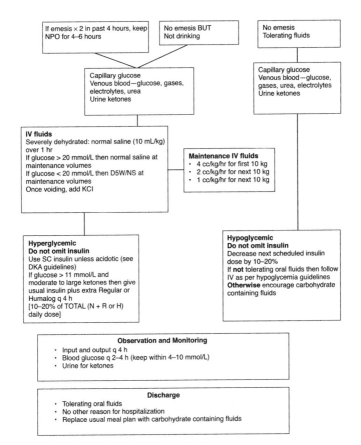

Source: Ontario Diabetes Strategy, Ministry of Health and Long Term Care. *Emergency guidelines for managing the child with Type 1 Diabetes.* http://www.health.gov.on.ca/english/providers/pub/diabetes/childguide.pdf.

▪ Figure 43.2   Emergency Guidelines for Intercurrent Illness

Mild, Moderate, or Severe

Mild: sweaty, tremor, palpitations, anxious, hungry, nausea, tingling

Moderate: confused, weak, inability to concentrate, drowsy, blurred vision, dizzy, difficulty speaking

Severe: requires external assistance to reverse hypoglycemia; confusion, seizures, unconscious

■ Severe events occur more frequently during sleep
■ Decreased serum glucose causes a rise in counter regulatory hormones
■ May have an inadequate hormonal response to hypoglycemia and lack normal warning signs: predisposes to severe attack
■ Treatment with insulin analogs or continuous subcutaneous insulin infusion pumps associated with lower incidence of hypoglycemia than conventional treatment

Clinical Presentation

■ Two types of symptoms:
  • Autonomic: shakiness, hunger, anxiety, palpitations, sweaty
  • Neuroglycopenic: dizzy, irritable, lethargic, headache, confused
■ Hypoglycemia with loss of consciousness may be followed by headache and vomiting, Todd's paralysis; usually resolves after several hours

Risk Factors

■ Young age or adolescence
■ History of prior hypoglycemic episodes
■ Male sex
■ Associated illness: hypothyroidism, celiac disease
■ Exercise

History		Clinical Signs
Recent hypoglycemic event requiring treatment by another person with glucagon or oral glucose especially if confusion ⇓ consciousness	and/or	Seizures Hemiparesis Any localizing neurological findings Altered state of consciousness

Obtain a blood glucose (capillary)
Electrolytes and gases not usually necessary

If child active, alert, and tolerating oral fluids well then encourage glucose-containing drinks at least at maintenance fluid rate

OTHERWISE

Start IV—at least 5% glucose in saline at maintenance rate, regardless of blood glucose level

If drowsy, and any neurologic impairment, localized or generalized: IV bolus of 0.25–0.5 grams/kg of 50% glucose (0.5–1.0 mL/kg) or 25% glucose (1–2 mL/kg)

Continue IV glucose until:
o No further neurologic signs and
o No longer drowsy, confused, irrational, or restless.

May take up to 12 hours if hypoglycemic encephalopathy is present
Aim to maintain blood glucose above 8 mmol/L
Then change to oral sugar-containing fluids

Discharge ONLY when child is
1) Fully alert
2) Tolerating oral fluids, and
3) Free of neurologic signs

Observation and Monitoring
Determine cause and arrange for follow-up
Decrease all insulin doses by 20% for next 24 hours
Renew prescription for glucagon if used

■ **Figure 43.3   Emergency Guidelines for Management of Hypoglycemia (moderate or severe)**

Prevention

■ Use of insulin pumps with subcutaneous insulin infusion may prevent hypoglycemia due to steady release of insulin
■ Eat carbohydrates or decrease short-acting insulin prior to exercise

Treatment

Severe hypoglycemia: confused, decreased level of consciousness, seizing, unresponsive, any localizing neurological findings
   • Check blood glucose
   • Give 0.25–0.5 g/kg IV glucose: 1–2 cc/kg D25W or
     0.5–1 cc/kg D50W, OR
     0.5–1 mg glucagon subcutaneously
   • Give oral glucose immediately after glucagon treatment

Mild–moderate hypoglycemia:
   • Treat with simple sugars (e.g., cookies and juice)
■ Posthypoglycemia hyperglycemia (Somogyi phenomenon) is a risk of overtreating hypoglycemia
■ Check blood glucose after treatment
■ Decrease insulin doses by 20% for next 24 hrs

References

Daneman D. Type 1 diabetes. *Lancet.* 2006;367:847–858.

Glaser N. Pediatric diabetic ketoacidosis and hyperglycemic hyperosmolar state. *Pediatr Clin North Am.* 2005;52(6):1611–1635.

Ontario Diabetes Strategy, Ministry of Health and Long Term Care. Emergency guidelines for managing the child with type 1 diabetes. Available at http://www.health.gov.on.ca/english/providers/pub/diabetes/childguide.pdf.

Ryan C, Gurtunca N, Becker D. Hypoglycemia: a complication of diabetes therapy in children. *Pediatr Clin North Am.* 2005;52(6):1705–1733.

44 ▪ Adrenal Crisis

WILLIAM MOUNSTEPHEN

Introduction

- Often presents with nonspecific complaints
- Requires high index of suspicion
- Adrenal cortex unable to produce enough glucocorticoid and mineralocorticoid in response to stress

Table 44.1	Adrenal Insufficiency
Primary	Glucocorticoid and mineralocorticoid production affected • Congenital (CAH) • Autoimmune • Adrenal hemorrhage • Infection: TB, histoplasmosis, meningococcemia
Secondary	Only glucocorticoid production affected • Suppression of ACTH in patients on pharmacologic dosages of glucocorticoids

Clinical Presentation

Primary Adrenal Insufficiency

- Gradual onset of symptoms/complaints such as weakness, fatigue, malaise, anorexia, weight loss
- Salt craving
- Hypotension
- Skin hyperpigmentation: lips, buccal mucosa, nipples, groin, palmar/axillary creases, areas of old scars or friction

Infancy

- Most common cause is congenital adrenal hyperplasia (CAH): failure to thrive, vomiting,

dehydration, hyperpigmentation of genitalia, ambiguous genitalia
* Rare before 5–7 days of life

Older Child/Adolescent
* Addison's disease (autoimmune): most common cause
* Onset prolonged, acute crisis may occur with infection
* If suspicious, consider other autoimmune endocrine disorders (often hypothyroid)

Secondary Adrenal Insufficiency
■ May have clinical signs of Cushing's syndrome ($\uparrow$BP, moon facies, central obesity, purple striae, acne)
■ Clinical adrenal insufficiency or acute adrenal crisis occurs upon withdrawal of steroids or with physiologic stress (surgery, infection, trauma) without appropriate increase in glucocorticoid dose

Investigations
■ Electrolytes: hyponatremia, hyperkalemia, hypochloremia
■ +/– Hypoglycemia
■ CBC: may be neutropenic
■ Plasma renin $\uparrow$
■ Urine sodium $\uparrow$, urine potassium $\downarrow$
■ Cortisol level $\uparrow$, aldosterone level $\uparrow$, ACTH level $\uparrow$
■ Save blood for other adrenal steroid metabolites (e.g., 17 hydroxyprogesterone in cases of suspected 21-hydroxylase deficiency)

Treatment
Fluids
■ Often present in shock: treat with bolus 20–40 mL/kg normal saline

- Once stable, fluid management:
  - D1OW/0.9 N/S for infants
  - D5W/0.9 N/S for children
- Add potassium after voiding: cortisol administration will cause potassium to fall rapidly

Adrenal Corticosteroid Replacement Therapy

Acute Crisis

- Hydrocortisone (Solucortef®) 100 mg/m^2 IV then 100 mg/m^2/day IV ÷ q 6 hrs
- Rough rule: infants 25 mg, small child 50 mg, larger child/adolescent 100 mg hydrocortisone IV
- Mineralocorticoid not necessary during acute crisis
- Treat underlying cause of stress: infection most common factor

Post Acute Crisis

- Hydrocortisone 20 mg/m^2/day ÷ tid PO, 12 mg/m^2/day ÷ q 6 hrs IV

Intercurrent Illness

For patients taking maintenance steroids (e.g., CAH or Addison's)
- For minor illness, double daily dose of hydrocortisone
- For serious illness, triple total daily dose and divide q 6 hrs

Surgical/Trauma Patient

- For patients with adrenal insufficiency who require surgery or emergent intubation or trauma patient: give hydrocortisone (Solucortef®) 100 mg/m^2 IV × 1 preop, then 100 mg/m^2/day IV divided q 6 hrs

Disposition

- Consult endocrinologist
- Admit acute adrenal insufficiency: Addisonian crisis

- Vomiting, inadequate oral intake, inability to take oral steroids, postural vital sign changes
- Uncertain compliance at home

References

Hale D. Endocrine emergencies. In: Fleisher G, Ludwig S, eds. *Textbook of Pediatric Emergency Medicine.* 4th ed. Philadelphia: Lippincott Williams & Wilkins; 2000:1101–1104.

Kowalczyk A, ed. *The 2005–2006 Formulary of Drugs, The Hospital for Sick Children.* 24th ed. Toronto: The Graphic Centre, HSC; 2005.

Schachner H, Silfen M. Endocrine emergencies. In: Crain E, Gerschel J, eds. *Clinical Manual of Emergency Pediatrics.* 4th ed. New York: McGraw-Hill; 2003:147–151.

PART XI

NEUROLOGIC EMERGENCIES

45 ▪ Headache

ABDULLAH AL-ANAZI

Introduction

- 60–70% of children experience headache by the age of 7–9 years
- Relatively unusual presentation in pediatric patients as an isolated complaint (0.7% to 1.3% of visits)
- Essential to rule out life-threatening causes
- Laboratory test and imaging modalities are rarely needed

History

- Mode of onset, pattern, duration, frequency, and location of headache
  - Abrupt onset with extreme pain: consider rupture of AV malformation
  - Occipital location: consider posterior fossa tumor
- Severity of pain, exacerbating and relieving factors
  - Headache that worsens with bending over or coughing: consider sinusitis or raised intracranial pressure
- Time and circumstances of headache
  - Early morning headache or one that awakens a child from sleep: consider brain tumor or increased intracranial pressure
- Associated symptoms (fever, vomiting, neck pain, photophobia, visual change, etc.)
  - Vomiting is the most commonly associated symptom in patients with intracranial pathology (present in 74%)
- Analgesia and response to therapy
- Any change from previous headache pattern
- Recent or remote trauma
- Exposure to medication or toxin
- Preexisting medical problems (VP shunt, malignancy, hematologic disease)

- Psychosocial history
- Family history of headaches or migraine

Examination

- Appearance (sick or well looking)
- Vital signs including blood pressure and temperature
- General physical exam, including sinus or dental tenderness, nuchal rigidity, lymphadenopathy, heart murmurs, cutaneous lesions, cranial bruits, and visual acuity
- Complete neurological examination

Clinical Classification

- Based on temporal pattern of headache
- Five patterns: acute, acute recurrent, chronic progressive, chronic nonprogressive, and mixed pattern

Acute Headache

- Single episode without prior history
- Usually secondary to an upper respiratory febrile illness (e.g., URTI, sinusitis, otitis media)
- In toxic-appearing patient with fever: consider meningitis (look for signs of meningeal irritation)
- Suspect subarachnoid hemorrhage if sudden onset and very severe headache

Acute Recurrent Headache

- Recurrent episodes of headache with symptom-free intervals
- Differential includes migraine and its variants, tension headache, cluster headache, and neuralgia

Migraine Headache

- Most prevalent form is migraine without aura (common migraine)
- Diagnostic criteria using International Headache Society classification:

A. At least five or more episodes fulfilling criteria B through D
B. Episodes last 1–48 hours
C. Two of the following: unilateral or bilateral, pulsating, moderate to severe intensity, aggravated by routine physical activities
D. Headache accompanied by one of the following: nausea and/or vomiting, photophobia, and/or phonophobia

Tension Headache
- Pain is symmetric with band-like distribution
- Often associated with emotional stress or fatigue, does not interfere with sleep, usually not associated with vomiting or photophobia

Chronic Progressive Headache
- Gradual increase in frequency and severity of headache
- Often includes serious diagnoses such as brain tumor, pseudotumor cerebri, hydrocephalus, chronic meningitis, brain abscess, AV malformation, subdural hematoma, hypertension
- History suggestive of intracranial pathology and increased intracranial pressure includes late night or early morning headache, headache that awakens child from sleep, and vomiting at night or early morning
- Abnormal neurological findings: papilledema, abnormal eye movements, ataxia, abnormal tendon reflexes, and visual examination defects

Chronic Nonprogressive Headache
- Frequent or constant headache without change in frequency or severity
- Causes: chronic sinusitis, post traumatic headache, and stress-related headache

Mixed Headache

■ Acute recurrent headache; usually migraine superimposed on a chronic daily headache

Investigations

■ Majority of patients with normal physical examination do not require investigation in the emergency department
■ Investigations should be based on suspected etiology
■ CBC and blood culture for suspected infection
■ Lumbar puncture for meningitis, subarachnoid hemorrhage, or pseudotumor cerebri
  • Consider CT prior to LP if evidence of increased ICP, altered level of consciousness, focal findings, or papilledema
■ CT head for:
  • Chronic progressive headache
  • Abnormal neurological examination
  • Focal neurological symptoms
  • Papilledema
  • Sudden onset severe headache: "thunderclap headache"
  • VP shunt
  • Headache or vomiting on awakening
  • Age < 3 years
  • Neurocutaneous syndrome

Treatment

Acute Headache

■ Treat underlying condition
■ Oral analgesics: acetaminophen or ibuprofen

Acute Recurrent Headache (Migraine)

General Measures

■ Identify and remove triggers: sleep disturbance, stress
■ Rest in quiet dark room is effective at onset of migraine

- Behavioral therapies: relaxation techniques and stress management
- Avoid caffeine: can precipitate headache in adolescents and may be associated with rebound headache
- Ketorolac efficacy and dosing have not been established in children for migraine headaches
- Migraine recurrence: common in first 24–48 hours, particularly if discharged from emergency without complete pain relief

Table 45.1   Rescue Medication for Migraines

1st line	Mild analgesics such as ibuprofen or naproxen	Acetaminophen may be effective
2nd line	Metoclopramide 0.1–0.2 mg/kg slow IV push; max dose 10 mg	
	Chlorpromazine 0.1–0.5 mg/kg IV push over 20 min; max dose 50 mg	Risk of hypotension: give fluid bolus 20 cc/kg and monitor BP
	Sumatriptan (5-hydroxytryptamine receptor agonist) 5 mg nasal spray > 12 years	Oral/subcutaneous: inadequate data to support use. Ongoing trials in children
3rd line	Dihydroergotamine 0.5–1 mg /dose IV/IM Pretreat with antiemetic to . decrease nausea and vomiting	Cannot be used in sequence or together with chlorpromazine
		Only use in consultation with neurology, dosing in children < 12 years not established
4th line	Consider dexamethasone 0.25 mg/kg IV/PO	For refractory cases Neurology consultation

Disposition and Referral

- Admit serious secondary causes (brain abscess, sinus venous thrombosis) for further treatment
- Outpatient follow-up with neurology referral
  - Chronic progressive headache
  - Children < 3 years
  - Recurrent migraine headache

References

Gorelick M. Neurologic emergency. In: Fleisher GR, Ludwig S, eds. *Textbook of Pediatric Emergency Medicine.* 4th ed. Philadelphia: Lippincott Williams & Wilkins; 2000:701–725.

Lewis DW, Ashwal S, et al. Practice parameter: pharmacological treatment of migraine headache in children and adolescents: report of the American Academy of Neurology Quality Standards Subcommittee and the Practice Committee of the Child Neurology Society. *Neurology.* 2004;63:2215–2224.

Plewa M, et al. Pediatric headaches. *Pediatr Emerg Med Reports.* 2004;9: 118–128.

Qureshi F, Lewis DW. Managing headache in the pediatric emergency department. *Clin Pediatr Emerg Med.* 2003;4:159–170.

46 ▪ Altered Level of Consciousness

D. Anna Jarvis

Introduction

Altered states of consciousness may vary from mild impairment to deep unresponsiveness and can signal present or impending life-threatening situations.

Definitions

Consciousness:	Awareness of self and environment
Confusion:	Slowed, impaired cognitive abilities
Delirium:	Succession of confused and unconnected ideas
Obtundation:	Awake but not alert
Stupor:	Aroused only with repeated, vigorous stimuli
Coma:	Unresponsiveness even to pain

- Accurate assessment of level of consciousness is essential, with serially repeated evaluations to track trends
- The Glasgow Coma Scale is accurate but lengthy (see Ch. 7, Head Injury)
- A valuable rapid quick assessment tool is the **AVPU** scale:
  A = Awake and aware (alert)
  V = Responsive to verbal stimuli
  P = Responsive to painful stimuli
  U = Unresponsive

Causes of Altered Level of Consciousness

- Numerous causes of altered level of consciousness
- A useful approach is "**TIPS from the Vowels**"
T	Trauma
I	Infection, inflammatory
P	Poison, psychiatric
S	Shock, stroke, shunt malfunction

A	Alcohol, anoxia, acidosis
E	Epilepsy, endocrine, electrolytes
I	Insulin (hypoglycemia), intussusception, inborn error of metabolism
O	Opiates
U	Urea/metabolic

Table 46.1 Common Causes by Age

INFANT	CHILD	ADOLESCENT
Infection	Toxin	Toxin
Metabolic	Infection	Trauma
Inborn error of metabolism	Seizure	Psychiatric
Seizure	Intussusception	Seizure
Maltreatment	Maltreatment	

Neurologic Findings

Focal Findings

Structural: tumor, abscess, hemorrhage, trauma, hydrocephalus

Medical: seizure, postictal state with Todd's paresis, poisoning

Nonfocal Findings

Structural: cerebral edema, hydrocephalus, hemorrhage, trauma, bilateral subdural hematomas

Medical: hypoxia, hypoglycemia, seizure, electrolyte abnormality, postictal state, DKA, poisoning, meningitis/encephalitis, inborn errors of metabolism, hypothermia, hyperthermia, intussusception, Reye's syndrome

Clinical Assessment

- ABCs, protect cervical spine
- Disability and examination

History

■ Onset, rate of progression, and fluctuation in altered neurological state
■ Associated symptoms particularly headache, seizures, weakness, changes in respiration, fever
■ Past medical history including growth and development
■ Allergies, medications, ingestants (or exposure to toxins)

Physical Examination

■ Vital signs
  • Cushing's triad (indicates increased intracranial pressure): hypertension (with widened systolic-diastolic gap), bradycardia, abnormal respirations
■ Level of consciousness
  • Document accurately and serially
  • Glasgow Coma Score

Table 46.2 Respiratory Pattern: Several Characteristic Patterns	
Hyperventilation	Metabolic acidosis or primary respiratory alkalosis
Hypoventilation	Metabolic alkalosis or respiratory acidosis
Cheyne-Stokes	Dysfunction deep in cerebral hemispheres or diencephalon
	Crescendo-decrescendo pattern
	Hyperpnea regularly alternating with apnea
	Common in metabolic encephalopathy
Central neurogenic hyperventilation	Midbrain dysfunction
	Regular rapid respirations despite normal oxygenation and low $PaCO_2$
	Sustained, regular, deep
Apneustic	Pontine infarction (anoxic encephalopathy or severe meningitis)
	Irregular, sporadic, varying amplitude

Pupillary size and reflexes:
- Invalid if eye-altering medications/ingestions present
- Reaction to light is most important feature to distinguish structural vs metabolic cause
- Metabolic conditions: pupils often constricted and reactive to light
- Structural conditions: depend on primary disorder and secondary effects of increased ICP
- Extraocular movements:

Table 46.3 Pupillary Response Associated with Structural Lesions

PUPILLARY SIZE AND REFLEX	STRUCTURAL LESION
Unilateral fixed dilated pupil	Mass lesion, uncal herniation with third nerve palsy
Fixed dilated pupils	Transtentorial herniation: pupils initially small, may become asymmetric with progressive herniation, then fixed and dilated
Midposition fixed pupils	Midbrain lesion
Pinpoint fixed pupils	Pontine lesion

Conjugate deviation of eyes at rest:
- Cerebral lesion: look toward side of lesion
- Brainstem lesion: look away from side of lesion
- Upper midbrain lesions and hydrocephalus: downward deviation (sunsetting sign)

Oculocephalic reflex (doll's eyes): normal response indicates intact brain stem
- Hold eyes open while head is rotated from side to side: normal response seen with conjugate deviation of eyes opposite to direction of head turning
- Contraindicated if suspected cervical spine injury

Oculovestibular reflex (cold calorics): normal response indicates intact brain stem
- Only indicated if absent doll's eye reflex
- More sensitive than oculocephalic reflex
- Normal response: nystagmus with quick phase *away* from side of stimulation and slow conjugate movement to irrigated side
- "COWS": **C**old **O**pposite **W**arm **S**ame
- Contraindicated if tympanic membrane perforated

■ Motor responses:
Assess muscle tone, strength, and deep tendon reflexes

Decorticate posturing:
- Indicates cerebral cortex and subcortical white matter dysfunction; intact brain stem
- Flexion of upper extremities, extension of lower extremities

Decerebrate posturing:
- Brain stem dysfunction
- Rigid extension of upper and lower extremities

Flaccid:
- No response to painful stimuli: indicates injury deep in brain stem

■ Fundoscopy
- Look for retinal hemorrhages (child abuse) or papilledema (late sign of increased ICP)

Management
■ ABCs and monitors
■ C-spine precautions
■ Intravenous access
■ Rapid bedside glucose
■ CBC, electrolytes, urea, creatinine, glucose, calcium, magnesium, blood gas, INR, PTT, liver function tests, lactate, ammonia

- Blood culture
- Toxicology screen, urinalysis
- ECG, chest X-ray
- CT head
- Consider sickle screen, amino acids, organic acids, LP, ultrasound (rule out intussusception)
- NG tube, Foley catheter
- ±Antibiotics/glucose/other medications (anticonvulsants)

Frequent reevaluation of ABCs and level of consciousness is essential.

References

Berger JR. Clinical approach to stupor and coma. In: Bradley WG, ed. *Neurology in Clinical Practice.* 4th ed. Philadelphia: Butterworth-Heineman; 2004:43–64.

Gausche-Hill M, Fuchs S, Yamamoto L, eds. *American Academy of Pediatrics and American College of Emergency Physicians: APLS The Pediatric Emergency Medicine Resource.* 4th ed. Sudbury, Mass: Jones and Bartlett; 2004:146–181.

Jones R, et al, eds. *Oxford Textbook of Primary Medical Care.* Oxford, England: Oxford University Press; 2004.

Plum F, Posner JB. *The Diagnosis of Stupor and Coma.* 3rd ed. Philadelphia: FA Davis; 1980:1–86.

47 ▪ Seizures and Status Epilepticus

KHALID AL-ANSARI

Introduction

- Seizures are a common presentation to the emergency department
- 4–10% of children have at least one seizure during childhood
- Majority of seizures during childhood are febrile seizures
- Status epilepticus: a seizure or series of seizures lasting for ≥ 30 minutes without return to full consciousness
- 12% of children present with status epilepticus as their first seizure

International Classification of Seizures

Generalized

- Tonic-clonic: most common type in children
- Tonic
- Clonic
- Myoclonic
- Atonic
- Absence

Partial

- Partial simple: no change in level of consciousness
- Partial complex
- Secondarily generalized

Febrile Seizure

- Benign seizures
- Occur in up to 5% of children
- Elevated body temperature lowers threshold for seizures

- Typical age: 6 months to 6 years
- Simple seizures: generalized, duration < 15 minutes, one episode in 24 hrs, developmentally normal child, no residual neurologic deficits
- Usually associated with viral illness
- Child often looks well in emergency department: can be discharged with reassurance and education for future episodes
- Clinical signs of meningitis may be absent in children < 12–18 months of age
- Consider septic workup including lumbar puncture in young child < 1 year, unwell appearance, or complex presentation (prolonged > 15 minutes, focal presentation, > 1 seizure in 24 hrs)
- Recurrence rate 30%
- Risk of epilepsy 2–4%

Afebrile Seizure

- First episode of afebrile seizure: consider workup including sodium, calcium, glucose
- Consider magnesium, ammonia, liver function tests, toxicology as indicated by history and examination
- CT head is rarely required for first afebrile seizure with nonfocal presentation unless prolonged or focal seizure, focal deficits, sick appearance, history of trauma or VP shunt, signs of increased ICP
- Outpatient CT head may be useful for identifying structural anomalies
- EEG should be arranged as an outpatient: usually abnormal in immediate postictal period
- Known seizure disorder: most common reason for recurrent seizures is subtherapeutic levels of anticonvulsants:
  - May be due to inadequate dose, noncompliance, or intercurrent illness
  - Measure anticonvulsant level in blood

Status Epilepticus

- 80% of status epilepticus have a focal onset and then secondarily generalize
- Mortality depends on underlying etiology
- Increased risk of subsequent epilepsy, cognitive neurological deficit, and movement disorders
- Refractory status epilepticus:
  - Sustained seizures that do not respond to medication and persist > 60 minutes
  - Requires ICU admission and continuous EEG monitoring
  - Duration correlates directly with increased mortality

Table 47.1 Etiology by Age		
NEONATES*	CHILDREN	ADOLESCENTS
Hypoxic ischemic encephalopathy	Febrile seizure	Epilepsy
Infection	Infection	Infection
Stroke	Metabolic disturbance	Drugs
Intraventricular hemorrhage	Epilepsy	Trauma
Trauma	Trauma	Tumor
Inborn error of metabolism	Tumor	Stroke
Congenital malformation	Congenital malformation	
Pyridoxine deficiency		

* See Ch. 11, Newborn Emergencies.

Phases

Compensatory Phase (< 30 minutes)

- Increased cerebral blood flow, catecholamine release, cardiac output, glucose concentration in the brain

- Cerebral energy requirements match supply of oxygen and glucose

Decompensation (> 30 minutes)
- Failure of cerebral auto regulation
- Falling cardiac output, blood pressure
- Rhabdomyolysis, hypoxia, acidosis, hypoglycemia

Complications
- Hypoxia
- Lactic acidosis
- Hypoglycemia, hyperkalemia
- Cerebral edema and raised intracranial pressure
- Cerebral venous thrombosis
- Cerebral hemorrhage and infarction
- Respiratory failure, cardiac failure, renal failure
- Hyperpyrexia, rhabdomyolysis, disseminated intravascular coagulation

Investigations
- Immediate Dextrostix®
- CBC and differential, electrolytes, glucose, calcium, magnesium, phosphate, urea, creatinine
- Blood gas
- Antiepileptic drug level if indicated
- Blood and urine cultures as indicated

Consider:
- Lactate, ammonium, liver function tests
- Lumbar puncture
- Quantitative serum amino acids and urine organic acids
- Toxicology screen

Consider CT if:
- Signs and symptoms of elevated intracranial pressure

- Focal seizure or persistent focal deficit
- History of head trauma
- Persistent seizure activity
- Ill-looking patient
- Before LP

Management

- General supportive care
- Stop and control seizure
- Assess cause and treat
- Prevent complications

General Supportive Care

- Position airway
- Suction, clear airway
- Oxygen, advanced airway management as indicated
- Bedside glucose check
- Continuous cardiorespiratory monitoring including BP and oxygen saturation

Treatment Guidelines for Convulsive Status Epilepticus

- Treatment should be started if still seizing after 5 minutes
- Longer seizures are more difficult to terminate
- Children who arrive seizing in the ED are considered to be in status epilepticus
- ICU admission and continuous EEG monitoring if patient:
- Requires assisted ventilation and neuromuscular blockade
- Remains unconscious following termination of seizure activity
- Requires prolonged treatment for refractory status epilepticus

Table 47.2 Emergency Management of Status Epilepticus

TIME FROM SEIZURE ONSET	DRUG	DOSAGE	ADMINISTRATION
5 min	Lorazepam	0.1 mg/kg, max 4 mg	PR/IV
For children under 18 months, consider pyridoxine 100 mg IV			
10 min	Lorazepam	0.1 mg/kg, max 4 mg	PR/IV
15 min	Phenytoin	20 mg/kg, max 1g	IV over 20 min, in normal saline

- Infusion of phenytoin limited by hypotension (1.5%) and arrhythmias (2.0%)
- The order of use of phenytoin and phenobarbital can be interchanged, except in:
  ○ Head injury when phenytoin is first line
  ○ Seizure due to toxic ingestion when phenobarbital is used
- If already on oral phenytoin, consider giving phenobarbital first
- If no IV access, administer rectal diazepam 0.5 mg/kg or midazolam 0.2 mg/kg IM/IN or paraldehyde 0.4 mL (undiluted)/kg, max 10 mL, PR (dilute in olive oil or normal saline)

35 min	Phenobarbital	20 mg/kg, max 1 g	IV over 20 min; if necessary, may be given IV push* over 5 to 10 min by MD only.

Table 47.2 Emergency Management of Status Epilepticus (continued)

If seizure persists > 10 min after administration of phenobarbital, treat as Refractory Status Epilepticus:
- Neurology and ICU consult
- Rapid sequence intubation if needed
- Admission to intensive care unit

45–50 min or on admission to ICU	Midazolam, IV infusion • Bolus 0.15 mg/kg followed by 2 mcg/kg/min infusion If seizure continues: • Increase by 2 mcg/kg/min q 5 min to max 24 mcg/kg/min • Bolus 0.15 mg/kg with increase in infusion as needed
1 hr 45 min	If seizures persist with midazolam, consider thiopental infusion: • Bolus 2–4 mg/kg followed by 2–4 mg/kg/h infusion • Stop midazolam and phenobarbital once infusion started • Maintain phenytoin at therapeutic level • Consider vasopressor support

* *Note:* Ensure airway support available; monitor blood pressure.

Source: With permission from: Kowalczyk A, ed. Status epilepticus guidelines. *The 2005–2006 Formulary of Drugs, The Hospital for Sick Children.* 24th ed. Toronto: The Graphic Centre, HSC; 2005.

References

Gorelick M, Blackwell CD. Neurologic emergencies. In: Fleisher G, Ludwig S, Henretig F, eds. *Textbook of Pediatric Emergency Medicine.* 5th ed. Philadelphia: Lippincott Williams & Wilkins; 2005:759–780.

Nolan M, Trope A, Weiss S, et al. Status epilepticus guidelines. In: Kowalczyk A, ed. *The 2005–2006 Formulary of Drugs, The Hospital for Sick Children.* 24th ed. Toronto: The Graphic Centre, HSC; 2005:292–293.

Reuter D, Brownstein D. Common emergency pediatric neurologic problems. *Emerg Med Clin North Am.* 2002;20(1):155–176.

Sabo-Graham T, Seay AR. Management of status epilepticus in children. *Pediatr Rev.* 1998;19(9):306–310.

Scott RC, Surtees RA, Neville BG. Status epilepticus: pathophysiology, epidemiology, and outcomes. *Arch Dis Child.* 1998;79:73–77.

The Status Epilepticus Working Party. The treatment of convulsive status epilepticus in children. *Arch Dis Child.* 2000;83:415–419.

48 ▪ Ventriculoperitoneal Shunts

ANGELO MIKROGIANAKIS

Introduction

- Hydrocephalus is one of the most common pediatric neurosurgical diseases
- Treated with mechanical shunting
- Shunt malfunctions significantly impact the quality of life of patients with shunted hydrocephalus

Shunts

The shunt apparatus usually consists of three parts:

1. A proximal end that is placed into the ventricle and is radio-opaque; this end has multiple small perforations
2. A valve to allow unidirectional flow: can be adjusted for various opening pressures and usually has a reservoir that allows for checking shunt pressure and sampling CSF
3. A distal end that is placed into the peritoneum or another absorptive surface by tracking the tubing under the skin

Shunt Malfunctions

The median survival of a shunt before it requires revision:

- < 2 years of age: 2 years
- > 2 years of age: 8–10 years

Clinical Presentation of Shunt Malfunction

- Headache, malaise, vomiting
- Cushing's triad: hypertension, bradycardia, irregular respirations
- Bulging fontanel, increased head circumference
- Sixth nerve palsy: horizontal double vision as the affected eye is unable to abduct (turn outward beyond midline)

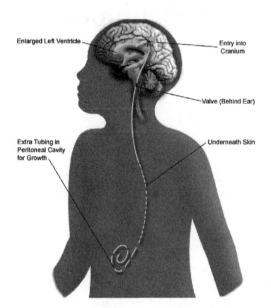

■ **Figure 48.1 Ventriculoperitoneal Shunt Placement**
Source: Used with permission from MCG Health. www.mcghealth.org.

- Changes in gait, mental status alterations
- Increased seizures
- Neck pain
- Change in school performance, personality changes

Obstruction

- The proximal tip may become obstructed with cells, choroid plexus, or debris
- Tubing may become kinked, or distal end may have migrated
- Diagnosis is based on signs and symptoms; confirmed by CT head

Infection

- Infection rates peak during the first few weeks after shunt insertion

- Late infection occurring years after shunt placement is *rare* unless skin is broken over tubing
- Signs and symptoms may be consistent with those of shunt malfunction and include fever, meningeal signs, vomiting, abdominal pain, and peritonitis
- Purulent material around shunt insertion site and redness along shunt tract may be signs of shunt infection
- Organisms are most commonly *Staphylococcus epidermidis* and *Staphylococcus aureus* (less common: Gram-negative organisms)
- Diagnosis is confirmed by positive blood cultures, shunt fluid cultures, and/or lumbar puncture cultures
- CSF > 10 WBC/hpf suggests infection

Tubing Problems
- Disconnection or breakage of the tubing; although less common than occlusion, can also lead to shunt malfunction
- Migration into scrotum, perforation of bowel wall, and intussusception are all rare complications

Investigations
- Shunt series: radiographs to look at tubing integrity
- CT head: check for enlarged ventricles
- Shunt tap: sterile tap of CSF from shunt reservoir; send for cell count, glucose, protein, culture, and sensitivity

Treatment
- Consult neurosurgeon
- Antibiotics including vancomycin and gentamicin
- May require external ventricular drainage and/or removal of shunt

References
Drake JM, Sainte-Rose C. *The Shunt Book.* University of Toronto, Canada: Blackwell Science Inc; 1995.

Iskander BJ et al. Pitfalls in the diagnosis of ventricular shunt dysfunction: radiology reports and ventricular size. *Pediatrics.* 1998;101(6):1031–1036.

Madikians A, Conway EE. Cerebrospinal fluid shunt problems in pediatric patients. *Pediatr Ann.* 1997;26(10):613–620.

PART XII

GYNECOLOGIC
EMERGENCIES

49 ■ Pelvic Inflammatory Disease

ANH DO

Introduction

■ Inflammatory disorders of upper genital tract:
  • Endometritis
  • Salpingitis
  • Oophoritis
  • Tubo-ovarian abscess
  • Pelvic peritonitis
■ Broad spectrum of clinical presentation
■ Highest rate of PID in adolescents 15–19 years

Etiology

■ Gonorrhea
■ Chlamydia
■ Anaerobes
■ Enteric Gram-negative bacilli
■ Mycoplasma
■ Ureaplasma

Risk Factors

■ Young age
■ Multiple sexual partners
■ Sexually transmitted infection (gonorrhea, chlamydia)
■ Nonuse of barrier methods
■ Prior history of pelvic inflammatory disease
■ Intrauterine device
Possible risk factors: douching, low socioeconomic status

Clinical Presentation

- May be asymptomatic to severe
- Symptoms include:
  Malodorous discharge, dyspareunia, irregular vaginal bleeding, dysuria, nausea, vomiting, fever

Exam

- Lower abdominal tenderness, peritoneal signs
- Pelvic exam:
  - Cervical, vaginal discharge
  - Uterine tenderness, adnexal tenderness, cervical motion tenderness

CDC Diagnostic Criteria

- Clinical diagnosis: need to consider in *all* sexually active adolescents with abdominal pain
- Minimal requirements:
  - Uterine or adnexal tenderness (unilateral or bilateral) OR
  - Cervical motion tenderness
- Additional criteria
  - Temperature > 38.3°C
  - Abnormal cervical or vaginal mucopurulent discharge
  - WBC on saline microscopy of vaginal secretions
  - Increased ESR or CRP
  - Positive chlamydia or gonococcus culture

Investigations

- Swabs for gonorrhea and chlamydia
- βHCG
- WBC, ESR, CRP
- Transvaginal ultrasound for tubo-ovarian abscess

Complications

- Recurrent infection

- Chronic pelvic pain
- Ectopic pregnancy
- Infertility: 10% > 1 episode, 50% ≥ 3 episodes

Inpatient Treatment Criteria

- Surgical condition not excluded
- Severe illness
- Tubo-ovarian abscess
- Pregnancy
- Compliance issues or intolerance of outpatient therapy, or no follow-up within 48–72 hrs (most adolescents)
- No response to outpatient treatment

Treatment Regimen

- Cefoxitin 2 g IV q8H *PLUS*
  Doxycycline 100 mg/dose PO/IV q12H
  OR
- Clindamycin 40 mg/kg/d IV divided q8H (max 900 mg/dose)
  PLUS
  Gentamicin 7.5 mg/kg/d IV/IM divided q8H (max 120 mg/dose)
  OR
  Alternative parenteral regimen:
- Levofloxacin 500 mg IV daily *PLUS*
  Metronidazole 500 mg IV q8H
- May stop parenteral therapy 24 hours after clinical improvement
- At discharge, need to complete 14 days of oral therapy with:
  Doxycycline 100 mg PO bid *OR*
  Clindamycin PO 30 mg/kg/d divided tid (max 450 mg/dose)

Outpatient Treatment

1. Levofloxacin 500 mg PO QD × 14 days *OR* Ofloxacin 400 mg PO bid × 14 days +/−

Metronidazole 500 mg PO bid × 14 days
OR

2. Ceftriaxone 250 mg IM × 1 dose *OR*
Cefoxitin 2 g IM × 1 dose with probenecid 1 g po × 1 dose
PLUS
Doxycycline 100 mg PO bid × 14 days WITH or WITHOUT
Metronidazole 500 mg PO bid × 14 days

■ Treat all partners regardless of cultures
■ Follow up in 48–72 hours, 1 week, 2 weeks
■ Do not use doxycycline in children < 8 years

References

2002 CDC Sexually Transmitted Diseases Guidelines. *MMWR.* 2002;51 (RR-6):1–80.

Beigi RH, Wiesenfeld HC. Pelvic inflammatory disease: new diagnostic criteria and treatment. *Obstet Gynecol Clin North Am.* 2003;30(4):777–793.

The Red Book. 2003 Report of the Committee on Infectious Diseases. 26th ed. Illinois: American Academy of Pediatrics:468–472.

Ressel GW. CDC releases 2002 guidelines for treating STDs: Part I. Diseases characterized by vaginal discharge and PID. *Am Fam Physician.* 2002;66(9):1777–1778.

50 ▪ Gynecologic Emergencies

ANH DO

Introduction

- Gynecologic problems are commonly seen in both prepubertal and adolescent age groups
- Speculum examination is contraindicated if no history of sexual intercourse

Developmental Changes by Age

Birth to 8 Weeks: Maternal Estrogen Effect

- Thickened, enlarged labia minora
- Large clitoris
- Vaginal discharge/bleed

8 Weeks to 7 Years

- Labia majora flat, minora thin
- No breasts, no pubic hair

7–10 Years: Premenarchal

- Labia majora filling out, labia minora thickening
- Leukorrhea

Adolescent

- Hormonal effects, adult genitalia

Vaginal Bleeding

History

- Pain, discharge
- Urinary symptoms
- Other sites of bleeding, family history blood dyscrasia

■ Trauma
■ Menarche and sexual history (adolescent)

Exam

■ Look for signs of hormonal stimulation:
  • Breast development, pubic hair, physiologic leukorrhea
■ Pelvic examination:
  • Frog-leg position (on parent's lap)

Differential Diagnosis

Premenarche	Postmenarche
Hormonal effect	Trauma
Neonatal	Tumor
Exogenous estrogen	Dysfunctional urine bleeding
Precocious puberty	Bleeding disorder
Urethral prolapse	Ectopic pregnancy
Vaginitis	Spontaneous abortion
Wart	Birth control pill
Trauma: accidental abuse	STD/PID
Foreign body	
Tumor	

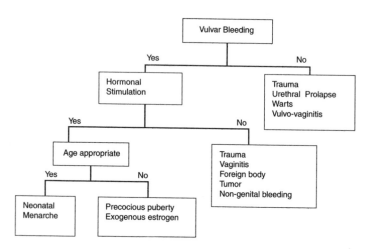

■ **Figure 50.1   Causes of Vaginal Bleeding**

- Inspect for hematoma, mass, active bleed, and foreign body (no speculum unless sexually active)
- Knee-chest position to examine posterior fourchette

Urethral Prolapse

- Protrusion of distal urethral mucosa beyond urethral meatus
- Cause: estrogen deficiency, intra-abdominal pressure, poor attachment of urethral mucosa to underlying smooth muscle
- Typical age 3–5 years
- African-American predominance

Clinical Presentation

- 90% present with painless vaginal bleeding/spotting
- Acute urinary retention
- Dysuria
- Edema of prolapsed tissue
- Vascular congestion: red/purple soft doughnut-shaped mass
- If persistent, necrosis may occur: surgical removal

Treatment

- Sitz baths several times daily
- Topical estrogen cream +/– antibiotics
- Medical treatment successful in up to 70% of cases

Straddle Injury

- Caused by a blow to the perineum due to falling on surface/object with force of one's own body
- Mechanisms of injury: fall from bicycle/furniture/playground equipment, climbing, running into object, water injuries (water skiing, water jets, jet skiing)
- Majority are minor lacerations/abrasions of genitalia, perineal body
- Majority do not require suture repair
- If repair required, consult gynecology

Emergency Assessment
- Rinse with warm water
- Tamponade with pressure: avoid packing vagina in prepubertal girl
- May require sequential assessments
- Frog-leg position, separation, and traction
- Assess hymen

Examination Under Anesthesia

Indications
- Active bleeding
- Penetrating injury even without bleeding (controversial)
- Cannot adequately assess extent of injury

Emergency Management
- Ice packs if actively bleeding
- Analgesia
- Foley catheter if needed

Discharge Instructions

Sitz baths, estrogen cream, reduction of activity for 24 hours

Child Abuse

Suspect if:
- Age < 9 months
- Perianal/hymenal/vaginal injury
- Extensive/severe injury
- Concurrent injury
- Multiple areas of bruising of perineum
- History/exam do not match

Abnormal/Dysfunctional Uterine Bleeding

- No identified cause
- 90% due to anovulation in adolescents
- Generally present with irregular, heavy, prolonged painless bleeding

Menarche

- Mean age: 12.8 years
- Cycle varies in adolescents 21–45 days

Investigations

- CBC, PT/PTT, βHCG, ferritin
- Pelvic ultrasound

Outpatient Workup

- FSH, LH, TSH, prolactin, testosterone, DHEAS, free androgen index, 17-OH progesterone

Management

- Minimal bleed: no hemodynamic compromise, no anemia
  - Reassure, educate, menstrual calendar, iron supplements, ensure follow-up
- Mild–moderate bleed: no hemodynamic compromise, varying degrees of anemia

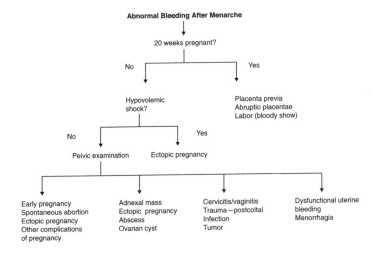

■ **Figure 50.2   Abnormal Bleeding After Menarche**

- Oral contraceptive pill (OCP): 30, 35, or 50 mcg ethinyl estradiol
■ Severe bleed: hemodynamic compromise, severe anemia
  - Admit, consult gynecology
  - IV premarin 25 mg q 6 h, max 4 doses or multidose 50 mcg ethinyl estradiol OCP
  - Blood transfusion if indicated
  - Antiemetic
  - Surgical management required rarely (e.g., D&C)

Vulvovaginitis

■ Present with discharge, pruritus, erythema, dysuria, pain, bleeding
■ Common in prepubertal girls due to combination of factors:
  - Poor hygiene, incorrect wiping technique, tendency to explore body
  - Thin vaginal mucosa and vulvar skin, lack of fat pads and pubic hair, close proximity to rectum
■ May present with erythematous vulvovaginal mucosa, with discharge and itching

Treatment

■ Correct wiping technique
■ Good hygiene
■ Cotton underwear, avoid tight constrictive clothing
■ Avoid irritants such as perfumed bath products or creams
■ Antibiotics only if pathogen identified
■ Reassurance

Acute Pelvic Pain

Differential Diagnosis

■ Ovarian torsion
■ Ruptured ovarian cyst
■ Hemorrhagic ovarian cyst

- Ectopic pregnancy
- Obstructive congenital anomalies
- Pelvic inflammatory disease (see Ch. 49, Pelvic Inflammatory Disease)

Ovarian Torsion

Clinical Presentation

- Abrupt onset of colicky pain
- Lower quadrant pain with radiation to flank or groin
- High incidence of nausea and vomiting
- Often a delay in diagnosis by 2–3 days: need high index of suspicion
- Some patients have intermittent torsion—up to 40%
- May occur in normal ovaries, usually unilateral

Physical Examination

- Palpable mass on abdominal-rectal exam in up to one-third of cases

Investigations

- WBC count may be increased
- Ultrasound: enlarged ovary in almost all cases
- May see complex mass with septation and debris, or cystic mass, or solid mass with peripheral cysts
- Doppler flow not reliable in torsion

Treatment

- Consult gynecology
- Early diagnosis: more likely successful detorsion
- Late diagnosis: may require oophorectomy

Ovarian Cysts

Physiologic Cysts

- Small although size varies with age, often incidental to presenting complaint

- Acute abdominal pain: consider rupture, torsion, hemorrhage, mass effect

Hemorrhagic Cyst

- Usually postmenarchal
- Abrupt onset pain, often midcycle, improves with time
- No fever or leukocytosis, negative βHCG
- If hemoperitoneum: may have peritoneal irritation and/or orthostatic hypotension
- Ultrasound: transvaginal if sexually active
- Conservative treatment

References

Kadir RA, Lee CA. Menorrhagia in adolescents. *Pediatr Ann.* 2001;30(9):541–546.

Paradise JE. Vaginal bleeding. In: Fleisher GR, Ludwig S, Henretig FM, eds. *Textbook of Pediatric Emergency Medicine.* 5th ed. Philadelphia: Lippincott Williams & Wilkins; 2006:669–676.

Rimsza ME. Dysfunctional uterine bleeding. *Pediatr Rev.* 2002;23:227–233.

Schroeder B, Sanfillipo JS. Dysmenorrhea and pelvic pain in adolescents. *Pediatr Clin North Am.* 1999;46(3):555–571.

Sugar NF, Graham EA. Common gynecologic problems in prepubertal girls. *Pediatr Review.* 2006;27:213–223.

■ PART XIII
DERMATOLOGY

51 ▪ Dermatology

ABDULLAH AL-ANAZI AND ELENA POPE

Introduction

Rashes presenting to the emergency department may be classified as follows:

- Morbilliform eruptions (maculopapular)
- Vesiculobullous eruptions
- Pruritic eruptions
- Life-threatening rashes
- Fungal infections
- Petechiae and purpura

Morbilliform Eruptions (Maculopapular Rashes)

Differential Diagnosis

- Viral: measles, rubella, roseola, erythema infectiosum
- Drug eruptions (usually antibiotics, anticonvulsants)
- Bacterial: scarlet fever
- Kawasaki disease
- Rocky Mountain Spotted Fever

Roseola Infantum

- Caused by human herpesvirus 6
- Common age 6 months to 2 years
- Well-looking child despite high fever
- Fever persists for 3–4 days
- Macular or maculopapular rash appears on 3rd–4th day of illness as fever subsides
- May be associated with febrile seizures (25% of cases)
- See Figure 51.1 in color insert

Erythema Infectiosum (Fifth Disease)

- Caused by parvovirus B19
- Common in spring months and school-age children
- Incubation period 6–14 days
- Rash starts on the cheek giving a "slapped cheek" appearance
- Maculopapular rash develops after 24 hours over trunk and extremities
- Rash clears with a lacy pattern
- Complications: transient arthritis, aplastic anemia in children with high bone marrow turnover (sickle cell disease, thalassemia, G6PD deficiency, spherocytosis)
- Pregnancy risk:
  - 50% of women are seropositive before pregnancy
  - Likelihood of transmission if exposed: 30–50%
  - 2–10% rate of fetal loss

Measles (Rubeola)

- Caused by measles virus (paramyxovirus)
- Highly contagious (transmitted by nasal and oral droplets)
- Incubation period: 1–2 weeks
- Contagious 3 days before until 4 days after appearance of rash
- Prodrome: cough, coryza, conjunctivitis, fever, photophobia
- Clinical presentation:
  - Koplik spots (white papules on buccal mucosa) present 2 days before until 2 days after rash appears
  - Morbilliform rash appears behind the ears spreading toward face, trunk, and then extremities
  - Rash fades after 3–7 days; fine desquamation is common with the exception of palms and soles
  - Complications: otitis media, pneumonia, encephalitis, subacute sclerosing panencephalitis
  - See Figure 51.2 in color insert

Rubella

- Generalized maculopapular rash with cervical, postauricular, and occipital lymphadenopathy
- 3–5 days of viral prodrome followed by a pink rash that spreads caudally from head to toes in 24 hours
- Palatal petechiae may be present
- Arthritis 1–2 weeks after the eruption (girls more commonly affected)
- See Figure 51.3 in color insert

Scarlet Fever

- Exotoxin-mediated rash secondary to group A β hemolytic Streptococcus infection of the pharynx, skin, or perianal area
- Generalized pinpoint papular eruption (sandpaper rash)
- Prominent in skin folds: Pastia's lines
- Strawberry tongue with circumoral pallor
- Resolves with desquamation
- Treatment: oral penicillin
- See Figure 51.4 in color insert

Rocky Mountain Spotted Fever

- Caused by *Rickettsia rickettsii*
- Incubation period: 2–10 days
- Clinical features:
  - Fever, headache, myalgias
  - Maculopapular rash erupts on day 3 of illness, may progress to hemorrhagic rash within 24–48 hours
- Treatment: doxycycline or chloramphenicol

Vesicullobullous Eruptions

Chickenpox

- Caused by varicella zoster virus
- Incubation period: 2–3 weeks

- Dual transmission: direct contact and airborne
- Clinical features:
  - Crops of lesions every 3–5 days
  - Starts with papules → vesicles → pustules that resolve with crusting
- Complications: secondary skin infection (particularly invasive GAS), necrotizing fasciitis, pneumonia, encephalitis
- Treatment: supportive
  - Acyclovir for immunocompromised or if significant complication
  - Varicella zoster immune globulin (VZIG) within 72–96 hours from contact for high-risk patients
  - See Figure 51.5 in color insert

Impetigo

- Bullous impetigo (see Figure 51.6 in color insert)
  - Caused by *Staphylococcus aureus*
  - Common in infants
  - Pustules evolving to bullae < 3 cm diameter on an erythematous base
  - Bullae are flaccid; slough and leave crusting
  - Commonly in diaper area or periumbilical
  - Treatment with oral antibiotics
  - Swab orifices
- Nonbullous impetigo:
  - Caused by group A β hemolytic streptococci or *S. aureus*
  - Forms pustules that exudate and dry with characteristic honey-colored crust
  - Treatment for localized, nonextensive: mupirocin 2% ointment
  - If extensive or associated with cellulitis or fever: dicloxacillin, erythromycin, or cephalosporins

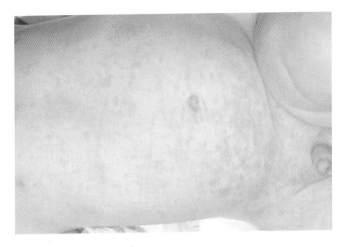

■ Figure 51.1   Roseola

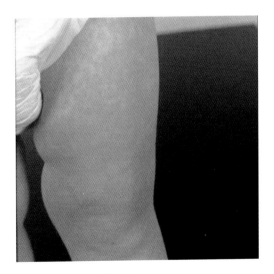

■ Figure 51.2   Measles

Source: Courtesy of Dr. Pope.

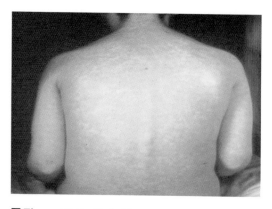

■ **Figure 51.3   Rubella**

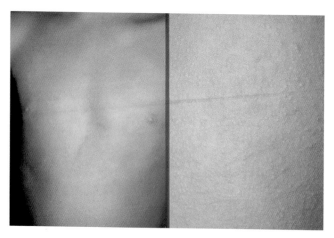

■ **Figure 51.4   Scarlet Fever**

Source: Courtesy of Dr. Pope.

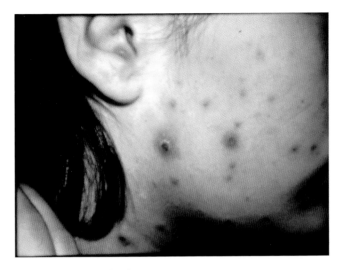

■ **Figure 51.5**   **Chickenpox**

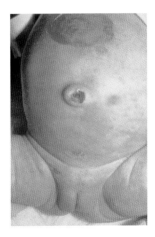

■ **Figure 51.6**   **Bullous Impetigo**

Source: Courtesy of Dr. Pope.

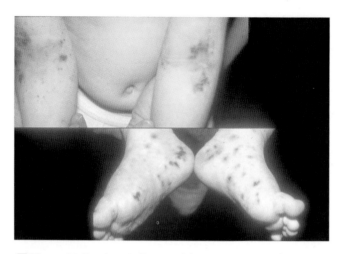

■ **Figure 51.7   Atopic Dermatitis**

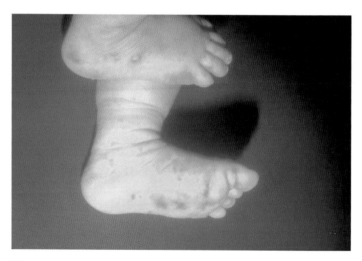

■ **Figure 51.8   Scabies**

Source: Courtesy of Dr. Pope.

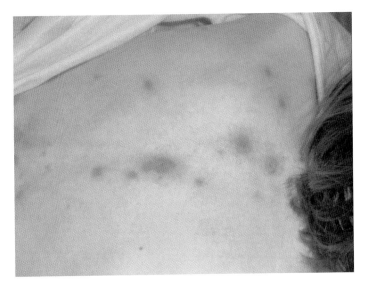

■ **Figure 51.9** **Erythema Multiforme**

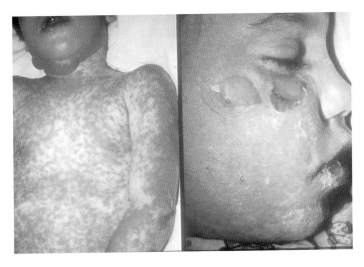

■ **Figure 51.10** **Toxic Epidermal Necrolysis**

Source: Courtesy of Dr. Pope.

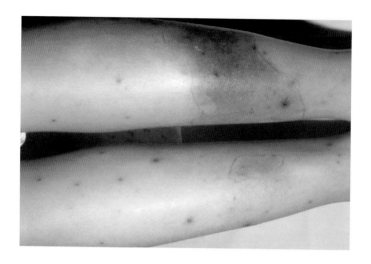

■ Figure 51.11   Necrotizing Fasciitis

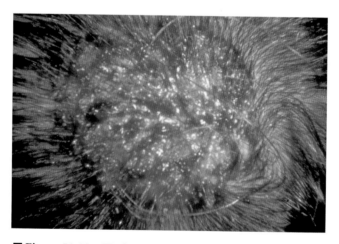

■ Figure 51.12   Kerion

Source: Courtesy of Dr. Pope.

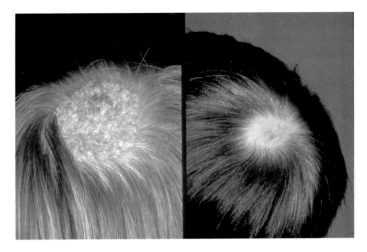

■ **Figure 51.13   Tinea Capitis**

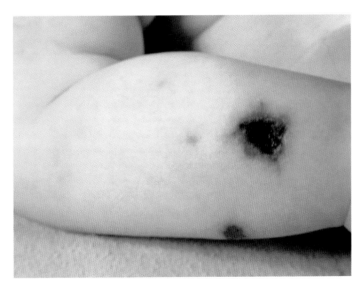

■ **Figure 51.14   Meningococcemia**

Source: Courtesy of Dr. Pope.

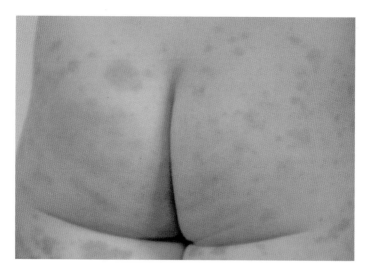

■ **Figure 51.15**   **Henoch-Schonlein Purpura**

Staphylococcal Scalded Skin Syndrome
- Caused by *Staphylococcus aureus* epidermolytic toxin
- Common < 5 years age
- Clinical presentation:
  - Diffuse tender erythema
  - Rapid progression to bullae and sloughing (positive Nikolsky sign)
  - Crusting around mouth and nose
  - Spares mucous membranes, palms, and soles
- Diagnosis:
  - Bullae culture usually sterile
  - *Staphylococcus aureus* may be recovered from orifices
- Treatment:
  - Treat fluid loss and electrolyte imbalance
  - Pain medication
  - IV antibiotics: cefazolin or oxacillin

Pruritic Eruptions
Differential Diagnosis
Acute: urticaria, scabies, insect bites, contact dermatitis
Chronic: atopic dermatitis, dermatitis herpetiformis

Urticaria
- Pruritic, erythematous wheals with pale center
- Transient and migratory (less than 24 hours)
- Self-limited
- Etiology: infectious (mostly viral) and drug
- Treatment: antihistamines

Serum Sickness
- Immune-mediated disease
- Common drugs: penicillin, sulfa, cephalosporin
- Occurs 1–2 weeks after exposure

- Fever, malaise
- Rash commonly urticarial, but also maculopapular or vasculitic
- Arthralgia, arthritis, nephritis, and angioedema
- Management:
  - Stop the predisposing agent
  - Antihistamines
  - Corticosteroids in severe cases

Contact Dermatitis

- Papulovesicular lesions
- Linear distribution
- Severe itching/burning
- Common cause: toxicodendron (Rhus dermatitis, poison ivy), nickel, neomycin, bacitracin, fragrances, latex, topical steroids
- Treatment: discontinue agent, mid to high potency topical corticosteroids (may need systemic steroids for several weeks for severe reactions), antihistamines

Atopic Dermatitis

- Chronic relapsing condition
- Acute manifestations: pruritic, erythematous, edematous rash
- Chronic manifestations: xerosis, lichenification
- Associated with history of atopy in affected children or family
- Diagnosis:
  - Chronic relapsing condition
  - Large areas of red, dry, excoriated, and/or crusted skin and chronic changes (lichenification)
  - Typical distribution: infant—forehead, cheeks, extensor surfaces; older children—flexor surfaces
- Treatment:
  - Environment control: avoid extreme temperatures and dryness
  - Avoid irritants: use mild/no soaps, mild detergents, no bleach or softeners

- Daily or twice daily baths with capful of emulsifier oil followed by emollient application (e.g., Vaseline®)
- Anti-inflammatories: mild corticosteroids for face and skinfolds, mid potency corticosteroids for body; use newer immunomodulators as a second-line treatment
- Antipruritics: hydroxyzine or diphenhydramine
- Complications : impetigo, cellulitis, eczema herpeticum
- See Figure 51.7 in color insert

Scabies

- Caused by a mite of *Sarcoptes scabiei*
- Transmitted by close contact
- Clinical features:
  - Severe itching
  - Papules/nodules in the axilla, wrist, web spaces
  - Infant may have scalp and face involvement or pustules on soles
- Treatment:
  - Treat child and all close contacts with 5% permethrin cream applied to body overnight and washes in the morning; repeat in 1 week
  - Wash clothing and bed linens
  - See Figure 51.8 in color insert

Life-Threatening Rashes

Erythema Multiforme

- Most commonly postinfectious: herpes simplex or *Mycoplasma pneumonia*
- Clinical features:
  - Target lesions: three concentric rings (dusky color or vesicles in the center, ring of pallor in the middle, and an erythematous ring at the edge) on the extremities, palms, and soles

- Evolves and resolves over 1–2 weeks (individual lesions are not migratory as in urticaria)
- 1–2 mucous membrane involvement
■ Treatment: symptomatic; oral steroids helpful for severe mucosal involvement
■ See Figure 51.9 in color insert

Stevens-Johnson Syndrome (SJS)/Toxic Epidermal Necrolysis (TEN)

■ Drug-related: anticonvulsants, sulfa drugs
■ Sick appearance; lesions develop over 1–2 days and progress rapidly
■ Atypical targets (1–2 rings) or flat petechial patches rapidly evolve to blistering
■ Severe mucosal involvement: mouth, conjunctivae, urethra, and vagina
■ < 10% BSA involvement: SJS; >30% BSA: TEN
■ Management:
  - Fluid resuscitation
  - Wound management
  - Ophthalmologic examination
  - IVIG: 3 g/kg/day in 1–2 divided doses over 1–2 days
■ Mortality rate 3–15%
■ See Figure 51.10 in color insert

Necrotizing Fasciitis

■ Deep soft-tissue infection
■ Involves fascia, muscle, skin, and subcutaneous tissue
■ Usually polymicrobial etiology: group A *Strept*, *S. aureus*, and anaerobic organisms
■ 40% of infections are preceded by varicella
■ Clinical features:
  - Febrile, unwell child
  - Rapid progression of erythema, edema

- Pain disproportionate to clinical findings
- Late-stage anesthesia of affected areas
■ Treatment:
  - Consider an emergency
  - Penicillin and clindamycin
  - IVIG
  - Urgent surgical consultation for debridement
  - See Figure 51.11 in color insert

Fungal Infection
Tinea capitis
■ Cause: *Trichophyton tonsurans* (most common)
        Microsporum canis (< 10%)
■ Seen in children 2–10 years of age
■ Five clinical patterns:
  - Diffuse scaling
  - Circular alopecia with scale
  - Kerion: boggy mass with pustules (see Figure 51.12 in color insert)
  - Black dots: alopecia with broken hairs at scalp level
  - Pustular type
■ Diagnosis: hair and scalp scraping for KOH and fungal culture
■ Treatment: Lamisil® (terbinafine) × 4 weeks; warn families about potential liver toxicity
■ See Figure 51.13 in color insert

Petechiae and Purpura
■ Infectious:
  - Meningococcemia (see Figure 51.14 in color insert)
  - Rocky Mountain Spotted Fever
  - *E. coli* sepsis
  - Enteroviruses (echo) and parvovirus

- Thrombocytopenic:
  - ITP
  - Leukemia
  - SLE
- Normal platelets:
  - Henoch-Schonlein Purpura and other vasculitides (see Figure 51.15 in color insert)
  - Coagulation disorder
  - Child abuse

References

Aditya K, et al. Superficial fungal infection. *Clin Dermatol.* 2003:417–425.

Honig PJ. Dermatology. In: Fleisher G, Ludwig S, eds. *Textbook of Pediatric Emergency Medicine.* 4th ed. Philadelphia: Lippincott Williams & Wilkins; 2000:1129–1157.

Sladden MJ, Johnston GA. Common skin infections in children. *BMJ.* 2004;329:95–99.

Strange GR, Ahrens W, Lelyveld S, Schafermeyer R. *Pediatric Emergency Medicine: A Comprehensive Study Guide.* 2nd ed. New York: McGraw-Hill; 2002.

■ PART XIV
ENVIRONMENTAL EMERGENCIES

52 ▪ Submersion Injuries

ADAM CHENG

Introduction

- Drowning: death within 24 hours of a submersion incident
- Near-drowning: survival for at least 24 hours following a submersion incident
- Near-drowning 2–20 times more common than drowning
- > 50% of drowning and near-drowning occur in children < 4 years of age
- Second leading cause of accidental death in children

Risk Factors for Near-Drowning

- Young age, particularly < 4 years
- Child maltreatment and neglect
- Alcohol intoxication: 40–50% of near-drowning associated with alcohol use
- Drug abuse
- Seizure disorder: 4- to 5-fold increased risk
- Cardiac disorder: prior history of arrhythmias
- Risk-taking behavior
- Residential swimming pool: most drownings < age 4
- Close proximity to rivers, lakes, canals, beaches: mostly adolescents

Pathophysiology

- Final common event: hypoxemia
- Dry drowning: water does not enter the lungs due to laryngospasm, but anoxia develops because of persistent laryngospasm

Accidental submersion
↓
Loss of normal breathing pattern
↓
Panic, struggle, breath holding
↓
Laryngospasm in 15% of cases = Dry drowning
Aspiration in 85% of cases = Wet drowning
↓
Hypoxemia

■ **Figure 52.1   Sequence of Events**

- Wet drowning can be divided into two categories, with different pathophysiologic consequences: fresh water and sea water drowning

Fresh Water Near-Drowning
- Hypotonic fresh water dilutes pulmonary surfactant and results in atelectasis and hypoxemia from ventilation-perfusion mismatch and intrapulmonary shunting
- Hyponatremia and hypokalemia occur in 15% of cases: hypotonic fresh water is rapidly reabsorbed into the systemic circulation from alveoli
- Hemolysis and hyperkalemia: large amounts of fresh water are aspirated, leading to hypotonic plasma and RBC hemolysis

Sea Water Near-Drowning
- Pulmonary edema: hypertonic sea water attracts fluid into alveoli
- Hypoxemia from shunting as fluid-filled alveoli continue to be perfused
- Intravascular hypovolemia may occur
- Electrolyte imbalances are uncommon

Table 52.1   Organ Systems Affected in Near-Drowning

Central nervous system	• Cerebral edema, increased intracranial pressure • Hypoxemic encephalopathy: hypothermia may be protective • Cord injury: from hypoxemia
Respiratory	• Decreased pulmonary compliance and increased airway resistance • Noncardiogenic pulmonary edema from damage to alveolar-capillary membrane in both fresh water and sea water aspiration • Gastric aspiration, impaired oxygenation • Infection in grossly contaminated water
Cardiac	• Dysrhythmias, hypovolemia, and hypotension
Metabolic	• Combined metabolic and respiratory acidosis: in 50% of near-drowning victims • Hyponatremia or hypokalemia in freshwater drowning (hyperkalemia in rare cases)
Renal	• Acute tubular necrosis, hemoglobinuria

Management of the Near-Drowning Victim: Prehospital Care

At the Scene

■ Remove from water immediately, Heimlich maneuver NOT indicated
■ Institute CPR
■ Obtain details of incident: submersion time, symptoms, vomiting

During Transport

■ Initiate PALS protocols and cardiorespiratory monitoring
■ Airway management, 100% oxygen

- Protect C-spine: jaw thrust if needed
- IV fluids: normal saline or Ringer's lactate
- Remove wet clothing and initiate rewarming: wrap in blankets

Management of the Near-Drowning Victim: Emergency Care

Airway and Breathing

- Intubate if indicated (e.g., apnea, severe respiratory distress, poor oxygenation, $PaCO_2$ retention, altered mental status, inability to protect airway)
- C-spine stabilization
- 100% oxygen to optimize oxygen saturation
- CPAP/PEEP: improves oxygenation and helps to correct ventilation-perfusion mismatch; may require PEEP 5–15 cm H_2O or greater
- Attempt to maintain normocapnia
- Chest X-ray: may show aspiration, pulmonary edema, atelectasis, pneumothorax, or may be normal (22%)

Circulation

- Cardiorespiratory monitoring
- Aggressive fluid resuscitation may be required for hypovolemia
- Normal saline or Ringer's lactate for fluid resuscitation
- Check bedside glucose
- Glucose-containing solutions not indicated as hyperglycemia is associated with poor neurologic outcome

Disability and Exposure

- Rapid neurologic assessment: AVPU or GCS, pupils
- Continuous reassessment of neurologic status
- Complete exposure and assessment for associated injuries and underlying comorbidity such as child abuse, drug abuse, etc.

Hypothermia

- Remove wet clothing
- Passive external rewarming if temp > 32°C: dry patient, warm blankets or towel
- Active internal rewarming if temp < 32°C: warmed humidified oxygen, warm IV fluids, lavage with warm fluids (gastric, rectal/colonic, bladder)
- Do not terminate resuscitation efforts until unresponsive to CPR and core temperature is > 32°C
- Avoid hyperthermia

Lab Investigations

- Blood gas, electrolytes, glucose, renal function, calcium, magnesium
- CBC, INR, PTT
- Toxicology screen, including alcohols
- 12-lead ECG
- Urinalysis

Adjunctive Therapy

- Bicarbonate: consider correcting severe acidosis (pH < 7.1) as metabolic acidosis will depress cardiac function
- Pulmonary physiotherapy
- Fluid therapy: fluid restriction to 50% maintenance after initial resuscitation
- Diuretic therapy: furosemide 0.5 to 1 mg/kg may improve gas exchange; forced diuresis required if hemoglobinuria present

Controversial Therapies

- Steroids: not indicated
- Antibiotics: not indicated for prophylaxis unless submerged in contaminated water, such as sewage. Therapy for pneumonia should be guided by clinical and radiographic signs: evolving/new infiltrates, leukocytosis, persistent fever, purulent secretions, etc.

- Bronchial lavage with saline: indicated when sand aspiration impairs adequate ventilation (radio-opaque particles seen on chest radiograph)

Disposition

Discharge when patient meets all the following criteria:
- Asymptomatic
- Normal physical examination
- Normal oxygenation by ABG and oxygen saturation
- Normal chest radiograph
- Guaranteed medical follow-up if required
- 6–12 hours of observation completed

Admission if:
- Symptomatic: chest pain, shortness of breath, cough, etc.
- Abnormal physical examination
- Abnormal chest radiograph
- Abnormal oxygenation, or requiring respiratory support
- Tachycardia or dysrhythmia
- Abnormal level of consciousness

Outcome

- Death in 25% of near-drowning victims brought to the emergency department
- 10–33% of near-drowning victims have permanent neurological sequelae

Poor Prognostic Factors

- Prolonged submersion > 25 minutes
- Resuscitation > 25 minutes
- Delay in initiation of CPR
- Severe metabolic acidosis; pH < 7.1
- Pulseless cardiac arrest on arrival in emergency department
- Elevated blood glucose level
- Fixed dilated pupils

- Abnormal initial CT scan of brain
- Glasgow Coma Score < 5

References

Baum CR. Environmental emergencies. In: Fleisher GR, Ludwig S, eds. *Textbook of Pediatric Emergency Medicine.* 4th ed. Philadelphia: Lippincott Williams & Wilkins; 2000:943–947.

Modell JH. Drowning. *N Engl J Med.* 1993;328:253–256.

Weinstein MD, Krieger BP. Near-drowning: epidemiology, pathophysiology, and initial treatment. *J Emerg Med.* 1996;14:461–467.

Zuckerman GB, Conway EE. Drowning and near drowning: a pediatric epidemic. *Pediatr Ann.* 2000;29:360–382.

53 ▪ Burns

ABDULLAH SHAMSAH, SUZAN SCHNEEWEISS, AND
AMINA LALANI

Introduction

- Burn injuries are commonly seen in the emergency department
- Scald injuries are more common in young children
- Older children are more likely to suffer from flame injuries
- Burn severity and depth may not be obvious on initial assessment
- Common to see different depths of injury in a burn; center usually demonstrates deeper burn
- Superficial burns may progress to deeper burns over the first 24 hrs
- Burns are classified as superficial, partial thickness, or full thickness
- Old terminology classified burns as first, second, third, or fourth degree

Table 53.1	Assessment of Burn Severity
Superficial (first degree)	• Erythema, dry, epidermal sloughing, painful • Blanches with pressure • Heal without scarring in 4–5 days • Not included in calculation of total burn surface area (TBSA) • Example: sunburn
Partial thickness (second degree) **1. Superficial partial thickness: < 50% of dermis**	• Red or mottled, epidermal sloughing or blisters, moist, and painful • Healing with minimal scarring in 7–10 days

Table 53.1	Assessment of Burn Severity (continued)
2. Deep partial thickness: > 50% of dermis	• Usually less painful as nerve fibers destroyed • White, pale appearance • Requires 2–3 weeks or more to heal • May be difficult to distinguish from full thickness burn • Scarring is common • Skin grafting is often necessary • Refer to plastic surgeon if burn does not heal within 7–10 days
Full thickness (third degree)	• Involves full dermis • White, leathery, waxy, dry, painless • Does not bleed, no capillary refill • High risk for infection and fluid loss • Cannot re-epithelialize; heals from periphery • Takes several weeks to heal • Refer to plastic surgery immediately • Most require skin grafting
Fourth degree	• Involve underlying fascia, muscle, and bone • Seen with severe electrical burns • Requires immediate plastic surgery consult

First Aid

■ Stop the burn and help dissipate heat
■ Run cool water or use saline-soaked gauze
  • Caution with large burns as risk of hypothermia
  • Avoid ice or submersion of wound in ice water
■ For large burns: cover with clean sheet during initial assessment of patient to provide pain control

Initial Assessment
Airway and Breathing

■ 100% oxygen
■ Look for signs of compromise: singed nasal hairs, eyebrows, or eyelashes; hoarse voice; stridor; carbonaceous sputum; perioral or perinasal burns

- Secure airway with intubation if any of above signs present
- Edema of airway may be delayed up to 48 hrs
- Delay in securing airway until signs of respiratory distress are present can lead to inability to secure airway and dismal outcome
- Do not rely on chest X-ray as it may be normal
- Consider bronchoscopy or laryngoscopy for direct visualization of airway
- Upper airway injury is usually secondary to direct thermal injury; lower airway injury is secondary to chemicals or toxins from smoke inhalation resulting in chemical pneumonitis

Circulation

- Assess location and depth of burn, total body surface area (TBSA), circumferential burns
- Assess TBSA using rule of 9s, or child's palm = 1% TBSA
- Adjust rule of 9s according to patient age

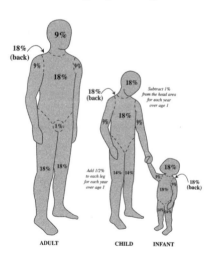

■ Figure 53.1   Body Surface Area Calculation
Source: With permission from: University of Michigan Trauma Burn Center, www.traumaburn.org.

- Start normal saline or Ringer's lactate at 20 cc/kg while assessing burn
- Use Parkland formula if TBSA > 10%:
  4 mL × weight (kg) × % TBSA partial and full thickness burns
  - Give half of volume in first 8 hrs, half in next 16 hrs
  - Add maintenance fluids containing 5% dextrose in children < 5 yrs
- Use warmed fluids for young children
- Vascular access may be difficult: if necessary use intraosseous access or cannulate through burned skin
- Foley catheter to closely monitor urine output

Criteria for Transfer to Burn Center/Admission

- Partial or full thickness burns > 10% TBSA in children < 10 years
- Partial or full thickness burns > 20% TBSA in children > 10 years
- Full thickness burns > 5% TBSA all ages
- Burns involving face, eyes, ears, hands, feet, genitalia, or over major joints
- Electrical burns including lightning injury
- Chemical burns
- Inhalational injury
- Burn injury in patients with preexisting medical condition
- Burn injury associated with major trauma (e.g., fractures)
- Burn injury to patients requiring social, emotional, and/or long-term rehabilitation including suspected child abuse and substance abuse

Management

Superficial Burn

- Moisturizer and acetaminophen/ibuprofen

Partial or Full Thickness Burn

- Clean with lukewarm saline
- Keep patient warm to avoid hypothermia
- Debridement of blisters is controversial
  - Blisters should be debrided if likely to rupture or large size
  - Small blisters may be left intact if they do not interfere with wound care
- Pain control often inadequate: covering burn with clean sheet significantly decreases pain; narcotic analgesia often necessary
- Topical antibiotic ointment for minor burns (e.g., Polysporin® or Bactroban®) plus nonadhesive dressing such as petroleum gauze, followed by dry gauze dressing
- Consult plastic surgery regarding use of other topical creams such as silver sulfadiazine (Flamazine®) or silver nitrate, or other synthetic occlusive dressings (e.g., Biobrane®)
- Dressing change every 2 days for superficial partial thickness; daily dressing changes for deep or full thickness burns
- Hand burns:
  - Dress fingers separately
  - Elevate limb (sling)
  - Volar slab to fingertips until seen by occupational therapy
- Tetanus toxoid: immunize if > 5 yrs since last immunization

Complications

- Wound infection
  - Difficult to differentiate from wound healing as erythema, edema, and tenderness may be present
  - If fever, malaise, or increasing symptoms, consider infection
  - May lead to sepsis and deeper burn damage
  - Requires admission and IV antibiotics
- Sepsis
- Burn shock
- Burn edema
- Escharotomy

- Rhabdomyolysis
- Inhalation injury
- Hypermetabolism

Chemical Burns

Acid Burns

- Coagulation necrosis: limits depth and penetration of burn
- Ingestion leads to gastric injury → strictures

Alkali Burns

- Liquefaction necrosis: deeper penetration, more significant burn
- Ingestion → significant GI injury and perforation, esophageal strictures

Management

- Remove all clothes
- Copious irrigation for minimum of 30 minutes
- Do not neutralize burn: leads to further exothermic reaction and burn injury
- Measure pH 15 minutes after irrigation to assess adequacy of irrigation (alkali substances less water soluble and take longer to neutralize)
- Ingestion: do not induce emesis; activated charcoal is contraindicated
  - Diagnostic endoscopy, followed by ingestion of milk or water

Electrical Burns

- Most injury due to contact with low voltage
- Thermal energy is released in proportion to amount of electrical current that passes through tissue
- Approach is similar to burn but with higher fluid requirement due to deep injury

- If electrical injury occurs to lips and mouth, bleeding from labial artery may occur 1–2 weeks later when eschar separates

See also Ch. 58, Electrical Injuries

Clinical Signs and Symptoms

- Cutaneous: flame burns, flash burns, arc burns, mottled cyanotic skin
- Cardiac effects: cardiac dysrhthymias, myocardial damage
- Musculoskeletal injury: tissue edema and necrosis, compartment syndrome
- Renal failure: hypoxic damage, renal tubular damage secondary to excess myoglobin deposition from extensive muscle damage
- CNS: painful sensation, loss of consciousness, respiratory center paralysis, confusion, motor paralysis, visual disturbances, deafness, sensory deficits, hemiplegia, quadriparesis, seizures, amnesia, disorientation, intracranial bleeds

References

Hettiaratchy S, Dziewulski P. ABC of burns: pathophysiology and types of burns. *BMJ.* 2004;328:1427–1429.

Reed JL, Pomerantz WJ. Emergency management of pediatric burns. *Pediatr Emerg Care.* 2005;21:2, 118–129.

54 ▪ Hyperthermia/ Hypothermia

SANJAY MEHTA

Introduction

- Heatstroke carries risk of significant mortality (14%), even with adequate treatment
- Hypothermia may require prolonged resuscitation to allow adequate rewarming

Heat-Related Illnesses

Hyperthermia vs fever
- Fever: elevation in hypothalamic set point
- Hyperthermia: thermoregulatory dysfunction

Thermoregulation
- Normal body temperature is 36.0–37.5°C

Hyperthermia

Predisposing Factors
- Age: infants and elderly
- Reactions (malignant hyperthermia), medications (anticholinergics, diuretics, β-blockers, Ca channel blockers), and drugs (alcohol, heroin, cocaine, amphetamines)
- Fever and infection
- Obesity, dehydration, skin abnormalities, cystic fibrosis
- Lack of acclimatization, fatigue, clothing
- Previous episode of heatstroke
- Metabolic disorders (hyperthyroidism, pheochromocytoma)

Differential Diagnosis
- Heat exhaustion
- Heatstroke

425

- Heat syncope
- Dehydration
- Cardiac syncope
- Ingestion

Minor Heat Illnesses

- Heat edema: cutaneous vasodilatation
- Heat cramps: severe cramps of heavily exercised muscles
  - Usually calves, arms, shoulders, and abdominals after exertion
- Heat syncope: syncopal episode during heat exposure in unacclimatized patient

Major Heat Illnesses

- Heat exhaustion: precursor to heatstroke
  Temperature regulatory mechanisms intact
- Heatstroke: life-threatening emergency
  Loss of thermoregulatory mechanism

Heatstroke

Exertional Heatstroke (e.g., Unacclimatized Athlete)

- Rapid onset
- Severe prostration
- Sweating intact

Classic/Nonexertional Heatstroke (e.g., Secondary to Confinement)

- More common in infants
- Slower onset
- Marked dehydration
- Sweating may be absent

Management of Heatstroke

- Give supportive care (e.g., oxygen) and cardiorespiratory monitoring
- Cooling measures
  - Ice packs to axillae and groin

Table 54.1 Heat Exhaustion versus Heatstroke

HEAT EXHAUSTION	HEATSTROKE
• T < 39.0°C	• T > 39.0°C
• Sweating	• Anhydrosis, dehydration
• Headache	• Headache
• Nausea/vomiting	• Nausea/vomiting
• Tachycardia	• Syncope/ataxia
• Intact mental status	• Mental status change or coma
	• Seizures

- Cool water spray and fan
- Antipyretics
- Fluid resuscitation 20 mL/kg NS or RL
  - Consider dobutamine (myocardial contractility and vasodilatation)
  - Consider internal cooling (gastric/rectal/bladder/peritoneal lavage)
- Investigations
  - Bedside glucose
  - CBC, electrolytes, Ca, PO_4, Mg, renal and liver function, coagulation studies, CPK, arterial blood gas
  - Urinalysis (i.e., myoglobin)
  - ECG
- Admit to monitored setting
  - Stop cooling when core temperature < 38.5–39.0°C

Prevention of Heatstroke
- Avoid exertion during warmest daytime hours
- Thin and light-colored clothing and frequent breaks
- Adequate intake of electrolyte solutions
- Avoid salt supplements

Cold-Related Illnesses

Hypothermia

- Core temperature < 34°C
- Classification: mild, moderate, or severe

Predisposing Factors

- Endocrine or metabolic derangements, hypoglycemia, hypothyroidism
- Infection: meningitis, sepsis
- Intoxication: alcohol, opiates
- Intracranial pathology
- Environmental exposure/submersion injury: water conducts heat 25 × faster than air
- Dermatologic: burns
- Iatrogenic

Management

- ABCs and cervical spine stabilization if indicated
  - Consider early ventilation with PEEP 5–10 cm H_2O to prevent acute respiratory distress syndrome
- IV: fluid resuscitate while rewarming to prevent cardiovascular collapse: "rewarming shock"
- Give initial bolus of 20 cc/kg NS
- Assess rectal temperature and remove wet clothing
- Bedside glucose and baseline bloodwork, blood gas, CXR, consider toxicology screen
- Begin rewarming: see below
- Goal: raise temperature by 1–2°C per hour
- Caution with rapid rewarming: may result in overshooting desired temperature
- Sinus bradycardia may occur with hypothermia: usually sufficient to maintain oxygenation and does not require pacing

Table 54.2   Classification of Hypothermia

MILD HYPOTHERMIA	MODERATE HYPOTHERMIA	SEVERE HYPOTHERMIA
• > 34°C	• 30–34°C	• < 30°C
• Shivering preserved	• Muscle rigidity	• "Appear dead," coma
• Tachycardia	• Cold diuresis	• Dilated unresponsive pupils
• Peripheral vasoconstriction	• Progressive loss of consciousness to coma	• Respiratory arrest and ventricular fibrillation
• Ataxia, slurred speech, inappropriate judgment, or mental slowing	• Difficult to detect vital signs	• Active rewarming to 30°C: lavage gives 3°C, while ECMO gives 9°C/hour
• Treat with passive rewarming	• ECG: J or Osbourne waves in inferolateral leads	
• Warm blankets	• Myocardium resistant to defibrillation and medications < 30°C	

- ■ "Not dead until warm and dead": continue CPR and active rewarming until temperature > 32°C for at least 30 minutes
- ■ Use clinical judgment in decision to terminate efforts as difficult to differentiate primary from secondary hypothermia
- ■ Admit moderate to severe hypothermic patients to intensive care unit

Warming Techniques

Mild Hypothermia

- ■ Passive rewarming: warm blankets, warm environment

Moderate Hypothermia

- ■ Active external rewarming: no invasive devices
- ■ Warm blankets, warm environment, warm IV fluids, warm forced air (e.g., Bair Hugger®), radiant heater

Severe Hypothermia

- Active external AND internal rewarming
- Core rewarming should precede external rewarming due to risk of vasodilation and "paradoxical undressing"
- Internal rewarming techniques:
  - Intubation and warmed humidified air to 44°C
  - Warmed IV fluids to 40–42°C via fluid rewarmer
  - Gastric lavage with NG tube or rectal lavage with enema tube and warmed saline
  - Peritoneal lavage with warmed saline
  - Bladder lavage via Foley catheter
- Consider ECMO
- Risk of afterdrop once rewarming has begun: cooler blood in extremities circulates to core
- Recent studies indicate that forced air rewarming is effective in some patients, even those with severe hypothermia

Cardiac Arrest

- Hypothermic heart may not respond to cardiac medications or defibrillation
- Repeated doses of vasoactive medications may lead to toxic accumulation
- If cardiac arrest, start CPR and active internal rewarming
- Passive or external rewarming is *not* adequate

Moderate Hypothermia

- Defibrillate once, continue CPR, give IV medications at longer intervals, and provide active internal rewarming

Severe Hypothermia

- Defibrillate once, continue CPR, *withhold* medications and further defibrillation until temp > 30°C
- May require prolonged rewarming

References

Barrow MW, Clark KA. Heat-related illnesses. *Am Fam Physican.* 1998;58(3):749.

Fleisher GR, Ludwig S, eds. *Textbook of Pediatric Emergency Medicine.* 4th ed. Philadelphia: Lippincott Williams & Wilkins; 2000.

Gausche-Hill M, Fuchs S, Yamamoto L, eds. *APLS: The Pediatric Emergency Medicine Resource.* 4th ed. Sudbury, Mass: Jones and Bartlett; 2004.

Giesbrecht GG. Emergency treatment of hypothermia. *Emerg Med Australasia.* 2001;13(1):5–6.

Glazer JL. Management of heatstroke and heat exhaustion. *Am Fam Physican.* 2005;71(11):2133–2140.

O'Neill KA, et al. The effects of core and peripheral warming methods on temperature and physiologic variables in injured children. *Pediatr Emerg Care.* 2001;17(2):138–142.

2005 American Heart Association guidelines for cardiopulmonary resuscitation and emergency cardiovascular care. Part 10.4: hypothermia. *Circ.* 2005;112:IV 136–IV 138.

Wexler RK. Evaluation and treatment of heat-related illnesses. *Am Fam Physican.* 2002;65(11):2307–2314.

55 ▪ Toxicology Part 1: Approach to Ingestions

SHAUNA JAIN

Introduction

- Young children are at risk for accidental poisonings
- Adolescents have higher morbidity and mortality because large amounts ingested and maybe multiple ingestants particularly in suicide attempts

Table 55.1   Epidemiology

Children < 6 years ingest substances in small quantities. Most commonly ingest:	Children > 6 years ingest toxins commonly involved in fatalities:
• Cleaning products	• Analgesics
• Analgesics (acetaminophen most common)	• Antidepressants
• Personal care products/cosmetics	• Cleaning products
• Cough and cold preparations	• Hydrocarbons and pesticides
• Plants	• Minerals (iron most common fatal ingestion)
• Topical agents	
• Pesticides, hydrocarbons	

- Acetaminophen is the most common ingestion
- Tricyclic antidepressants are the most common *fatal* ingestion

Toxins associated with adolescent fatalities:

- Analgesics
- Antidepressants
- Sedatives, hypnotics, psychotics
- Street drugs (especially stimulants)
- Cardiac medications
- Toxic alcohols

432

Approach to a Toxic Ingestion

■ ABCDs of toxicology:
  • Stabilize: Airway, Breathing, Circulation, Disability/dextrose
  • Consider: Decontamination/elimination/antidote
■ Complete history including amount and timing of ingestion, possibility of co-ingestants and significant past medical history
■ Key physical exam findings: vitals and evidence of toxidrome (level of consciousness, pupils, skin, bowel/bladder abnormalities)
■ Key laboratory tests: glucose, electrolytes, anion gap, osmolar gap, CBC, ECG, U/A, toxicology screen, drug level
■ Call poison control, consult Poisindex® or toxicologist for advice

The Toxicologic Exam

Toxidromes

■ May not be helpful in the face of multiple ingestions
■ All signs and symptoms may not be present in every toxidrome
■ Considerable overlap of all toxidromes

Table 55.2 Toxidromes	
Sympathomimetics	• Fight or flight response • Hypertension, tachycardia, tachypnea, hyperthermia, diaphoresis, mydriasis, altered mental status • Risks: rhabdomyolysis, myocardial infarction, stroke • Management: benzodiazepines, cooling • Toxins: cocaine, PCP, XTC, amphetamines

(continues)

Table 55.2   Toxidromes (continued)

Anticholinergics	• Similar to sympathomimetic toxidrome except skin is dry • Tachycardia, hyperthermia, dry, hot flushed skin, mydriasis, altered mental status, urine and stool retention • Hot as a hare, dry as a bone, red as a beet, blind as a bat, mad as a hatter, plugged as a pig • Risks: arrhythmias, seizures, rhabdomyolysis • Toxins: TCA, jimsonweed, antihistamines, phenothiazines • Treatment: $NaHCO_3$ for TCA

Cholinergics	• Secretions from all sites
	• Clinical findings include: **SLUDGE**
	    Salivation, small pupils, Lacrimation, Urination, Diarrhea, diaphoresis, GI cramps, Emesis
	    And the **B**'s: Bradycardia, Bronchorrhea, Bronchoconstriction
	• Toxin: organophosphate
	• Management:
	    ◦ Protective clothing
	    ◦ Decontaminate patient
	    ◦ Supportive treatment
	    ◦ Atropine, pralidoxime

Opioids	• Depression of pulse, blood pressure, respiratory drive, miosis • Cause of death is respiratory arrest, risk of pulmonary edema • Treatment: naloxone, supportive care • Toxins: morphine, codeine
Sedatives	• Depression of blood pressure, pulse, respiratory rate • Benzodiazepine clinical picture is of depressed mental status with normal vital signs • Treatment: supportive, flumazenil in some benzodiazepine cases but increased risk of seizures; contraindicated in multidrug ingestion

Table 55.3 Clues to the Toxins

Pupils and toxins	Miosis 　　Cholinergics, clonidine 　　Opiates, organophosphates 　　Phenothiazines, pilocarpine 　　Sedative-hypnotics Mydriasis 　　Antihistamines 　　Anticholinergics 　　Antidepressants 　　Sympathomimetics
Skin findings and toxins	Diaphoresis (**SOAP**) 　　**S**ympathomimetics 　　**O**rganophosphates 　　**A**SA 　　**P**CP Red skin: carbon monoxide Blue skin: methemoglobinemia
Bradycardia/ hypotension and toxins	Antihypertensives: 　　ß-blockers and Ca channel blockers 　　Digoxin, narcotics
Seizures and toxins	(**OTIS CAMPBELL**) **O**rganophosphates **T**ricyclic antidepressants **I**soniazid **S**ympathomimetics **C**amphor **A**mphetamines **M**ethylxanthines **P**CP, phenol, propanolol **B**enzodiazepine withdrawal **E**thanol withdrawal **L**ithium **L**idocaine, lead, lindane

Decontamination Methods

Ipecac

- Limited use as must be given immediately post ingestion
- Contraindicated in ingestion of hydrocarbons, caustics, absent gag reflex

Gastric Lavage

- Efficacy is variable and difficult to remove large pill fragments
- For maximum effectiveness should be within 1 hour ingestion
- Best suited for intubated patients with life-threatening ingestion

Whole Bowel Irrigation

- Best for toxins not adsorbed by charcoal, sustained release toxins, street drug packers and stuffers (e.g., cocaine)
- Contraindicated if ileus or obstruction

Activated Charcoal (AC)

- Adsorbs most toxic ingestions
- Little adsorption for **PHAILS**:
  Pesticides, **H**ydrocarbons, **A**cids, alkali, alcohols, **I**ron, **L**ithium, **S**olvents
- Dose is 10:1 charcoal:drug or children 1 g/kg, adults 50–100 g
- Multiple dose AC useful for phenobarbitol, phenytoin, carbamazepine, theophylline, ASA, valproic acid, TCA, digoxin, dapsone, sustained-release medications
- Do not use if absent airway reflexes
- Cathartics with AC have no proven efficacy and should not be used more than once

Elimination

Urinary Alkalinization

- Urine pH 7–8 traps toxic ions for elimination
- Maintain normokalemia and serum pH < 7.55 to facilitate elimination
- Use for ASA, phenobarbital, formate, MTX

Hemodialysis and Hemoperfusion

- Use when evidence of end organ toxicity or certain toxic drug levels
- Hemodialysis used for methanol, ethylene glycol, lithium, ASA
- Hemoperfusion used for theophylline
- Forced diuresis, cholestyramine, and continuous arterial-venous hemofiltration dialysis have limited use

Table 55.4 Antidotes

Toxin	Antidote
Opioid	Naloxone
Cholinergic	Atropine, physostigmine
Ethylene glycol	Fomepizole
Acetaminophen	N-acetylcysteine
β-blocker	Glucagon
INH	Pyridoxine
Sulfonylureas	Octreotide
Cyanide	Sodium nitrite, sodium thiosulfate
Benzodiazepines	Flumazenil
Iron	Deferoxamine
CO	Oxygen
Warfarin	Vitamin K
Digoxin	Fab fragments
Methemoglobinemia	Methylene blue
TCA	$NaHCO_3$

Investigations

Anion Gap

Anion gap = $Na - (Cl + HCO_3)$, normal gap is 12 +/− 4

Elevated anion gap found in: **MUDPILES**

Methanol, **U**remia, **D**KA, **P**araldehyde, phenformin/metformin, **I**ron, isopropanol, INH, **L**actic acid (CO, cyanide, sepsis), **E**thanol/ethylene glycol, **S**alicylates, solvent (toluene)

- If metabolic acidosis with elevated anion gap:
  - Determine if urine ketones present
  - If acidosis and ketones present, consider DKA or salicylate poisoning
- Check for uremia and lactic acid levels
  - If no ketones and no lactic acid, calculate osmol gap and consider toxic alcohols

Note: A decreased anion gap is found in poisoning by bromide, iodine, and lithium

Osmol Gap

Osmol Gap = measured osmolality – calculated osmolality

Osmolality = $(2 \times Na)$ + glucose + urea

(normal osmolality = < 10)

- Causes of an elevated osmol gap:
- Ethanol, methanol, ethylene glycol, isopropanol
- Acetone, mannitol, renal failure, lactic acid, paraldehyde

Note: A normal osmol gap does not exclude a toxic ingestion

Toxicology Screen

- Does not affect immediate management as not immediately available
- Toxins screened vary between institutions
- Serum levels of certain drugs are useful because they will affect outcome and treatment:
  - ASA, acetaminophen
  - Ethylene glycol, methanol
  - Carbon monoxide, methemoglobin
  - Iron, lithium

Abdominal X-ray

- Mainly used in iron ingestions due to high toxicity
- Other medications seen on X-ray but limited use in these ingestions (**CHIPS**):
  Chloral hydrate, **H**eavy metals, **I**ron, **P**henytoin, **S**low-release medications

ECG

- Important to rule out abnormalities such as arrhythmia or widened QRS (e.g., TCAs)

Table 55.5 Single Pill or Sip Toxicity

TOXIN	EFFECT
Antihistamines	Seizures
Methylsalicylate oil	Pulmonary and cerebral edema
Atropine	Apnea
Benzocaine	Methemoglobinemia
Camphor	Seizures
Clonidine	Hypotension, bradycardia
Ethylene glycol	Renal failure
MAO inhibitors	Autonomic instability
Methanol	Blindness
Opioids	Apnea
Sulfonylureas	Hypoglycemia
Tricyclic antidepressants	Seizures, arrhythmias
Sustained-release or long-acting meds (α or Ca channel blocker)	Hypotension

References

Erikson TB. Toxicology: ingestions and smoke inhalation. In: Gausche-Hill M, Fuchs S, Yamamoto L, eds. *American Academy of Pediatrics and American College of Emergency Physicians: APLS The Pediatric Emergency Medicine Resource.* 4th ed. Sudbury, Mass: Jones and Bartlett; 2004: 235–262.

Nelson L, Hoffman R, Howland MA, et al. New York City Poison Control Center and Bellevue Hospital Center and Metropolitan College and St. John's University: An Intensive Review Course in Clinical Toxicology (syllabus). New York: March 13–14, 2003.

Osterhoudt KC, Shannon M, Henretig FM. Toxicologic Emergencies. In: Fleisher GR, Ludwig S, et al, eds. *Textbook of Pediatric Emergency Medicine.* 4th ed. Philadelphia: Lippincott Williams & Wilkins; 2000:887–942.

56 ▪ Toxicology Part 2: Specific Toxins

Introduction

- Acetaminophen is the most common toxic ingestion seen in the emergency department
- Tricyclic antidepressants are the most common *fatal* ingestion in children

Acetaminophen

- Acetaminophen is metabolized by the liver; 5% is metabolized by cytochrome P450 to a toxic metabolite, N-actyl-para-benzoquinoneimine (NAPQI), which is reduced by glutathione to a nontoxic metabolite
- In an overdose, glutathione stores are depleted and NAPQI causes liver toxicity
- N-acetylcysteine (NAC) is given to eliminate NAPQI directly and indirectly by increasing glutathione levels

Clinical Presentation

1–24 hours:	Nausea, vomiting, anorexia
24–48 hours:	RUQ pain, elevated liver enzymes and functions
48–96 hours:	Peak hepatotoxicity, renal insufficiency, cerebral edema, coma, acidosis
4–14 days:	Resolution of symptoms

Evaluating Patients for Acetaminophen Toxicity

Acute Ingestion

- Toxic dose: > 150 mg/kg acetaminophen

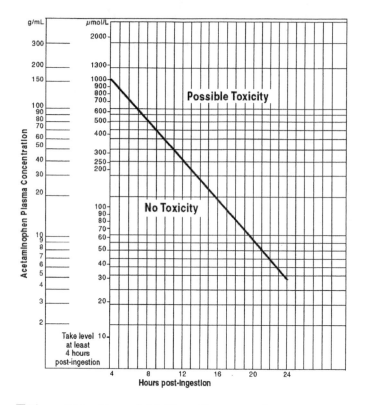

■ **Figure 56.1   Rumack-Matthew Nomogram for
Acetaminophen Toxicity**
Source: With permission from: Rumack-Matthew. Modified from:
Rumack BH, Matthew H. *Pediatrics* 55, page 871 copyright 1975.

- Measure serum level at 4 hours and evaluate on Rumack-
  Matthew nomogram
- If patient presents 6–8 hours post ingestion, give NAC loading
  dose while waiting for level and continue NAC if
  acetaminophen level is toxic on nomogram

Chronic Ingestion

- Toxic dose: > 120 mg/kg/day acetaminophen
- If a patient presents late and has detectable acetaminophen levels or elevated liver enzymes, consider to be at risk for a toxic ingestion

Treatment

- Charcoal is given if the patient presents within 4 hours of ingestion and no contraindications
- N-acetylcysteine (NAC) IV is given for a toxic ingestion:
  - Significant benefit of NAC even > 24 hours post toxic ingestion
  - Risk of anaphylactoid reaction, likely dependent on IV infusion rate
  - Two protocols available: 20- and 48-hour protocols
  - Oral NAC is available and has less risk of an allergic reaction
- Supportive therapy

Salicylates

- Salicylate toxicity results in uncoupling of oxidative phosphorylation and disruption of the Krebs cycle; decreases ATP production
- Result is glycogenolysis, lipolysis, and anaerobic metabolism leading to hyperglycemia and *metabolic acidosis*
- Respiratory alkalosis results from salicylates stimulating medulla to increase respiratory drive
- Salicylate toxicity presents as a respiratory alkalosis with metabolic acidosis and initial hyperglycemia, then hypoglycemia

Clinical Presentation

- Mild toxicity (150–300 mg/kg salicylates): vomiting, gastritis, tinnitus, tachypnea

- Moderate toxicity (300–500 mg/kg salicylates): hyperthermia, diaphoresis, renal and liver dysfunction
- Severe toxicity (> 500 mg/kg salicylates): coma, seizures, pulmonary edema

Evaluation

- Toxic salicylate dose: 150 mg/kg
- Done nomogram has limited use due to variable absorption rates of salicylates: should not be used as a marker of toxicity
- Presents as a respiratory alkalosis with anion gap metabolic acidosis and hyperglycemia followed by hypoglycemia
- Treatment is based on evidence of clinical and/or laboratory toxicity or an absolute salicylate level > 40 mg/dL

Management

- Charcoal: within 4 hours of ingestion, consider multiple-dose charcoal since salicylates delay gastric emptying and form bezoars
- Fluid resuscitation
- Urinary alkalinization with $NaHCO_3$ to a pH of 7.8–8.0 will enhance ASA elimination
- Maintain normokalemia to promote urine alkalinization
- Hemodialysis if:
  - End organ salicylate toxicity (severe acidosis, renal failure, pulmonary edema)
  - Deterioration despite alkalinizing urine
  - Serum level >100 mg/dL acute ingestion

Tricyclic Antidepressants (TCAs)

- Multiple pharmacological effects in overdose:
  - Anticholinergic effects: toxidrome
  - Sodium channel blockade: dysrhythmias
  - α-Adrenergic receptor blockade: vasodilation
  - Antihistamine effects: sedation
  - GABA antagonism: seizures

■ Anticholinergic toxidrome
  • Mad as a hatter: altered mental status
  • Hot as a hare: tachycardia, hyperthermia
  • Dry as a bone: dry skin and secretions
  • Red as a beet: hot flushed skin
  • Blind as a bat: mydriasis
  • Plugged as a pig: urine and stool retention
■ Danger: seizures, coma, arrhythmias

Evaluation: ECG

■ Key to diagnosing toxicity
■ QRS prolongation (limb leads):
  • > 100 msec: 33% risk of seizures
  • > 160 msec: 50% risk of ventricular arrhythmias
  • Treatment indicated for QRS > 100 msec
■ Right axis deviation:
  • avR: terminal 40 msec RAD, R wave > 3 mm
  • RAD may be normal in children
■ QT prolongation
■ Sinus tachycardia
■ If normal rate, QT, QRS, and axis: negative predictive value for cardiac toxicity = 100%

Treatment

■ Decontamination if protected airway (intubated or awake):
  • Gastric lavage within 1 hour
  • Activated charcoal within 4 hours (consider multi-dose)
■ Sodium bicarbonate
  • Bolus if QRS > 100 msec
  • Maintain serum pH 7.45–7.55
■ Fluids and norepinephrine for hypotension
■ No role for physostigmine
■ May be medically cleared if observed for 6 hours, no clinical toxicity signs and normal ECG

Toxic Alcohols

- Most common: methanol, ethylene glycol, isopropanol
- Toxic alcohol ingestions present as a delayed anion gap metabolic acidosis
- May have an elevated osmol gap, but a normal osmol gap does not rule out alcohol toxicity
- Patients present as if "drunk"

Methanol

- Sources: gasoline, antifreeze, windshield washer fluid, paint, varnish remover
- Toxicity from metabolite—formic acid
- Retinal toxicity: ask about visual changes

Ethylene Glycol

- Sources: car coolant and antifreeze, solvents, deicers
- Toxicity from metabolite—oxalic acid
- Renal toxicity: from calcium oxalate precipitates

Toxic Alcohol Management

- Little role for decontamination: no role for charcoal; gastric lavage must be within 30 minutes of ingestion
- Determine toxic alcohol and ethanol levels
- Sodium bicarbonate for serum alkalinization to help eliminate toxic metabolites
- Ethanol and fomepizole block metabolism of methanol/ethylene glycol to toxic metabolites
  - Ethanol is difficult to titrate and there are risks associated with CNS sedation
  - Fomepizole is preferred although more expensive
- Indications for hemodialysis: evidence of end organ toxicity and absolute levels of methanol or ethylene glycol > 25 mg/dL
- Vitamins help eliminate toxic metabolites:
  - Methanol: folate
  - Ethylene glycol: thiamine and pyridoxine

Iron

- Common fatal overdose in children as readily available and looks like candy
  - Mild–moderate ingestion: 20–60 mg/kg
  - Severe ingestion: > 60 mg/kg
- History of vomiting > 4 times suggests serious ingestion

Clinical Stages

1–6 hours:	Vomiting, diarrhea, abdominal pain
6–24 hours:	Latent stage, patient asymptomatic
> 24 hours:	Hepatocellular dysfunction, myocardial depression, hypotension, metabolic acidosis, altered mental status, seizures
4–6 days:	Pyloric outlet obstruction from scarring

Diagnosis

- Serum iron levels within 4–6 hours ingestion may be helpful
- Iron seen on abdominal radiograph implies a significant ingestion, but nonvisualization does not rule out toxicity
- May see leukocytosis and hyperglycemia

Management

- Decontamination with gastric lavage if present within 1 hour ingestion; otherwise whole bowel irrigation is preferable
- Supportive therapy, particularly fluid resuscitation
- Discharge if asymptomatic at 6 hours post ingestion, normal radiograph, and serum level < 350 mcg/dL

Indications for Deferoxamine (IV)

- Signs of clinical toxicity, acidosis
- Iron visible on abdominal X-ray
- Elemental iron level > 20 mg/kg
- Serum iron level > 500 mcg/dL
  Deferoxamine challenge test: urine color changes to *vin rose* after dose of IM deferoxamine

References

Erikson TB. Toxicology: ingestions and smoke inhalation. In: Gausche-Hill M, Fuchs S, Yamamoto L, eds. *American Academy of Pediatrics and American College of Emergency Physicians: APLS The Pediatric Emergency Medicine Resource.* 4th ed. Sudbury, Mass: Jones and Bartlett; 2004:235–262.

Nelson L, Hoffman R, Howland MA, et al. New York City Poison Control Center and Bellevue Hospital Center and Metropolitan College and St. John's University: An Intensive Review Course in Clinical Toxicology (syllabus). New York: March 13–14, 2003.

Osterhoudt KC, Shannon M, Henretig FM. Toxicologic emergencies. In: Fleisher G, Ludwig S, eds. *Textbook of Pediatric Emergency Medicine.* 4th ed. Philadelphia: Lippincott Williams & Wilkins; 2000:887–942.

57 ▪ Street Drugs

Introduction

- Use of street drugs may not be reported, may be denied, or underestimated
- Reported drugs may have been adulterated, substituted, or combined with other drugs

Initial Management

- Assess airway, breathing, and circulation
- Assess vital signs
- Supportive treatment and resuscitation as necessary
- Consider DONT antidotes: Dextrose, Oxygen, Naloxone, Thiamine
- Consider decontamination if indicated: activated charcoal, whole bowel irrigation
- Consider other diagnoses
- Look for toxidromes

Sympathomimetic Ingestion

- Toxidrome: tachycardia, hypertension, hyperthermia, mydriasis, diaphoresis, increased bowel sounds
- Common street drugs: ecstasy, cocaine, ketamine, amphetamine, methamphetamine

Ecstasy

- Hyponatremia: SIADH, marathon dancing, sweating, water ingestion
- Jaw clenching, bruxism

Cocaine

- Arrhythmias: blocks sodium channels (wide QRS), QT prolongation
- Myocardial ischemia/infarction: coronary artery vasospasm and/or thrombosis
- Pneumothorax, pneumomediastinum, aortic dissection

Ketamine

- Dissociation with hallucinations, vivid dreams

Complications

- Hyperthermia, seizure, arrhythmia, rhabdomyolysis, acute renal failure, end organ damage, ARDS, DIC, intracranial hemorrhage, circulatory collapse

Investigations

- Electrolytes (hyponatremia), CPK, and urine (rhabdomyolysis)
- ECG: ischemia, arrhythmia, QRS, QT intervals
- Drug screen
- Others as indicated: CXR, CT head, etc.

Anticholinergic Ingestion

- Anticholinergic toxidrome: flushed, dry skin, mydriasis, hyperthermia, hallucinations, tachycardia, hyper- or hypotension, decreased bowel sounds
- Common street drugs: jimsonweed, abuse of over-the-counter medication (Benadryl® and Gravol®)
- Complications: similar to sympathomimetic ingestion

Management

- Similar to sympathomimetic ingestion
- QRS widening and hypotension from sodium channel blockade, consider sodium bicarbonate

Table 57.1 Management of Sympathomimetic Ingestion

Tachycardia and hypertension	• IV fluid for dehydration • Sedation with benzodiazepines • Avoid pure β-blockers (paradoxical hypertension) • First choice: phentolamine, nitroprusside
Arrhythmias	• Routine treatment • Cocaine related: consider sodium bicarbonate
Hyperthermia	• IV fluid for dehydration • Sedate with benzodiazepines: prevent further heat generation • Rapid cooling: mist and fan • Prevent shivering: paralyze if necessary
Rhabdomyolysis	• Hydration • Alkalinize urine
Seizures	• Routine treatment
Electrolyte imbalance	• Routine treatment
Chest pain	• Benzodiazepines • Nitroglycerin • Phentolamine, avoid β-blocker alone (paradoxical hypertension) • Consider calcium channel blockers • Thrombolytics controversial
Agitation	• Benzodiazepines

■ Physostigmine may worsen arrhythmias and seizures
■ Jimsonweed seeds: consider whole bowel irrigation up to 24 hours

Opioid Ingestion

■ Toxidrome: miosis, respiratory depression, CNS depression

- Common street drugs: heroin, prescription narcotic abuse, methadone
- Complications: hypothermia, bradycardia, death from respiratory arrest

Management

- Opioid antagonist naloxone 0.4 mg–2 mg IV q 3 min; titrate to response
- Naloxone: half-life of 60 minutes, signs of opioid overdose may reappear
- Can start naloxone infusion: two-thirds initial dose per hour

Gamma Hyroxybutyrate (GHB)

- Alternating agitation and coma, bradycardia, respiratory depression, hypothermia, amnesia
- Potential "date rape" drug: highly soluble, colorless and tasteless, rapid onset of coma, no hangover effect, difficult to detect
- Prodrug versions: gamma butyrolactone (GBL), 1,4 butanediol (1,4BD)

Management

- Supportive treatment
- ABCs, may require intubation
- Recover quickly < 6–8 hours

Psychedelics

- LSD, PCP, psilocybin, mescaline, MDMA, ketamine
- May present as sympathomimetic toxidrome and complications

LSD

- Psychedelic effects, panic attacks, acute psychotic reaction, depression, paranoia
- Risk of physical trauma and suicide
- "Flashbacks": hallucinogen persisting perception disorder

PCP
- Clouds sensorium, not heightened awareness
- Cholinergic, anticholinergic, and sympathomimetic effects
- Violence, delusions

Psilocybin, mushrooms Psilocybe semilanceata (Liberty Cap) and Mescaline, Mexican peyote cactus Lophophora williamsii
- Often adulterated (PCP, LSD)
- Hallucinogenic effects similar, but milder than LSD
- Drug screen will not detect, but will identify adulterant PCP

Marijuana
- Leaves and flowers of *Cannabis sativa*
- Dried resin hashish
- Drowsiness, euphoria, heightened sense of awareness
- Distortions of time and space, paranoia, panic reactions, brief toxic psychosis

Management
- Similar to sympathomimetic ingestion
- Quiet, low-stimulation environment
- Ensure safety of patient and staff
- Reassurance
- Benzodiazepines, haloperidol for sedation and agitation
- May require restraints
- Admit if 8–12 hrs continued psychiatric symptoms

References
Graeme KA. New drugs of abuse. *Emerg Med Clin North Am.* 1997; 15(2):365–379.

Lange RA, Hillis LD. Cardiovascular complications of cocaine use. *N Engl J Med.* 2001;345(5):351–358.

Olson KR. *Poisoning and Drug Overdose.* 3rd ed. Stamford, Conn.: Appleton & Lange; 1999.

Schwartz RH, Miller NS. MDMA (ecstasy) and the rave: a review. *Pediatrics.* 1997;100(4):705–708.

Tintinelli JE. *Emergency Medicine: A Comprehensive Study Guide.* 5th ed. New York: McGraw-Hill; 2000.

Winickoff JP, et al. Verve and jolt: deadly new Internet drugs. *Pediatrics.* 2000;106(4):829–830.

58 ▪ Electrical Injuries

MICHAL MAIMON

Introduction

- Electrical burns account for 2–3% of pediatric burns assessed in the emergency department
- Low-voltage injuries account for 60–70% of electrical injuries, usually < 6 yrs with oral or hand contact on electrical cord or sockets
- High-voltage injuries: children > 12 yrs with risk-taking behavior

Factors Determining Severity of Electrical Injuries

Resistance of tissue:

- Mucous membranes, nerve tissue, and moist skin have very low resistance

Type of current:

- Low voltage (< 600 volts)
  - Alternating current (AC) causes tetanic contraction and "locking on" extending duration of contact
  - Direct current (DC) will cause single contraction that may throw the victim
- High voltage (600–1,000,000 volts): causes single contraction in AC and DC

Current intensity:

- 3–5 mA: maximum current at which a child can "let go"
- 20–50 mA: paralysis of respiratory muscles
- 50–100 mA: ventricular fibrillation
- > 2 A: asystole

Pathway taken by the current:
- Vertical pathway: parallel to axis of body, involves all vital organs, 20% mortality from cardiac arrhythmias
- "Hand to hand": involves heart, respiratory system, spinal cord C4–C8 (most dangerous, 60% mortality)
- "Leg to leg": usually not lethal (< 5% mortality)

Clinical Manifestations
Cardiovascular
- *Dysrhythmias*
- Asystole: high voltage and lightning; sinus rhythm may spontaneously return due to automaticity of the heart
- Ventricular fibrillation: low voltage
- Other: sinus tachycardia, atrial fibrillation, SVT
- *Conduction defects*: AV block, bundle branch block
- *Myocardial necrosis* may occur when the current passes through the heart
- *Cardiac ischemia* secondary to anoxia

Note: Degree of injury to heart depends on voltage; at any given voltage, AC is worse than DC

CNS
- Most brain injuries are secondary to anoxia or blunt head trauma
- Direct passage of current through brain may cause injury to respiratory center
- Other injuries: coma, transient LOC, amnesia, seizures, cranial nerve deficit
- Hemiplegia/quadriplegia due to transection of spinal cord at C4–C8 in "hand to hand" injuries
- Transient paralysis and autonomic instability in lightning injuries secondary to massive catecholamine release
- Intracranial hemorrhage: secondary to damage to blood vessels

Cutaneous

Low-Voltage Injuries

- Severity of burn depends on intensity, surface area, and duration
- Mostly superficial burns
- In low resistance (e.g., wet skin), severity of burn is not predictive of internal injury
- Oral burns may be full thickness: eschar forms within hours and detaches within 2–3 weeks
- Injury to labial artery may cause significant bleeding when eschar detaches

High-Voltage Injuries

- Three types of burns: flash from heat, electrothermal from electrical current, flame from burning of clothes
- Lightning: 89% have burn, 5% full thickness
- Lichtenberg figure: pathognomonic for lightning, appears 1 hr after strike and fades in 24–36 hrs

Respiratory System

- Tetanic contraction of respiratory muscles
- Respiratory arrest secondary to CNS injury

Musculoskeletal

- Rhabdomyolysis: increased CPK, potassium
- Fractures: most commonly upper limb and vertebrae
- Risk of compartment syndrome (rare in lightning strike)

Renal

- Acute tubular necrosis secondary to myoglobinuria

Eyes/Ears

- 50% of lightning victims sustain eye injuries, > 50% have ruptured tympanic membranes

- Most serious eye injuries include cataracts, retinal detachment, retinal hemorrhage, optic nerve degeneration, may occur years after the event
- Risk of hearing loss, chronic infections, tinnitus

Investigations

- CBC, electrolytes, BUN, creatinine, CPK, cardiac enzymes, ALT, AST, amylase
- ECG
- Urinalysis for myoglobin
- X-rays for musculoskeletal injury
- CT head: for severe lightning injuries, falls, and persistent abnormal neurological findings

Management

- ABCs with spinal cord precautions
- Triage: lightning injury—priority to pulseless victims
- Assess parameters determining severity of injury (voltage, AC or DC, wet skin, entry and exit site)
- Consider blunt thoracic or abdominal trauma in high-voltage injuries
- Fluid management: high fluid requirement in severe electrical injuries (use Parkland formula)
- If significant muscle damage, risk of renal failure: Foley catheter to monitor urine output, IV fluids to keep urine output at 2 mL/kg/hr, alkalinize urine with $NaHCO_3$, monitor for hyperkalemia
- Oral burns: consult plastic surgery
- Ophthalmology follow-up

Note: Internal burns may be present in absence of visible external burns

Disposition

Cardiac monitoring indicated for:

- High-voltage injury
- Loss of consciousness
- Abnormal ECG on arrival in emergency
- Previous cardiac problem
- Cardiopulmonary arrest
- Abnormal neurological findings
- Severe burns
- Visceral or blood vessel injury

Low-Voltage Injuries (< 200 V)

- Observe in emergency × 4 hours with cardiac monitoring
- If only minor wounds present, no arrhythmia and no loss of consciousness, may be discharged and managed as outpatient

High-Voltage Injuries (> 1,000 V)

- Admit and observe on cardiac monitor × 24–72 hrs

References

Bailey B, et al. Experience with guidelines for cardiac monitoring after electrical injury in children. *Am J Emerg Med.* 2000;18:671–675.

Cherington M, et al. Lightning and Lichtenberg figures. *Injury.* 2003;34: 367–371.

Garcia C, et al. Electrical injury in the pediatric emergency department. *Ann Emerg Med.* 1996;26:604–608.

Koumbourlis AC. Electrical injuries. *Crit Care Med.* 2002;30(suppl): s424–s430.

■ PART XV
MINOR TRAUMA

59 ▪ Foreign Bodies

AMINA LALANI

Introduction
- If early attempts at foreign body removal are unsuccessful, consider referral and/or procedural sedation

Nose
- Usually history of putting object into nose
- Persistent, unilateral, foul-smelling, purulent rhinorrhea: nasal foreign body until proven otherwise
- Usually visible in anterior nares; may have to suction purulent secretions
- Radiographs not helpful; most foreign bodies are radiolucent

Techniques for Removal
- Standard: curette, alligator forceps, suction, right-angle hook
- Alternative methods for removal:
  - Nasal positive pressure techniques
  - Magnetic removal
  - Glue

Removal of Nasal Foreign Bodies
- Adequately restrain child
- Apply topical anesthetic and vasoconstrictor
  - 2% lidocaine
  - Phenylephrine or xylometazoline
- Use nasal speculum and headlight
- Equipment: curette, alligator forceps, suction, or hook
- Do not push/irrigate into posterior nasopharynx in case of aspiration
- Consider amoxicillin to prevent/treat infection after removal of long-standing FB

- Complications: rhinosinusitis, laceration, epistaxis, aspiration, incomplete removal

Nasal Positive Pressure Techniques
- Older child: ask child to blow nose while occluding unaffected side
- Apply self-inflating bag-valve mask over *mouth* only and give positive pressure ventilation
- Parent blows into child's mouth: 80% success rate in one study

Magnetic Removal of Nasal Foreign Bodies
- Magnet can be applied to nostril to remove metallic FB
- Avoids need for anesthetic, easy and safe

Ear
- Mostly solid objects: stones, beads, erasers
- Live insects may also enter canal
- Round objects can be removed with warm water irrigation
  - Not if suspected perforation, ear tube, or object has potential to swell (e.g., vegetative matter)

Methods of Removal
- Ear curette, alligator forceps, irrigation, suction, glue

Soft Tissue
- Earrings, lip and tongue studs
- Grasp and remove earring stud from posterior, mucosal, or inferior aspect
- Thread front of earring forward through soft tissue to remove
- May require local anesthesia and small incision

Digit
Strangulating Ring
- Three removal techniques: ring cutting, string compression, string pull

Ring Cutting

- If minimal edema distal to ring, try other techniques first
- Digital block, insert ring-cutter guard
- Place blade on ring and apply pressure while rotating blade of ring cutter
- If hard metal, watch for heating with friction
- After ring is cut through, pull apart manually or use hemostat to remove
- Complications: vascular compromise, trauma to digit

String Compression (Thread Wrap)

- Consider digital block
- Wrap string or 3-0 silk suture around finger starting at distal edge of ring
- Cover PIP joint, place proximal end of string under ring
- Twist and pull ring over suture
- If fails, pull on string under proximal end in circular unwrapping fashion

String Pull

- Consider digital block
- Use string or heavy suture, lubricate distally
- Place one end of string under ring and pull through
- Grasp both ends of suture 10 cm from ring and pull in a circular motion
- Continue slipping suture around the ring as it moves along the finger

Subungual Splinters

- Restrain hand with fingers extended, consider digital block
- If visible, pull directly with tweezers or hemostat
  - Complications: bleeding, infection
- If embedded, use No. 11 blade held perpendicular to direction of splinter
- Scrape nail from proximal to distal to make U-shape

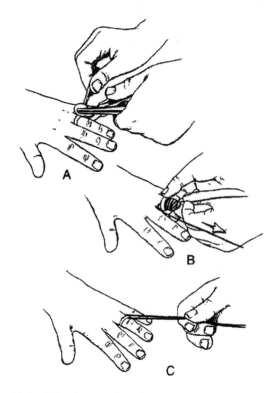

■ **Figure 59.1   Ring Removal Technique**
Source: With permission from: Fleisher GR , Ludwig S, Henretig F, eds. *Textbook of Pediatric Emergency Medicine.* 4th edition. Philadelphia: Lippincott Williams and Wilkins; 2000:1868.

- Use small forceps to grasp splinter and remove from nail bed
- Alternate method: cut V-shaped piece of nail and remove with nail elevator and forceps
- Avoid pushing splinter farther into the nail bed
- Soak finger several times daily to decrease risk of infection

Hair Tourniquet

- Strangulation of digit or penis by hair or fine thread

- Hair winds around a digit during bath, drying, or moving toes in clothing
- Most likely due to hair shed from a parent; higher risk in first three months postpartum when excessive maternal hair loss
- Impairs blood flow causing ischemic pain and distal swelling
- Hair can be unwound from the digit intact or cut with scissors
- If unsuccessful, use fine-tipped forceps and thin loupe or probe
- May need nerve block and a perpendicular incision over the hair
- Make incision on lateral aspect of digit to avoid neurovascular damage
- Hair removal creams (e.g., Nair®) can also be effective

Fish Hooks

- Most commonly used technique requires local/regional anesthesia:
  Drive hook forward through skin with forceps, cut off hook end, and thread remaining hook backward through skin to remove

Airway

- Foreign bodies may cause acute upper airway obstruction
  - Severe cough, hoarseness, respiratory distress
- If crying/talking then only *partial* obstruction:
  - Back blows or Heimlich contraindicated, need urgent bronchoscopy
- If unable to speak, may be *total* obstruction:
  - Perform back blows (infant) or Heimlich maneuver (child)
- Usually history of coughing/choking on food or toy
- Often no acute distress except mild cough or wheeze
  - Tracheal: inspiratory and expiratory stridor
  - Mainstem bronchus: unilateral wheeze
- If bronchus completely occluded: volume decrease, atelectasis and infiltrate on involved side

Chest X-ray

- Inspiratory and expiratory films show air trapping from ball-valve effect
  - Obtain right and left lateral decubitus films in young child
- Hyperaeration on involved side, contralateral volume loss from atelectasis
- Any radiographic asymmetry signals possible foreign body
- Most foreign bodies are radiolucent, not seen on radiographs
  - Normal chest X-ray does not rule out foreign body

GI Tract

- Most serious consequence of foreign body ingestion is esophageal impaction
- Lodge at sites of natural narrowing: cricopharynx, thoracic inlet, arch of aorta, gastroesophageal junction
- Most esophageal FB are round and radio-opaque
- Coins: 50–75% of esophageal foreign bodies, one-third asymptomatic
- Presentation: gagging, vomiting, drooling, pain with swallowing, and refusal to eat
- Unexplained dysphagia or drooling may indicate unwitnessed ingestion
- Impacted esophageal FB may cause secondary airway symptoms
- Check oral cavity: if no FB seen, obtain foreign body X-ray survey
- Radiographs will not show plastic FB or food bolus
  - Need barium swallow to rule out FB

Management

- If no FB on radiograph or exam, management determined by symptoms:
  - If significant pain, consult ENT for endoscopy

- If mild pain, able to swallow, no respiratory distress: FB sensation may be secondary to mucosal scratch; consider discharge and return if sensation persists
- If positive symptoms and suspect non-radio-opaque object, obtain barium swallow
- Disc batteries: need to remove immediately if in esophagus
■ Remove impacted FB immediately if in esophagus, especially sharp objects and disc batteries
■ Risks: respiratory distress, upper airway compromise, esophageal perforation, mediastinitis, fistula
■ Wait 24 hours for spontaneous passage of round, noncorrosive objects if asymptomatic and good follow-up
■ Handheld metal detectors can be used to follow patients with coin ingestions
■ Once FB has passed to stomach, follow-up radiographs not required
■ No role for glucagon in children due to risk of vomiting

Vaginal

■ Presentation: intermittently bloody, foul-smelling vaginal discharge
■ Most commonly toilet paper (not radio-opaque)
■ For optimal view of vagina, use knee-chest position
■ Rectal exam can be helpful to palpate FB in vagina
■ High index of suspicion if vagina cannot be properly inspected
■ Rigid foreign bodies (erasers, pins, beads, nuts) more likely palpable on rectal exam
■ If FB not seen, gentle vaginal lavage with saline, 50 cc syringe with plunger removed, catheter, and gravity
■ If large or sharp object, or unsuccessful, need sedation or examination under anesthesia

References

Botma M, et al. A parent's kiss: evaluating an unusual method for removing nasal foreign bodies in children. *J Laryngol Otol.* 2000;114(8):590–600.

Douglas SA, et al. Magnetic removal of a nasal foreign body. *Int J Pediatr Otorhinolaryngol.* 2002;62(2):165–167.

Lichenstein R, et al. Nasal wash technique for nasal foreign body removal. *Pediatr Emerg Care.* 2000;16(4):307.

Schunk J. Foreign body ingestion/aspiration. In: Fleisher GR, Ludwig S, Henretig F, eds. *Textbook of Pediatric Emergency Medicine.* 4th ed. Philadelphia: Lippincott Williams & Wilkins; 2000:267–273.

60 ▪ Wound Management

GRAHAM JAY

Introduction

- Mechanism of injury predicts healing and outcome
- Shear injuries have a better outcome
- Poorer outcomes found in blunt injuries over a large area
- Factors affecting healing include diabetes, obesity, nutritional status, and steroids
- Children have lower infection rates than adults

History and Examination

- History: time of injury, crush component, location, mechanism, tetanus status
- Examination: location, size, depth, shape of wound, contamination
- Perfusion of distal limb, neurological status, position of limb, and local tendon function
- Consider taking photographs

Definitions

- Laceration: secondary to blunt injury; skin is torn with irregular edges and adjacent skin usually crushed
- Incised wound (or cut): caused by a sharp object; wound has clean-cut edges
- Abrasions (or grazes): superficial blunt injury in which force has been applied tangentially
- Puncture wound: often caused by a sharp object but may be secondary to a blunt object if sufficient force; often small diameter but may be deep

Investigations

- X-ray may detect radio-opaque structures > 1–2 mm and any associated fractures
  - Wood and aluminum do not show up on X-ray (ultrasound may be useful)
- Bloodwork often not required unless in the setting of more major trauma

Management

Anesthesia

- Only a gentle cleanse before administering local anesthetic
- Topical: LET = Lidocaine, Epinephrine, Tetracaine
  - Soak cottonball with 3 mL of LET and apply to wound with moderate pressure for 20–30 minutes
  - Do not repeat
  - Works well for facial lacerations
- Injectable lidocaine 1%
  - Lidocaine with epinephrine is ideal for many wounds especially mouth and facial lacerations
  - Plain lidocaine (without epinephrine) to be used with lacerations of tips of digits, ears, nose (i.e., end organs)
  - Onset of action: approximately 3 min
  - Dosage   5 mg/kg of a 1% lidocaine solution
                 7 mg/kg of a 1% lidocaine with epinephrine solution
  - Addition of epinephrine in low concentrations (1:200,000 to 1:100,000) extends the effect of lidocaine to 3 hrs
- Bupivacaine: if more prolonged anesthesia required, maximum dose is 2 mg/kg of 1% solution

Wound Preparation

- Detergent-containing antiseptics may be harmful to tissue
- Most important step is decontamination with pressure irrigation

- Irrigation of normal saline through an 18G angiocath will generate sufficient pressure; for each 1 cm of wound, irrigate with at least 10 mL
- Keep hair away from edges of wounds with Vaseline, clipping is not recommended
- Do not shave eyebrows: regrowth may be unpredictable
- Debride obviously nonviable tissue from wound edges
- Remove foreign material from abrasions to prevent tattooing
- Do not close wound if suspect retained foreign body

Hemostasis

- Fingertip: tourniquet around proximal finger is helpful but avoid prolonged use (longer than 30 minutes)
- Direct pressure if nonpulsatile: closure of wound will usually cause hemostasis
- If visible bleeding vessels, ligation may be beneficial but use extreme caution
- If extensive bleeding, elevate, apply pressure, and refer for immediate surgical consultation

Wound Closure

- Apply minimum tension to close and evert edges of wound
- Golden period:
  - Low-risk wounds: primary closure of wounds up to 12–24 hrs after injury (face—24 hrs, other—12 hrs)
  - High-risk wounds: primary closure of contaminated wounds, in locations with poor vascular supply, and in immunocompromised patients within 6 hrs
- Closure of dead space advised although controversial
- Sutures placed in fat contribute no strength to repair and fail to prevent hematoma and infection
- Place only enough subcutaneous sutures to restore anatomic and functional integrity
- Perform delayed primary closure in 3 to 5 days on wounds left open due to high risk of infection

- Avoid deep sutures in highly contaminated wounds because of increased risk of infection
- If history of keloid formation, skin should be closed with minimal tension; consider use of pressure dressing for 3–6 months

Instruments and Lighting
- Toothed forceps required as less likely to crush tissue
- Ensure adequate lighting available before suturing

Sutures
- Absorbable vs nonabsorbable:
  - Absorbable have higher reactivity and can produce an inflammatory reaction
  - Concern with poorer cosmetic appearance unsupported by evidence; however, many clinicians do not use on facial wounds
  - Useful for intraoral and lip lacerations
- Alternatives to sutures:
  - Staples useful for injuries to scalp
  - Cyanoacrylates (glue): use on low-tensile wounds, low mobility < 3 cm in length

Suture Techniques
- General principles:
  - Ensure wound eversion
  - Avoid excess tension to avoid devascularization
  - Width between sutures should be equal to width of each bite
  - Use mattress sutures to provide eversion
- Simple interrupted: use for simple lacerations
- Interrupted mattress: use when wound is long, useful for providing eversion
- Vertical mattress: provides eversion and good tensile strength

- Half-buried mattress: useful for T- and V-shaped wounds
- Continuous running: use on superficial incised wounds

Preparation

- Be organized and well prepared
- Give reassurance and build rapport with child
- Use parents as allies and keep them in the room
- Do not draw up medication in front of patient

Administering Anesthetic

- Consider warming the local anesthetic (40–42°C)
- Buffer 1:10 with 8.4% sodium bicarbonate
- Inject slowly using a smaller, longer needle (27 gauge, 1.5 cm)
- Initiate puncture closest to nerve supply if possible and at apices of wound allowing needle to travel the length of the wound edge as you inject
- A field block created by directing the needle outward at an angle from the apices provides a wide rectangular zone anesthetic with minimal number of punctures
- Local nerve blocks where possible: especially useful for hand, foot, ear, face

Uncooperative Child

- Consider nonpharmacological techniques (e.g., distraction)
- Use mild to moderate sedation in selected patients

Prophylactic Antibiotics

- Wound infection rates 1–3% overall
- Most important factor in preventing infection is early and adequate cleaning and irrigation
- Prophylaxis rarely required for more than 3 days
- Consider for cat, human, dog bites as well as open fractures and exposed joints or tendons for 3–5 days

Specific Wounds

- Intraoral: seldom require sutures
- Lip: need to exactly oppose vermillion border
- Scalp:
  - May be closed using staples if superficial; defects in galea closed using absorbable sutures
  - Hair tie technique can help avoid use of sutures
- Bites: antibiotic use inconsistently supported in the literature; may use antibiotics for higher risk wounds (e.g., bites to hand), wounds over underlying structures such as joints and tendons
  - Clavulin is antibiotic of choice

Dressings

- Keep wounds clean
- Epithelialization occurs at 24–48 hours after repair
- Consider nonadherent dressing during first 48 hours to keep wound dry and protect from contamination
- After this period, can wash wound, but do not scrub or soak
- Maintaining moist environment (e.g., petrolatum-impregnated mesh dressing initially) around wound has been shown to speed the rate of epithelialization
- For abrasions and burns: use petrolatum-impregnated mesh dressing covered by dry gauze
- Restrict movement of affected limb
- Topical antibiotic ointment to reduce infection rate and prevent scab formation
- Observe wound for erythema, warmth, swelling, or drainage that may indicate infection; seek medical advice early if this occurs
- Review heavily contaminated wounds within 48 hours
- Timing of suture removal:
  - Sutures or staples can be removed from most areas of the body in 7 days

Table 60.1   Tetanus Prophylaxis

PRIOR TETANUS TOXOID IMMUNIZATION (DOSES)	CLEAN MINOR WOUND	ALL OTHER WOUNDS ("DIRTY")
Uncertain or < 3	DTP or Td	DTP or Td and TIG
3 or more (most recent > 10 years ago)	Td	Td
3 or more (most recent 5–10 years ago)	None	Td
3 or more (most recent < 5 years ago)	None	None

Key: DTP: diphtheria, tetanus, pertussis toxoid; Td: adult diphtheria, tetanus toxoid; TIG: tetanus immunoglobulin
Source: Adapted from: Fleisher GR, Ludwig, S, Henretig, F, eds. *Textbook of Pediatric Emergency Medicine.* 4th ed. Philadelphia: Lippincott Williams & Wilkins; 2000:786.

- • Facial sutures 3–5 days
- • Sutures under tension (e.g., over joints and on hands) 10–14 days
- ■ Advise parents that appearance of scar may change substantially during the first year after repair
- ■ Avoid exposing wound to sun to prevent excess scarring
- ■ Tetanus prophylaxis

References

Kanegaye JT. A rational approach to the outpatient management of lacerations in pediatric patients. *Curr Probl Pediatr.* 1998; 28:210–234.

Quaba O. A users guide for reducing the pain of local anaesthetic administration. *Emerg Med J.* 2005;22:188–189.

61 ▪ Bite Wounds

JONATHAN PIRIE

Introduction

- Human and animal bite wounds are common: ~1% of all emergency department (ED) visits
- Most bite wounds are minor, but may cause significant morbidity
- Management requires an understanding of the microbiology of wound infections, assessment of low- versus high-risk wounds, treatment strategies, and tetanus and rabies prophylaxis
- Notify local public health department for *all* animal bite wounds

Frequency and Infection Rates

- Dog bites are most common type of animal bite but have low infection rates
- Younger children are most susceptible to significant morbidity and occasional mortality
- Cat bites less frequent but have much higher infection rate
  - Cats tend to inflict deep puncture wounds; they are hard to clean and tend to occur on hands and upper extremities
- Human bites are least common yet have a relatively high infection rate
- Beware of closed-fist injuries affecting area around the metacarpal-phalangeal joints

Microbiology

- Bite wounds often involve multiple species:
  - *Pasteurella* species: dog and cat bite wounds
  - *Eikenella corrodens:* human bites
  - *Capnocytophaga canimorsus:* dog or cat bites, can cause septicemia and shock in patients with asplenia or immunosuppression

478

Table 61.1   Bites and Infection Rates by Species

SPECIES	FREQUENCY OF BITE (%)	FREQUENCY OF INFECTION (%)
Dog	80–90	2–20
Cat	5–15	30–50
Human	3.6–23	10–50

- Other common organisms: streptococci, staphylococci, oral anaerobes
- Amoxicillin/clavulanic acid is antimicrobial of choice: covers all potential pathogens in bite wound infections

Bite Wound Management

- Copious irrigation: normal saline with a 20-mL or larger syringe and 19G angiocath
- Cautious debridement if indicated
- Prophylactic antibiotics (high risk: see below)
- Therapeutic antibiotics if signs of infection
- Primary closure: low-risk lacerations
- Immobilization in position of function
- Elevation
- Tetanus toxoid if indicated +/– tetanus immune globulin as necessary
- Rabies prophylaxis if indicated

Note: Antibiotics alone not sufficient

Prophylactic Antibiotics

- Controversial; limited studies
- If present to ED within 24 hours, without signs of infection, *and* have high-risk criteria, consider for antibiotic prophylaxis
- Give first dose in emergency department

- Duration 3–5 days
- Antibiotic of choice: amoxicillin-clavulanic acid
- Alternatives: penicillin V + (cephalexin or cloxacillin)
- Penicillin allergic: clindamycin + TMP-SMX

High-Risk Wounds: Indications for Antibiotic Prophylaxis

Wound Type or Location

- Deep puncture wounds
- Bites over tendons, joints, bone
- Hand: closed-fist injury (CFI)
- Bites on the face: lower infection rates, but higher cosmetic and serious complication risk if infection occurs

Offending Species

- Cat bites, human bites (unless minor)
- Some dog bites depending on location and wound type

Other Factors

- Immunocompromised host
- Delayed presentation (> 8 hours)
- Primary laceration repair

Low-Risk Wounds: No Prophylaxis

- Superficial abrasions and lacerations
- Areas of good blood supply and away from vital structures
- Presentation shortly after incident
- Dog bites that do not meet above high-risk criteria

Management of Infected Bite Wounds

- Majority with early infection can be managed with outpatient oral antibiotics
- Antibiotic choice: as for prophylaxis, duration 7–10 days
- Limited studies, management controversial

Indications for Admission

- Systemic manifestations of infection (fever, chills)
- Severe cellulitis
- Penetration of a joint, nerve, bone, tendon, or central nervous system
- Likelihood for noncompliance
- Immunocompromised by disease or drugs
- Significant bites to the hand
- Head injuries
- Infection refractory to oral or outpatient therapy

Intravenous Antibiotic Choices for Inpatients

- First choice: penicillin V + (cefazolin or cloxacillin)
- Alternative choices: cefuroxime +/– metronidazole, ceftriaxone
- Penicillin allergic: clindamycin + TMP–SMX

Tetanus

- Saliva and puncture wounds are both criteria for "dirty wounds" in the tetanus management of bite wounds
- Recommendations depend on previous immunization history

Table 61.2   Tetanus Prophylaxis

PRIOR TETANUS TOXOID IMMUNIZATION (DOSES)	CLEAN MINOR WOUND	ALL OTHER WOUNDS ("DIRTY")
Uncertain or < 3	DTP or Td	DTP or Td and TIG
3 or more (most recent > 10 years ago)	Td	Td
3 or more (most recent 5–10 years ago)	None	Td
3 or more (most recent < 5 years ago)	None	None

Key: DTP: diphtheria, tetanus, pertussis toxoid; Td: adult diphtheria, tetanus toxoid; TIG: tetanus immunoglobulin
Source: Adapted from: Fleisher GR, Ludwig, S, Henretig, F, eds. *Textbook of Pediatric Emergency Medicine.* 4th ed. Philadelphia: Lippincott Williams & Wilkins; 2000:786.

Rabies

- Rare in North America
- < 20% chance of contracting rabies from bite of a rabid animal but almost uniformly fatal once contracted
- Principal vectors : foxes, skunks, bats, and raccoons
- Uncommonly transmitted by domestic animals (cats > cattle, dogs)
- Bites from rabid bats may go undetected: bite may not be felt, may not leave visible marks
- Indications for post-exposure prophylaxis:
  - Bats found in a room with young children
  - Incapable of giving history of bat bite
  - Sleeping unattended, bat in room
- Important historical features: animal species, type of exposure, circumstances (provoked, etc.), animal available for quarantine and testing
- Prompt thorough wound irrigation can reduce incidence of rabies by up to 90%

Rabies Prophylaxis

- Need passive and active prophylaxis
- Immunoprophylaxis is considered 100% protective if given appropriately and prior to symptoms
- Passive immunization: human rabies immune globulin (HRIG)
  - Day 0 as a single 20 IU/kg dose, half infiltrated around site of exposure, other half given intramuscularly
- Active immunization: human diploid cell vaccine (HDCV) or rabies vaccine adsorbed (RVA):
  - Administered IM in a series of five 1-mL injections given on days 0, 3, 7, 14, and 28
  - Deltoid muscle of adolescents and anterolateral thigh of small children are recommended injection sites for HDCV and RVA; administration into gluteal region has been associated with treatment failure

References

Anderson CR. Animal bites: guidelines to current management. *Postgrad Med.* 1992;92:134–136, 139–146, 149.

Callaham M. Prophylactic antibiotics in dog bite wounds: nipping at the heels of progress. *Ann Emerg Med.* 1994;23:577–579.

Canadian Immunization Guide 1998. 5th ed. Canada: Canadian Medical Association.

Cummings P. Antibiotics to prevent infection in patients with dog bite wounds: a meta-analysis of randomized trials. *Ann Emerg Med.* 1994;23:535.

Davies D. When your best friend bites: a note on dog and cat bites. *Paediatr Child Health.* 2000;5:381–383.

Dire D. Emergency management of dog and cat bite wounds. *Emerg Med Clin North Am.* 1992;10:719.

Garcia V. Animal bites and Pasteurella infections. *Pediatr Rev.* 1997;18:127.

Griego R, et al. Dog, cat, and human bites: a review. *J Am Acad Derm.* 1995;33:1019–1029.

LeBer C. Rabies post-exposure treatment (PET): Ontario, April 1 to June 30, 1998. *PHERO.* 1999;16–19.

Leung AK, Robson WL. Human bites in children. *Pediatr Emerg Care.* 1992;8:255–257.

Talan DA, et al. Bacteriologic analysis of infected dog and cat bites. *N Engl J Med.* 1999;340:85–92.

62 ▪ Common Emergency Procedures

ANGELO MIKROGIANAKIS AND CHRISTINA RICKS

Procedures

- Orthopedic splints
- Laceration repair: suturing and glueing
- Lumbar puncture
- Chest tube insertion

Orthopedic Splints

Materials

- Stockingette, webril, plaster, kling wrap, flannel, water (cast setup)

Instructions for All Splints

- Position patient
- Place stockingette over extremity (measurements should be taken on unaffected side)
- Wrap extremity in webril: extra padding is needed over bony prominences
- Dip measured plaster (10 layers) in water and squeeze out excess
- Place plaster over affected extremity, wrap with kling and mold into proper position. If second layer of plaster (tong or stirrup) needed for reinforcement around joints, mold first layer, then apply stirrup, wrap in kling, and mold second layer.
- Finally, wrap completed splint in flannel. Secure with tape for a nice-looking cast.

Table 62.1   Orthopedic Splints

TYPE OF SPLINT	INDICATION
Volar (short arm)	Nondisplaced distal forearm and wrist fractures
Sugar tong, forearm	Nondisplaced distal radio-ulnar fractures
Sugar tong, humerus	Stable distal humeral fractures (e.g. supra-condylar)
Thumb spica	Stable fracture of metacarpal/proximal phalanx of thumb and scaphoid fractures
Ulnar gutter	4th and 5th metacarpal and proximal pha-langeal fractures
Long arm	Stable fractures around elbow joint
Short leg	Stable distal tibia/fibular fractures, and ankle injuries
Long leg	Stable fractures of proximal tibia/fibula, distal femur fractures, and knee injuries

Instructions for Specific Splints
Volar Splint
- Begins at MCP joints and courses along volar surface of forearm to mid forearm, covering ulna and radius
- Position child supine on bed with elbow at 90° or child may sit with fingers pointing up and elbow flexed 90°
- Mold plaster with wrist in neutral position and fingers flexed at all joints

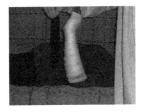

■ **Figure 62.1   Volar Splint**

Sugar Tong, Forearm Splint

- Should cover ulnar and radial edges of forearm and course along dorsal surface from MCP around elbow to palmar crease
- Place child prone with affected arm hanging toward floor and elbow flexed 90°, or sitting with elbow flexed 90°

Sugar Tong, Humeral Splint

- First place long arm splint
- Sugar tong: splint from acromioclavicular joint around elbow, ending just distal to axilla
- Place child in sitting position, elbow flexed 90°, and humerus internally rotated

Thumb Spica Splint

- Position arm with elbow resting on bed
- Splint should wrap around thumb and extend along radial side of arm to mid forearm
- Wrist should be in neutral position with thumb abducted and MCP and PIP in slight flexion as if holding a cup

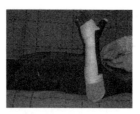

■ Figure 62.2   Thumb Spica Splint

Ulnar Gutter Splint

- Position arm with elbow resting on bed at 90°
- Splint wraps around ulnar surface from DIP of 5th digit to mid forearm.
  Cotton padding should wrap around 4th and 5th digits. Place additional cotton padding between digits for comfort.

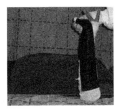

■ Figure 62.3   Ulnar Gutter Splint

■ Splint should be molded with wrist in neutral position and MCP and PIP in 70° and 30° of flexion, respectively

Long Arm Splint

■ Should extend from dorsal surface of upper arm, down around elbow, along ulnar surface of forearm to palmar crease
■ Child may lie prone with arm hanging over bed and elbow at 90°, or sitting on bed with elbow at 90°
■ Mold plaster with elbow at 90° and wrist in neutral position
■ To reinforce splint, place humeral sugar tong splint over long arm splint

Short Leg Splint

■ Should extend from fibular neck to proximal toes, covering dorsum of lower leg
■ Position child prone on bed with knee flexed and foot extended toward ceiling
■ Mold splint with ankle at 90°. May strengthen splint by applying a stirrup (sugar tong) splint. Stirrup should wrap around heel of foot and extend up to mid lower leg, bilaterally
■ Give crutches to those 6 years and older, with instruction

Long Leg Splint

■ Consider orthopedic consult as growth disturbances are common around knee

- Should cover posterior aspect of upper and lower leg extending from proximal thigh to heel distally
- Place child prone on bed with leg in position of comfort, or supine with someone supporting leg
- Mold plaster with knee in slight flexion and ankle in neutral. May need reinforcement around knee to prevent cast from cracking
- Give crutches to those 6 years and older, with instruction

Laceration Repair: Suturing

Superficial: a superficial laceration is restricted to the epidermis
Deep: a deep wound extends beyond epidermis into dermis

Sutures

- Absorbable:
  - Two most commonly used are surgical gut and Vicryl
  - Absorbable sutures should be used in subcutaneous closure
  - Rapidly absorbing sutures may be used on certain facial lacerations, especially in small children, and if difficult removal of sutures
- Nonabsorbable:
  - Commonly used sutures are nylon, polyester, and polypropylene
  - Nonabsorbable sutures used for cutaneous/superficial closures
- In general, smaller diameter sutures (5-0 and 6-0) are used on the face and neck, while larger sutures (3-0 and 4-0) are used on the extremities
- Needle holder should be appropriate size for needle
  - Holder may be flat or curved
  - Holder should grasp needle 1/3 to 1/2 distance from the swaged end

Suturing Techniques

Simple Interrupted Suture

- Clean and anesthetize (see Ch. 60, Wound Management)
- Sutures are placed 2–4 mm apart and ~ 3 mm from wound edge
- Always enter skin with needle at 90°
- Pass through subcutaneous tissue and emerge directly across from entrance point 3 mm from wound edge
- To tie knots, wrap suture around needle driver twice, then clasp free end of suture and pull so that tie is square to skin
- Repeat wrapping suture around driver only once for subsequent 3 knots

Running Suture

- Begin with simple suture at one end of wound
- Tie suture and cut only one free end
- Continue with running suture along the laceration, taking perpendicular bites across wound (suture will lie diagonally above skin)
- Last loop is placed just beyond laceration; use this loop as free suture end to tie knot

Horizontal Mattress Suture

- Use for gaping wounds or everting skin edges
- Begin with simple suture on far side of wound, pass through subcutaneous tissue, exit on the other side
- Reenter skin on same side 2 mm apart from exit point, back through subcutaneous tissue, and exit on starting side

Triangular Flap Laceration Repair

- A horizontal mattress suture that is partially buried in the subcutaneous tissue of the flap
- Start at tip/point of wound approximately 3 mm from the point of wound and 3 mm from wound edge

- Enter skin on near side of wound, then proceed through subcutaneous portion of flap, such that suture is partially buried in the flap
- Exit again on the near side of the wound 3 mm from the point and 3 mm from the wound edge
- Repeat process for each edge of flap

Laceration Repair: Glueing

- 2-octylcyanoacrylate (Dermabond®) is a tissue adhesive used for repair of superficial lacerations
- Possesses antibacterial properties particularly against Gram-positive organisms
- Similar cosmetic outcome when compared with suturing; less painful and takes less time
- Adhesive can be stored at room temperature (< 30°C)

Indications

- Superficial lacerations of any length and width, generally < 4 cm in length and 0.5 cm in width (must be able to easily approximate wound edges)
- Can be used for skin closure of deep wounds if deep absorbable sutures are applied

Not Recommended For

- Contaminated wounds requiring heavy debridement
- Bites
- Wounds in motion (e.g., hands, joints); bond can fracture and adhesive can wear off
- Hair-bearing surfaces (e.g., scalp)
- Wounds crossing mucocutaneous junctions
- Tissue adhesive must not come in contact with conjunctival sac as conglutination may occur

Technique

- Clean and dry wound in sterile fashion
- LET or topical anesthetic may be helpful for providing hemostasis for vascular wounds and decreasing any discomfort with use

Superficial Wound

- Appose wound edges avoiding gaps and bumps with edges slightly everted using forceps, fingers, or steristrips (two pairs of hands will be needed, unless the wound is very small and superficial in which case tweezers may be used)
- Hold applicator in a vertical position and squeeze ampule to break seal
- Turn ampule over and allow adhesive to enter cotton tip; invert and squeeze applicator until tip is saturated with colored solution and almost drips from end
- Paint a thin film of adhesive over apposed skin edges and extend at least 1/2 cm beyond each end of wound
- Appose wound edges for at least 30–60 seconds to allow polymerization
- Apply approximately 3–4 layers over wound waiting approximately 20 seconds between layers
- Hold edges together for 2 minutes after application of final layer to allow glue adhesive to reach maximum tensile strength

Deep Laceration

- Place absorbable subcutaneous sutures in deep tissue
- Apply superficial adhesive as described above

Considerations

- Avoid runoff of glue by placing wound in a flat, level plane
- Laceration close to the eye:
  - Position wound so that any runoff is directed away from the eye

- Hold dry gauze over the eye and apply a line of petroleum jelly around the eye to provide a barrier
■ Care must be taken that no instruments, cloths, swabs, or gloves come in contact with the adhesive as they will adhere to the surface being glued
■ Instruments contaminated with adhesive can be cleaned with acetone
■ Misalignment can be corrected by picking off glue with forceps and starting again
■ Cyanoacrylate can be removed from skin by applying Vaseline® or petrolatum

Discharge Instructions
■ Do not pick or scratch
■ Wound may be covered with a dry dressing if likely to be abraded
■ Wound should be kept dry for 3–5 days (may get wet after 24 hours but do not scrub or soak)
■ No swimming for 5–7 days
■ Do not use polysporin or topical creams or ointments
■ Glue will slough off spontaneously in 5–10 days
■ No follow-up necessary
■ Follow up with family doctor or emergency department if evidence of wound infection

Lumbar Puncture
Materials
■ Sterile gloves, gown, mask
■ Spinal needle 22G adequate for all lengths: 1″ for infant, 1″ or 2″ for toddler, 2.5″ for school age child, 2.5″ or 3″ for teenager
■ Lumbar puncture tray
■ Betadine and cleansing sponges
■ Sterile drapes
■ Lidocaine 1%, NO epinephrine
■ EMLA® patch

General Procedure

■ Place EMLA® patch on patient's back at L4/L5 or L3/L4 60 minutes prior to LP
■ Position child lying or sitting
■ If lying, neck and knees should be flexed toward abdomen with shoulders and hips perpendicular to bed
■ Holder supports shoulders if child in sitting position. Back should be rounded with hips and shoulders square
■ Landmark entrance point by drawing an imaginary line between posterior superior iliac crests (L4) and enter space below (L4/L5). Never enter above L3, as the spinal cord in infants ends at L3
■ Place sterile drape under patient, clean with betadine. Drape patient with remaining towels
■ Consider 1% lidocaine injection into subcutaneous tissue if topical anesthetic not used, taking care not to inject lidocaine into the spinal canal
■ Using correct spinal needle, approach entrance site with needle pointed toward the umbilicus, bevel pointing up. If patient is in sitting position, bevel should be vertical. Advance needle until you feel a "pop" (may not always be present), or a decrease in resistance
■ Remove stylet and look for fluid. A "traumatic tap" occurs when there is blood in the cerebrospinal fluid (CSF). If the blood clears while collecting the fluid, you are in the correct space
■ Collect 0.5–1 mL in CSF tubes. Reinsert stylet, and remove needle. Apply pressure with sterile gauze to stop any bleeding
■ Send CSF for Gram stain, culture, protein, glucose, cell count, +/– viral studies

Contraindications to Lumbar Puncture

■ Cellulitis over entrance site
■ Increased intracranial pressure with focal neurological deficits
■ Uncorrected coagulopathy

- Cardiopulmonary compromise
- Known spinal abnormality or trauma
- Evidence of cerebral herniation

Chest Tube/Tube Thoracostomy

Indications for Insertion

- Drainage of large hemothorax, pneumothorax (> 25%), or pleural effusion
- Penetrating trauma to chest
- Flail chest segment on ventilator
- Severe pulmonary contusion
- For purpose of air transport of trauma patient

Contraindications

- No contraindications in trauma situation
- Infection over site
- Uncontrolled bleeding diathesis

Materials

- Chest tube
- Suction device (Pleuravac®) with tubing, suction, water for creating underwater seal
- Suture tray (needle driver, 0-silk) and scalpel
- Tape (waterproof) and gauze for dressing
- Lidocaine, 10-cc syringe, 25G needle
- Sterile prep (gown, glove, mask)

Table 62.2   Chest Tube Size by Age

PATIENT	CHEST TUBE SIZE
Adult/teen male	28–32 Fr
Adult/teen female	28 Fr
Child	18 Fr
Newborn	12–14 Fr

Elective Placement of Chest Tube

- Always obtain informed consent from patient or primary caregiver
- Need for serial X-rays to follow

Procedure

- Select site for insertion: mid-axillary line, between 4th and 5th ribs (usually on a line lateral to the nipple)
- Don mask, gown, and gloves; prep and drape area of insertion. Have patient place ipsilateral arm over head to "open up" ribs
- Widely anesthetize area of insertion with 2% lidocaine; infiltrate skin, muscle tissues, and down to pleura

Note: Moderate sedation is an option for patients who are clinically stable

Chest Tube Insertion

- After infiltrating insertion site with local anesthetic, make a 3–4 cm incision through skin and subcutaneous tissues between the 4th and 5th ribs, parallel to the rib margins
- Continue incision through the intercostal muscles down to the pleura
- Insert Kelly clamp through the pleura and open the jaws, parallel to the direction of the ribs (this "creates" a pneumothorax, and allows the lung to fall away from the chest wall)

Opening the Incision with a Kelly Clamp

- Insert finger through incision and into the thoracic cavity. Make sure you are feeling lung (or empty space) and not liver or spleen
- Grasp end of chest tube with Kelly forcep (convex angle toward ribs), and insert chest tube through the hole you made in the pleura. After tube has entered thoracic cavity, remove Kelly, and manually advance the tube

Using a Kelly Clamp to Guide Insertion of the Chest Tube

- Clamp outer tube end with Kelly clamp
- Suture and tape tube in place
- Attach tube to suction unit
- Obtain post-procedure chest X-ray for placement; tube may need to be advanced or withdrawn slightly

Complications, Prevention, and Management

- Puncture of liver or spleen: entirely preventable; insertion site is in the nipple line, between 4th and 5th ribs
- Bleeding; usually ceases
- Cardiac puncture: preventable, carefully control the tube during insertion, and remove trochar early (or do not use trochar set)
- Passage of tube along chest wall instead of into chest cavity. In this case, widen and deepen the dissection between the ribs and make sure the insertion of the tube follows this path

Documentation in the Medical Record

- Consent if obtained
- Indications and contraindications for procedure on this patient
- Procedure used (trochar vs nontrochar)
- Complications
- Who was notified of complication (family, attending physician)

References

Algren JT, Algren CL. Sedation and analgesia for minor procedures. *Pediatr Emer Care.* 1996;12(6):435–441.

Kanegaye J. A rational approach to the outpatient management of lacerations in pediatric patients. *Curr Probl Pediatr.* 1998;210–234.

Quinn J, Wells G, Sutcliffe T, et al. A randomized trial comparing octyl-cyanoacrylate tissue adhesive and sutures in the management of lacerations. *JAMA.* 1997;277(19):1527–1530.

Singer AJ, Hollander JE, Quinn JV. Evaluation and management of traumatic lacerations. *N Engl J Med.* 1997;337:1142–1148.

Yaster M, Tobin JR, et al. Local anesthetics in the management of acute pain in children. *J Pediatr.* 1994;124(2):165–176.

63 ▪ Intraosseous Access

D. ANNA JARVIS

Introduction

- Used to rapidly secure vascular access in critically ill children with circulatory collapse or difficult IV access
- Can be used in all ages (consider battery-powered E-Z IO™ for older children and adolescents)

Indications

- If unable to establish peripheral or central access in a timely fashion in a critically ill child, intraosseous route may be lifesaving
  - Guideline: three peripheral stabs unsuccessful, OR 90 seconds
- Usually children < 6 years of age
  - May be used in older children if no other route available
- Can use to administer all fluids, blood products, and drugs that can be administered intravenously

Contraindications

Absolute Contraindications

- Recent fracture in bone
- Recent intraosseous infusion in bone
- Osteogenesis imperfecta
- Osteopetrosis

Relative Contraindications

- Cellulitis
- Burns
- Bleeding disorders

Equipment

- Cleaning and antiseptic fluids and supplies
- Sterile gloves
- 3–5 mL syringe with saline
- Intravenous tubing and fluid
- Tape and board (or other means of securing the limb)
- T-piece and 3-way stop-cock are optional
- Intraosseous needle:
  - Several commercial choices, all with a stylet
  - If no intraosseous needle is available, use 14–18G hypodermic needle, 18–20G 2-inch spinal needle, bone aspiration needle, 16–18G scalp vein needle

Sites

- Proximal tibia: preferred site for ease of access and safety
  - Flat medial surface is punctured 1–2 cm below tibial tuberosity in order to avoid growth plate
- Distal femur: more difficult site to landmark because of overlying fat and muscles
  - Lower third of femur is punctured ~ 3 cm above lateral condyle
- Distal tibia: may be used in older children or adults
  - Medial surface of tibia is punctured proximal to medial malleolus

Technique

- Prepare skin with antiseptic and secure leg
- Holding the needle perpendicular to the bone *or* at a 60° *away* from the adjacent growth plate, advance firmly with a rotatory motion until a soft pop indicates entry into the marrow cavity
- Attempt aspiration of marrow to confirm placement
- If no aspirate in syringe, ensure needle stands firmly in the bone and gently syringe in 10 mL of normal saline. If this flows freely *and* a hand below the limb does not feel a "cold flush"

and there is no obvious swelling, the site may be used for infusion

■ Tape needle securely using H-type bridge technique (allows for constant observation of the needle puncture site for signs of extravasation)

Note: A pump may be needed to ensure adequate flow

References

Carlson DW, et al. Illustrated techniques of pediatric emergency procedures. In: Fleisher G, Ludwig S, eds. *Textbook of Pediatric Emergency Medicine.* 4th ed. Philadelphia: Lippincott Williams & Wilkins; 2000:1809.

Gausche-Hill M, Fuchs S, Yamamoto L, eds. *American Academy of Pediatrics and American College of Emergency Physicians: APLS The Pediatric Emergency Medicine Resource.* 4th ed. Sudbury, Mass: Jones and Bartlett; 2004:736–738.

■ PART XVI
PAIN AND SEDATION

64 ▪ Pain Management

SUZAN SCHNEEWEISS

Introduction

- Treatment of pain should be priority for all clinicians; pain as fifth vital sign
- Children often endure unacceptable levels of pain during hospitalization
- Children generally receive analgesia less frequently than adults in the emergency setting
- When inadequate analgesia is given, children and neonates often experience more distress with subsequent procedures

Pain Assessment

- Pain history: location, intensity, quality, duration, frequency, aggravating, and relieving factors
- Regular assessment based on presence and severity of pain: self-report, behavioral observation, and physiologic measures
- Self-report is considered "gold standard":
  - Children can report degree of pain by 3–4 yrs
  - Children > 6 yrs can provide detailed descriptions of pain intensity, quality, and location

Pain Scales

FLACC (Face, Legs, Activity, Cry, Consolability)

- For infants and children ages 2 months to 7 yrs and cognitively impaired

Pain Word Scale

- For children ages 3–7 yrs and older, children unable to use numerical rating scale
- Categories: none, a little, medium, a lot

Table 64.1   FLACC Scale

CATEGORY	0	1	2
Face	No particular expression or smile	Occasional grimace or frown, withdrawn, disinterested	Frequent to constant quivering chin, clenched jaw
Legs	Normal position or relaxed	Uneasy, restless, tense	Kicking, or legs drawn up
Activity	Lying quietly, normal position, moves easily	Squirming, shifting back and forth, tense	Arching, rigid, or jerking
Cry	No cry (awake or asleep)	Moans or whimpers; occasional complaint	Crying steadily, screams or sobs, frequent complaints
Consolability	Content, relaxed	Reassured by occasional touching, hugging or being talked to, distractable	Difficult to console or comfort

*Each of the five categories is scored from 0–2, which results in a total score of 0–10.
Source: With permission from: Merkel SI, Voepel-Lewis T, Shayevitz JR, Malvyia S. The FLACC; a behavioral scale for scoring postoperative pain in young children. *Pediatric Nursing.* 1997;23(3):293–297.

Faces Pain Scale-Revised (FPS-R)

For ages 5–12 yrs

■ Figure 64.1   Faces Pain Scale
Source: With permission from: International Association for the Study of Pain. In: Hicks CL, von Baeyer CL, Spafford P, van Korlaar I, Goodenough B. Faces Pain Scale Revised: toward a common metric in pediatric pain management. *Pain.* 2001;93:173–183.

Numerical Rating Scale

- For children > 7 yrs
- Numerical scales from 0–10 or 0–100

Psychological Aspects of Pain

- Uncertainty, anxiety, and fear of procedures
- Expectations of pain to be experienced
- Previous experiences of pain
- Parental anxiety

Behavioral Approach to Pain

- Avoid using medical jargon
- Talk to children using age-appropriate language
- Distraction techniques: tell a story, music, mobiles during a procedure
- Guided imagery

Pharmacologic Management of Pain: General Principles

- Systematic approach to the administration of analgesics for pain
- Use "analgesic ladder" for escalation of analgesics: 90% effective in relieving pain
- Acetaminophen or NSAIDs for mild pain
  - NSAIDs have ceiling effect; no additional analgesic effect beyond maximum dose
  - Oral NSAIDs equally effective to IV NSAIDs
- Add oral opioid if persistent or increasing pain
  - Separate dosage form of opioid and non-opioid if higher doses required
  - Oral morphine preferable to oral codeine; codeine metabolized to small amount of morphine for analgesic effect

- Codeine is ineffective in 10% of population who are "nonmetabolizers"
■ Add parenteral opioid for moderate to severe pain
  - Avoid IM injection
  - Titrate to effectiveness, no ceiling effect
  - Half-life of morphine varies with age: 6.5 hrs in neonate, 2 hrs in older children and adults
  - Use appropriate monitoring
■ Use regularly scheduled dosing for persistent pain ("around the clock")
■ Treating pain does not lead to psychologic dependence/addiction

Table 64.2 Analgesics for Mild Pain

ANALGESIC	DOSAGE	ADVANTAGES	DISADVANTAGES
Acetaminophen	15 mg/kg q 4–6 h PO/PR (max 75 mg/kg/day or 4 g/day if > 12 yrs, whichever is less)	Well tolerated Safe	Liver toxicity if overdosed
Ibuprofen	5–10 mg/kg PO q 6–8 h (max 40 mg/kg/day or 2,400 mg/day adult)	Longer duration of action	GI irritation Increased risk of bleeding after tonsillectomy
Naproxen	10–20 mg/kg/day PO divided bid Dose limit 1 g/day	Long duration of action Oral suspension	GI irritation
Codeine	0.8–1.5 mg/kg PO/IM q 4–6 h Usual adult dose: 30–60 mg/dose	Potent analgesic No renal or hepatic toxicity Low addiction potential	Nausea Constipation

Table 64.3   Analgesics for Moderate to Severe Pain

ANALGESIC	DOSAGE	ADVANTAGES	DISADVANTAGES
Morphine	Intermittent dosing: 0.2–0.4 mg/kg PO/PR q 4 h (> 50 kg: 10–20 mg PO q 4 h) 0.05–0.1 mg/kg IV/SC q 2–4 h Dose limit: 15 mg/dose IV/SC Continuous infusion: 0.1–0.2 mg/kg loading dose 10–40 mcg/kg/hr IV/SC (calculate: 1/2 body weight (kg) as mg of morphine in 50 mL NS, then 1 mL/hr = 1 mcg/kg/hr)	Rapid onset Potent, analgesic Hypotension	Respiratory depression
Meperidine	1–1.5 mg/kg IV/SC/IM/ PO q 3–4 h Dose limit 100 mg/dose	Potent analgesic	Respiratory depression Seizures
Fentanyl	0.5–1.0 mcg/kg IV; titrate slowly in incremental doses q 1–2 min to effect (max 3 mcg/kg; max initial dose 100 mcg)	Potent analgesic Less hypotension	Respiratory depression Apnea, chest wall rigidity

Note: Naloxone is opioid antagonist for overdose. (See Ch. 65, Procedural Sedation).

Management of Procedural Pain: General Principles

- Setting: equipment set up before child enters room, visual distractions on walls and ceilings
- Parental availability for comfort and support
- Anticipate potential problems before beginning procedure

Address before any procedure:
- Explanation of need and importance of procedure
- Accurate description of procedure

- Expectation of intensity and duration of pain the child may experience
- Possible need for repeated procedural attempts
- Measures to be used for alleviation of pain
- Parental guidance as to how child may react to pain

Procedural Sedation

- Often employed in children, particularly < 5 yrs of age to help alleviate anxiety related to procedures
- Potential for airway compromise always exists; appropriate skilled personnel and equipment for airway management and resuscitation should be available
- See Ch. 65, Procedural Sedation

Local Anesthetics

Lidocaine Injection

- Use lowest concentration of lidocaine (1% vs 2%)
- Addition of epinephrine facilitates hemostasis; extends duration of anesthesia
- Buffering with 8.5% sodium bicarbonate reduces pain of anesthetic preparation (1:9 or 1:10 ratios)
- Use 27–30G needle to control rate and volume of injection
- Injecting through wound edges is less painful than through intact skin for subcutaneous and intradermal injections
- Maximum dosage: 5 mg/kg (7 mg/kg with epinephrine); 1% solution = 10 mg/mL
- Toxicity: CNS—seizures, CV—arrhythmias

LET (lidocaine 4%, epinephrine 0.1%, tetracaine 0.5%)

- Topical anesthetic for laceration repair
- Dosage: 3 mL (or 1 mL per cm laceration, maximum 3 mL)
- Onset of action: 20–30 minutes
- Avoid use on mucosal surfaces and end organs (penis, pinna, tip of nose, fingers)

- Guidelines for use: apply LET to cottonball and press onto wound; cover with gauze pad and apply pressure for 20–30 minutes

EMLA (Eutectic mixture of lidocaine 2.5% and prilocaine 2.5%)

- Topical anesthetic oil in water emulsion that penetrates intact skin
- Apply generously to dermal surface to be anesthetized and cover with air-tight occlusive dressing for at least 45–60 minutes; effects persist for 1–2 hrs
- Side effects: local itching, pallor, or erythema
- May be used in neonate, but caution due to potential for prilocaine-induced methemoglobinemia

Ametop® (4% tetracaine)

- Topical anesthetic for intact skin
- Equally effective as EMLA
- Apply with occlusive dressing for 30–45 minutes; effects last 4–6 hrs
- Side effects: erythema

ELA-max®/Maxilene® (liposomal lidocaine 4%)

- Topical anesthetic for intact skin; may be used for temporary relief of pain with minor cuts, burns, and abrasions
- Apply to skin 30 minutes prior to procedure; does not require occlusive dressing
- Not for use on mucous membranes
- Minimal vasoactive properties: less blanching or erythema at site
- Equally effective as EMLA

Glue (N-2-butylcyanoacrylate or octylcyanoacrylate)

- Tissue adhesives indicated for repair of superficial lacerations < 4 cm length and 0.5 cm width

- Good cosmetic result
- Advantages: no needles/injection required
- Avoid in:
  - Deep wounds requiring layered closure
  - Contaminated wounds requiring heavy debridement including bites
  - Wounds in motion (e.g., hands, joints)
  - Hair-bearing surfaces
  - Wounds crossing mucocutaneous junctions

References

Berde C, Sethna NF. Analgesics for the treatment of pain in children. *N Engl J Med.* 2002;347(14):1094–1103.

Brent AS. The management of pain in the emergency department. *Pediatr Clin North Am.* 2000;47(3):651–679.

Hicks CL, von Baeyer CL, Spafford P, van Korlaar I, Goodenough B. Faces Pain Scale Revised: toward a common metric in pediatric pain management. *Pain.* 2001;93:173–183.

Krauss B. Management of acute pain and anxiety in children undergoing procedures in the emergency department. *Pediatr Emerg Care.* 2001;17(2):115–122.

Merkel SI, Voepel-Lewis T, Shayevitz JR, Malyvia S. The FLACC; a behavioral scale for scoring postoperative pain in young children. *Pediatr Nurs.* 1997;23(3):293–297.

O'Brien L, Taddio A, Lyszkiewicz DA, Koren G. A critical review of the topical local anesthetic amethocaine (Ametop™) for pediatric pain. *Pediatr Drugs.* 2005;7(1):41–54.

Quinn J, Wells G, et al. A randomized trial comparing octylcyanoacrylate tissue adhesive and sutures in the management of lacerations. *JAMA.* 1997;277(19):1527–1530.

Schechter NL, Blankson V, Pachter LM, et al. The ouchless place: no pain, children's gain. *Pediatrics.* 1997;99:890–894.

Zempsky WT, Schecter NL. What's new in the management of pain in children. *Pediatr Rev.* 2003;24(10):337–348.

65 ▪ Procedural Sedation

SAVITHIRI RATNAPALAN AND SUZAN SCHNEEWEISS

Introduction
- Ensure patient safety and welfare
- Minimize physical discomfort or pain during the procedure
- Minimize negative psychosocial responses to treatment
- Enhance cooperation
- Return patient to a state whereby safe discharge is possible

Procedural Sedation
- Procedural sedation in the emergency setting allows patients to:
  - Tolerate unpleasant procedures while maintaining cardiorespiratory function
  - Maintain airway independently and continuously
  - Maintain protective airway reflexes

Levels of Sedation
- Sedation is a *continuum*, not easily divided into discrete stages
- Not drug specific
- Individual patient responses vary so careful titration of drugs is essential

Sedation Guidelines for Non-Anesthesiologists
Patient Selection
- Only ASA I and II status
- Consider other risk factors such as obesity, nonfasting status, previous sedation complications

Facilities
- Dedicated space with appropriate resuscitation equipment

Table 65.1   Levels of Sedation

Minimal sedation	Impaired cognitive function and coordination with: • Normal response to verbal commands • Normal cardiorespiratory function
Moderate sedation	Depressed state of consciousness associated with: • Maintenance of protective airway reflexes • Ability to maintain patent airway • Appropriate responses to stimulation/verbal commands
Deep sedation	Depressed state of consciousness/unconsciousness from which patient is not easily aroused: • Partial or complete loss of protective reflexes • May not maintain a patent airway independently • Inability to appropriately respond to physical stimulation or verbal commands
General anesthesia	State of unconsciousness associated with: • Loss of protective reflexes • Inability to independently maintain a patent airway • Inability to appropriately respond to physical stimulation or verbal commands
Dissociative state	Trancelike cataleptic state induced by ketamine and characterized by: • Profound analgesia and amnesia • Usually with retention of protective airway reflexes • Spontaneous respiration and cardiopulmonary stability

■ Equipment: oxygen, bag-valve-mask setup, suction, monitoring equipment, emergency cart, drugs for sedation and resuscitation including reversal agents

Personnel

■ Designated physician to sedate and observe child

- Physician performing procedure
- Nurse

Preparation of Patient/Family

- Consent
- Verbal explanation of drug(s) to be used, expected behavior, and potential complications
- Written discharge instructions and 24-hour contact number

Table 65.2 American Society of Anesthesiology Classification

ASA CLASS	DESCRIPTION
I	Healthy, no underlying organic disease
II	Mild or moderate systemic disease that does not interfere with daily routines (e.g., well-controlled asthma, essential hypertension)
III	Organic disease with definite functional impairment (e.g., severe steroid dependent asthma, IDDM, uncorrected congenital heart disease)
IV	Severe disease that is life threatening (e.g., head trauma with increased ICP)
V	Moribund patient, not expected to survive
E (suffix)	Physical status classification appended with an "E" connotes a procedure undertaken as an emergency (e.g., an otherwise healthy patient presenting for fracture reduction is classified as ASA status I E)

Pre-Sedation Assessment

- Age, weight, fasting status, ASA status
- Bromage sedation score
- Consent and assent
- History
  - Underlying medical conditions, allergies
  - Current medications

Table 65.3	Bromage Sedation Score
0	Awake and alert
1	Occasionally drowsy, easy to arouse
2	Frequently drowsy, easy to arouse
3	Somnolent, difficult to arouse, inappropriate response to physical stimulation or verbal command
4	Unresponsive to verbal command or physical stimulation
S	Asleep, easy to arouse

Sedation score 0–2 = minimal to moderate sedation
Sedation score 3 = red flag, bordering on deep sedation
Sedation score 4 = deep sedation/general anesthesia

- Past experience with anesthesia or sedation
- Family history of anesthesia problems
■ Exam
  - Baseline vital signs including temperature, saturation
  - Cardiorespiratory exam
  - Focused airway assessment: face shape, facial trauma, large central incisors, loose or absent teeth, receding mandible, size and configuration of palate, evidence of upper airway obstruction such as stridor, voice change, neck mobility
  - Mallampati classification

NPO Guidelines for Children

Elective Non-Emergency Procedures
■ 8 hours: solids
■ 6 hours: milk or formula
■ 4 hours: breast milk
■ 2 hours: clear fluids

Emergency Procedures
■ Use clinical judgment; risks vs benefits

- Use lightest sedation possible
- At minimum, solids 4 hours, clear fluids 2 hours

Monitoring

- Minimal sedation such as with oral midazolam requires no special monitoring or fasting
- Moderate sedation
  - Pre-procedure vital signs
  - Continuous monitoring during procedure (ECG, pulse oximetry)
  - Vital signs q 5–10 minutes during procedure including HR, RR, BP, sedation score

Discharge

Discharge Criteria

- Cardiorespiratory function and airway patency satisfactory
- Easily arousable and protective reflexes intact
- Can talk/walk/sit as developmentally appropriate
- State of hydration is adequate

Discharge Instructions

- Drugs, contact person and number, common problems, appropriate activity, when and what to eat/drink

Sedative Agents

Benzodiazepines—Midazolam

- Short acting, no active metabolites
- Sedation, anxiolysis (no analgesia)
- PO, IV, IM, IN (intranasal), buccal
- Minimal hemodynamic effects: mild hypotension and compensatory tachycardia
- Dose-dependent and infusion-dependent respiratory depression and apnea especially if administered with opioids

Barbiturates—Pentobarbital

■ Most commonly used barbiturate to produce immobility in pediatric patients who must remain still for nonpainful procedures (e.g., diagnostic imaging studies)
■ Mechanism of action unknown; CNS depressant
■ Side effects: respiratory depression, apnea, airway obstruction, coma, paradoxical excitement, residual hangover effect

Chloral Hydrate

■ Not commonly used in emergency department
■ Indicated for nonpainful procedures: EEG, CT scans
■ Less effective than pentobarbital; inadequate immobility in 30–40% of patients
■ May cause airway obstruction, rarely cardiac dysrhythmias
■ Use cautiously in newborn and preterm infants; accumulation of active metabolites

Ketamine

■ Synthetic phencyclidine
■ Hypnosis, immobility, amnesia, profound analgesia
■ May rapidly induce general anesthesia
■ Difficulty in assessing level of sedation because inability to use eye signs, degree of pain, or muscle movement (dissociative state)

Side Effects

CNS   Increased ICP, nystagmus/diplopia, dream-like state, muscle hypertonicity, myoclonic jerks, emergence reactions (hallucinations)

CVS   Tachycardia and hypertension (in catecholamine—depleted patients—myocardial depressant)

Resp   Laryngospasm, transient apnea or respiratory depression with rapid IV

GI   Hypersalivation, emesis

Skin   Erythema or measles-like rash

Contraindications
- Head injury
- Cardiovascular disease
- Glaucoma or acute globe injury
- Psychosis, porphyria, thyroid disorder
- Age < 3 months
- History of airway instability, tracheal surgery, or tracheal stenosis
- Procedures with stimulation of posterior pharynx
- Active pulmonary infection or disease

Ketamine—Adjunctive Agents
- To reduce salivation, especially in young children: atropine 0.01 mg/kg (minimum 0.1 mg, maximum 0.6 mg) OR
  glycopyrrolate 0.005–0.01 mg/kg (maximum 0.2 mg)
- To reduce emergence reactions in older children and for muscle relaxation: midazolam 0.025 mg/kg

Nitrous Oxide
- Odorless, colorless gas
- Provides anxiolysis, amnesia, and mild analgesia in concentrations of 20–50%
- Dose-dependent depression of the central nervous system
- Self-administration of Entenox® requires cooperative child
- 100% oxygen during recovery for 3–5 minutes to prevent diffusion hypoxia
- Recovery is rapid with little residual sedation (no "hangover")
- Adjuvant agent for painful procedures (e.g., fracture reductions)

Contraindications/Caution
- Bowel obstruction
- Pneumothorax
- Oxygen requirement > 40%
- Middle ear obstruction

Propofol

- Nonopioid, nonbarbiturate, short-acting, potent sedative-hypnotic agent with amnestic properties
- Rapid and pleasant recovery
- Lacks inherent analgesic properties and may have to be combined with an opioid agent for painful procedures
- Used primarily for *deep sedation*: ultra-rapid onset and high potency of propofol makes it difficult to titrate; substantial risk of overshooting resulting in deep sedation or even general anesthesia
- Adverse effects: upper airway obstruction, hypoventilation, and apnea leading to hypoxemia and hypotension
- Do not give to patients allergic to soybean oil or egg phosphatide
- May need to decrease dose by 20–30% in hypovolemic patients
- Make sure patient is well hydrated, bolus normal saline 20 mL/kg if necessary
- Routine use of oxygen mask recommended

Analgesic Agents

- Used in conjunction with sedative agents for analgesic effects
- Morphine, fentanyl, and meperidine
- Equipotent doses produce similar degrees of nausea, vomiting, biliary tract spasm, pruritis, constipation, and respiratory depression

Risk Factors for Complications

■ Infants < 3 months, premature infants up to 20 weeks corrected age
■ History of apnea or disordered control of breathing
■ Cardiorespiratory disease
■ Hemodynamic instability
■ Neuromuscular disease
■ Chronic neurologic condition
■ Intracranial hypertension
■ Renal or liver disease

Table 65.4	Relative Potencies of Intravenous Opioids		
DRUG	IV DOSE (MG/KG)	FREQUENCY (HRS)	RATIO OF EQUIVALENCE TO MORPHINE
Morphine	0.1	2–4	1
Fentanyl	0.001	1–2	80–100
Meperidine	1.0	2–4	0.1

Source: From Yaster M, Krane JE, eds. *Pediatric Pain Management and Sedation Handbook.* St. Louis: Mosby–Yearbook Inc; 1997.

Morphine

■ Active metabolite; caution in renal insufficiency
■ Adverse reactions
  • Respiratory and CNS depression
  • Induces histamine release; caution in asthma and children who are hypovolemic
  • Synergistic with other respiratory depressants (e.g., benzodiazepines)

Fentanyl

- Synthetic opioid with no active metabolites
- Few cardiovascular effects other than bradycardia; ideal in patients with congenital heart disease and trauma (neurosurgical) victims
- Short duration of action (< 60 minutes); excellent for short, painful procedures
- Adverse reactions
  - Respiratory depression (synergistic effect when administered with benzodiazepines)
  - Chest wall and glottic rigidity may occur with high (> 5 mcg/kg) doses but may occur even with low doses (1–2 mcg/kg); can be treated with naloxone or neuromuscular blockade and controlled mechanical ventilation

Meperidine

- Toxicity prevalent with prolonged use
- Normeperidine (metabolite): half potency of meperidine but twice the CNS excitation effects → seizures, myoclonus, and agitation
- Avoid use of monoamine oxidase inhibitors → CNS depression, hyperpyrexia, hypo- or hypertension
- Tachycardia: avoid in heart disease, conduction abnormalities (SVT)

Reversal Agents

Naloxone

- Opioid antagonist
- For reversal of opioid side effects such as respiratory depression, apnea, chest wall rigidity, hypotension, dysphoria, itching, and biliary spasm
- May only have partial effect on hypotension
- Observe patient for at least 3 hours following administration

Table 65.5   Sedative, Analgesic, and Reversal Agents

DRUG	DOSAGE	ONSET OF ACTION/ TIME TO PEAK EFFECT	DURATION OF ACTION
Sedatives			
Midazolam	Oral 0.5–0.75 mg/kg (Wt < 20 kg) 0.3–0.5 mg/kg (Wt > 20 kg) Intravenous 0.05–0.15 mg/kg (slowly titrate to effect) Intranasal 0.1–0.2 mg/kg (max 1 mL)	Oral Onset 10–30 min Peak effect 30–60 min Intravenous Onset 1–3 min Peak effect 3–5 min Intranasal Onset 5–10 min Peak effect 5–12 min	Oral 60–90 min Intravenous 45–60 min
Ketamine	Intravenous 0.5–1.5 mg/kg/dose May repeat 0.5 mg/kg in 10 min (max 100 mg) Intramuscular 4 mg/kg/dose May repeat ½ the total dose in 10 min	Intravenous Onset 1 min Intramuscular Onset 5 min	Intravenous 10–15 min Intramuscular 15–30 min

(continues)

Table 65.5 Sedative, Analgesic, and Reversal Agents (continued)

Drug	Dosage	Onset of action/ time to peak effect	Duration of action
Pentobarbital	4–6 mg/kg IV (max 200 mg) Slow titration	Onset 1–10 min	3–4 hours
Nitrous oxide	50% nitrous/50% oxygen	Peak effect 3–5 min	
Propofol	0.5–1 mg/kg IV (max 40 mg) over 1–2 min Supplemental doses 0.5 mg/kg (max 20 mg) allowing a minimum of 60 sec between each subsequent dose or 50–100 mcg/kg/min for continued sedation (infusion) (deep sedation dose)	Onset within seconds Peak effect Children 1–3 min Adults 1–2 min	5–10 minutes with IV bolus Full recovery: 10–15 min after discontinuing infusion
Chloral Hydrate	Sedation 80–100 mg/kg PO/ PR May repeat with 40 mg/kg in 1 hr Dose limit 2 g/dose PO/PR Hypnotic 50 mg/kg/dose PO/PR Dose limit 1 g/dose	Onset 30–60 min (administer 20–45 min prior to procedure)	2–8 hrs

Table 65.5 Sedative, Analgesic, and Reversal Agents (continued)

Drug	Dosage	Onset of action/ time to peak effect	Duration of action
Analgesics			
Morphine*	0.05–0.1 mg/kg IV (max 15 mg/dose)	Onset 1–5 min Peak effect 10–20 min	2.5–7 hrs (prolonged effect in neonates)
Fentanyl*	0.5–1 mcg/kg IV Titrate to effect (max dose 3 mcg/kg or 100 mcg initial dose)	Onset 2 –3 min Peak effect 5–15 min	30–60 min
Reversal Agents			
Naloxone	Partial reversal dose 0.001 mg/kg IV, IM titrate to max of 0.01 mg/kg or 1 mg/dose May need to repeat dose every 30–60 min	Onset 1–2 min	45 min (varies with route of administration)
Flumazenil	0.01 mg/kg IV, repeat q 1–3 min to max of 5 doses (max total dose 1 mg)	Onset 1–3 min	30–60 min

*Reduce dose of analgesic agent if combined with sedative as synergistic effect and may result in respiratory depression.

Flumazenil

- Reverses respiratory depression, sedative, amnestic, and anti-seizure effects of *benzodiazepines*
- Reserve for emergency use
- May precipitate seizures particularly in patients taking benzodiazepines for seizure control or in patients with tricyclic antidepressant overdose
- Observe patient for at least 3 hours following administration

References

American Academy of Pediatrics Committee on Drugs. Guidelines for monitoring and management of pediatric patients during and after sedation for diagnostic and therapeutic procedures: addendum. *Pediatrics.* 2002;110(4):836–838.

American Academy of Pediatrics Committee on Drugs. Guidelines for monitoring and management of pediatric patients during and after sedation for diagnostic and therapeutic procedures. *Pediatrics.* 1992;89:1055–1115.

American College of Emergency Physicians. Clinical policy: evidence-based approach to pharmacologic agents used in pediatric sedation and analgesia in the emergency department. *Ann Emerg Med.* 2004;44(4):342–377.

American Society of Anesthesiologists Task Force on Sedation and Analgesia by Non-Anesthesiologists. Practice guidelines for sedation and analgesia by non-anesthesiologists. *Anesthesia.* 1996;84:459–471.

Godwin SA, Caro DA, Wolf SJ, et al. American College of Emergency Physicians. Clinical policy: procedural sedation and analgesia in the emergency department. *Ann Emerg Med.* 2005;45(2):177–196.

Green SM, Krauss B. Clinical practice guideline for emergency department: ketamine dissociative sedation in children. *Ann Emerg Med.* 2004;44(5):460–471.

Krauss B, Brustowicz RM, eds. *Pediatric Procedural Sedation and Analgesia.* Baltimore: Lippincott Williams & Wilkins,1999.

Krauss B, Green SM. Sedation and analgesia for procedures in children. *N Engl J Med.* 2000;342(13):938–945.

Pershad J, Godambe SA. Propofol for procedural sedation in the pediatric emergency department. *J Emerg Med.* 2004;27(1):11–14.

Yaster M, Krane JE, eds. *Pediatric Pain Management and Sedation Handbook.* St. Louis: Mosby-Year Book Inc; 1997.

Zempsky WT, Cravero JP, Committee on Pediatric Emergency Medicine and Section on Anesthesiology and Pain Medicine. Relief of pain and anxiety in pediatric patients in emergency medical systems. *Pediatrics.* 2004;114(5):1348–1356.

■ PART XVII

PSYCHOSOCIAL EMERGENCIES

66 ▪ Child Maltreatment

D. ANNA JARVIS

Introduction

- Child maltreatment is a complex syndrome that includes deliberate injury, inappropriate sexual contact, neglect, failure to provide the necessities of life, and/or emotional maltreatment of a child
- Occurs in all segments of population, frequently undetected until a child dies
- In US: ~ 2.5% of all children are abused or neglected annually
- Adult surveys: 20% of women and 5–10% of men report childhood sexual abuse
- Must be alert to the possibility of child maltreatment at each clinical encounter
- If suspect child abuse, required by law to report to Child Protection Services for investigation

Note: Child maltreatment is the current preferred descriptive terminology for child abuse

Types of Maltreatment

- Physical: varies from harsh discipline to torture
- Sexual
- Neglect: 70% of failure to thrive in infancy is nonorganic
- Emotional

Munchausen Syndrome

- Deliberate injury of a child by poisoning, physical means, or interference with medical care so that the child presents sick or unwell or with "repeated life-threatening events"
- Result is repeated and escalating medical investigation and intervention

Various Presentations

- Unexplained electrolyte disturbances
- Sepsis and unusual infecting organisms
- Positive toxicology tests without history of ingestion

Vulnerable Child: Risk Factors

- Premature
- Colic
- Physical/emotional challenges
- Special needs
- Demanding child
- Delayed bowel/bladder control

Note: Only one child in a family may be victimized

Predicting Child Maltreatment

- A very high proportion of children who experience abuse grow up to be *abusers:* the "cycle of abuse"

Social and Environmental Factors

- History of childhood maltreatment in perpetrator
- Alcohol/substance dependency
- Crisis situation in perpetrator's life
- Spousal and domestic violence
- Mental illness/depression in caregiver

Suspected Child Maltreatment

- Consider possibility of maltreatment with all injuries
- Explore exact mechanism and circumstance of injury
- Ask, "Does the story make sense?" given the age and development of the child
- Check past records for repeated or unusual injuries
- Consider possibility of neglect or inappropriate supervision
- Accident prevention information and teaching should be an integral part of acute injury care

Suspicious History

- No history on mechanism of injury
- Partial history
- History changes
- History is developmentally unrealistic
- Delay in seeking care
- Unrealistic expectations of child

Can Bruises Be Accurately Dated?

- Color of bruises does *not* accurately reflect age
- "Timing of bruises" charts are inaccurate
- Document exactly what is seen including description of shape, size, color, texture, and level of discomfort or pain; photographs may be useful for visible injuries

Suspicious Injury Patterns for Nonaccidental Trauma

Head/CNS Injuries

- Torn frenulum
- Dental injuries
- Bilateral black eyes
- Traumatic hair loss
- Diffuse/severe CNS injury
- Retinal hemorrhage
- Shaken baby syndrome:
  - Diffuse brain injury
  - Subdural or subarachnoid hemorrhage
  - Retinal hemorrhage
  - Minimal or no evidence of external trauma
  - Associated bony fractures

Skin Injuries

- Bites
- Bruises, burn in shape of an object

- Burns: glove/stocking distribution
- Bruises of various ages
- Bruises in protected areas

Bone Injuries

- Rib fractures without major trauma
- Femur fractures in children < 1 year of age
- Spiral fractures of long bones in nonambulatory children
- Metaphyseal fractures in infants—"bucket handle" sign
- Multiple fractures of varied ages
- Complex/multiple skull fractures

Genitourinary/Gastrointestinal

- Chronic abdominal/perineal pain
- Injury to genitalia/rectum
- Sexually transmitted disease/pregnancy
- Recurrent vomiting or diarrhea

Sexual Abuse

- Sexual abuse may present with nonspecific abdominal pain or recurrent urinary tract infections
- Each child who presents with pregnancy or a sexually transmitted disease should be questioned about possible sexual abuse
- Other presentations include a wide range of psychological, self-destructive, and somatic behaviors including substance abuse

Medical Evaluation of Sexual Abuse: Immediate

- Sexual abuse within 72 hours
- Presence of injuries or symptoms
- Psychosocial concerns
- Parental distress

Medical Evaluation of Sexual Abuse: Nonacute

- No acute symptoms or injuries

- Time from last episode > 72 hours
- Child in a safe environment

Sexual Assault Evidence Kit (Rape Kit)

- Must observe legal protocols to preserve "chain of evidence"
- Improperly collected, labeled, or transferred specimens are *not* admissible as evidence in court
- Swab samples from mouth, vagina, anus, sites contaminated with secretions
- Oral and vaginal washings
- Saliva sample
- Samples of hair (scalp and pubic)
- Blood group and drug screen
- Collection of clothing

Sexual Assault: Prophylactic Medication

- Prevention of pregnancy: Levonorgestrel (Plan B®), pregnancy test
- Sexually transmitted infections

Table 66.1	Sexual Assault Prophylactic Medication
Gonorrhea	Cefixime 400 mg orally single dose or Ciprofloxacin 500 mg orally single dose
Chlamydia trachomatis	Azithromycin (Zithromax®) 1g orally single dose or Doxycycline 100 mg orally bid × 7days
Hepatitis B	+/– Hepatitis B virus vaccine +/– Hepatitis B immune globulin
Human immuno-deficiency virus (HIV)	Contact child abuse specialist for recommendation

Note: Refer to most recent national or state health guidelines for antibiotic recommendations.

Summary

- Any suspected child maltreatment issues must be reported to the appropriate Child Protection Services
- Keep detailed records
- Investigations depend on history, pubertal development, physical findings, consent
- Findings may be: normal/nonspecific, suspicious, suggestive, definitive
- *All* suspicious cases should be discussed with the Suspected Child Abuse and Neglect/Child Protection team prior to investigations or discharge from the emergency department

References

American Academy of Pediatrics Committee on Child Abuse and Neglect. When inflicted skin injuries constitute child abuse. *Pediatrics.* 2002;110(3):644–645.

Block RW, Krebs NF, Committee on Child Abuse and Neglect, Committee on Nutrition. American Academy of Pediatrics Clinical Report. Failure to thrive as a manifestation of child neglect. *Pediatrics.* 2005;116(5):1234–1237.

Dubowitz H, Giardino A, Gustavson E. Child neglect: guidance for pediatricians. *Pediatr Rev.* 2000;21(4):111–116.

Huyer D. Proper evaluation can help sexually abused adolescents. *Can J Cont Med Educ.* 1997;9:85–97.

Kellogg N, Committee on Child Abuse and Neglect. American Academy of Pediatrics Clinical Report. The evaluation of sexual abuse in children. *Pediatrics.* 2005;116(2):506–512.

Mudd SS, Findlay JS. The cutaneous manifestations and common mimickers of physical child abuse. *J Pediatr Health Care.* 2004:18(3):123–129.

Sirotnak AP, Grigsby T, Krugman RD. Physical abuse of children. *Pediatr Rev.* 2004;25(8):264–277.

67 ▪ Psychiatric Emergencies

SANJAY MEHTA

Introduction

- Children often present to the emergency department in crisis
  - Suicidality, behavioral crisis/aggression, acute psychosis, or anxiety
- Crisis: acute emotional upset (normal response to abnormal life events) arising from situational, developmental, or sociocultural sources resulting in temporary inability to cope through usual problem-solving devices
- Psychiatric emergencies: acute behavioral disturbances related to severe mental or emotional instability or dysfunction that requires medical intervention (e.g., medication or admission)
- Rule out organic etiologies for change in behavior before psychiatric consultation
- Determine if agitated and withdrawn children are psychotic
- Need to conduct a risk assessment to determine risk of self-harm or harm to others

Clinical Assessment of Psychiatric Emergencies

- Identifying complaint
  - Source and reason for referral, who patient lives with, and source of information
- Chief complaint and history of present illness
  - Time of onset, duration, predisposers, precipitators, perpetuators, and severity
- Mood symptoms
  - Depression: irritable or depressed mood, loss of interest/pleasure (anhedonia), reactivity, feeling sad, change in appetite or weight, sleep disturbance, loss of energy and

535

    fatigue, social isolation and withdrawal, poor concentration and indecisiveness, worthlessness, and feelings of guilt, low self-esteem, or feeling hopeless
- Mania: agitation, mood elevation, pressured speech or grandiosity
■ Anxiety symptoms
- Isolated or generalized worries, age-inappropriate phobias, panic, obsessions, compulsions, dissociations, flashbacks, and avoidance
■ Psychotic symptoms
- Circumstantiality, loosening of associations, delusions, auditory or visual hallucinations, communicating telepathically, thought broadcasting or insertion, catatonia or changed affect (e.g., flat, inappropriate, or incongruent)
■ Psychiatric history
- Psychiatric hospitalizations, outpatient treatment, psychiatric diagnoses, psychiatric medications, involvement with child protection services, counselors
■ Medical and developmental history
- Pregnancy, birth, delivery, milestones, medical illnesses, hospitalizations, or diagnoses, past and current medications
■ Personal history
- Previous level of adjustment, social (family and peer relations), academic performance, areas of interest and special competences, behavioral functioning, abuse (sexual or physical), substance abuse, aggression, violence, body image, eating problems, sexual preference or orientation
■ Family history
- Psychiatric disorders and medications, relationships, suicides in extended family, substance abuse

Suicidality and Homicidality Assessment

■ Past or present suicidal/homicidal behaviors
- Suicidal or homicidal thoughts, thoughts about death or dying, or hurting or killing, and for how long, or previous

attempts or rehearsals (method, severity, impulsivity, suicidal or homicidal note or notification of others)
- • Red flags: plan and means available (pills, knives, poison, and especially firearms)
■ Risk factors for suicidality (often attempting to escape dysphoria)
- • Disciplinary or amorous crises, circumstances leading to shame (e.g., bullying, coming out), males, family history, "contagion effect," mood or conduct disorders, impulsiveness, and certain personality factors, substance use, isolation, or alienation
■ Self-harm or mutilation (often attempting to seek euphoria)
- • Can have significant tissue damage, usually fixed and rhythmic, often superficial from carving, cutting, burning, etc.
■ Threat of self-harm supercedes right of confidentiality
- • Guardians have right to be informed of risk to their wards

Table 67.1   Features of Agitated or Withdrawn Child

THE AGITATED CHILD	THE WITHDRAWN CHILD
• Anxious, upset, unresponsive	• Unresponsive, quiet, non-rapport
• Pacing, loud, abusive, disoriented	• Clinging, whining, crying
• Tantrums, crying, violent	• Sullen, apathetic
• Distraught, sullen, angry	• Different from *shyness*
• Improve in ED with structure	○ Temperamental quality within
○ Sense of forthcoming help	range of normal behavior

Disturbed Child: Differential Diagnosis

Psychosis

■ Major disturbances in *thinking, relating, and reality testing*
- • Unclear expression, difficulty with direct questions, suspicious, hostile, suicidal or parasuicidal, self sleep deprivation, self-malnutrition

Medical Causes

- Trauma, CNS lesions, cerebral hypoxia
- Metabolic/endocrine, collagen vascular diseases (e.g., SLE)
- Infections (e.g., malaria, typhoid fever)
- Miscellaneous (e.g., Wilson's)

Toxins

- Hallucinogens, marijuana, PCP, cocaine, amphetamines
- Anticholinergics, heavy metals
- Corticosteroids
- Opioids
- Alcohol, barbiturates
- Antipsychotics

Depression Precipitants

- Parental divorce or separation
- Loss of a parent through death
- Recent devaluation of personal abilities (e.g., poor academic performance)
- Peer rejection
- Onset of significant physical illness

Conduct Disorder

- Significant behavioral disruption
- Features include: aggressiveness, stealing, fire-setting, truancy, other forms of delinquency
- Angry and resentful (may improve when behaviors not tolerated)

Post-traumatic Stress Disorder (PTSD)

- Recurrent nightmares or flashbacks, lack of involvement in usual friendships or activities, fluctuating behavior with episodes (e.g., excitement, fearfulness, irritability)
- Can be upset or guilty, may refuse to discuss

Adjustment Reaction

- Deterioration of functioning from a previously higher level in the presence of some precipitating event or situation (patient can usually explain problem)
  - Developmental trigger
  - New school, peer pressure, emergence of secondary sexual characteristics during puberty
  - Acute trigger (e.g., loss of a parent through death or divorce)

Attention Deficit Disorder

- Impulsivity
- Associated distractibility
- Learning difficulties

Medical Considerations

- Thyrotoxicosis
  - Tachycardia
  - Appetite and sleep disturbances
  - Weight loss
  - Exophthalmos
- Temporal lobe epilepsy: seizures, auras, abnormal neurologic findings

Evaluation

- Determine if behavior is caused by a medical condition
- Assess psychiatric manifestations of presenting condition
- Assess family system and social supports

Examination

- Pupils, vitals
- Complete neurological exam

Table 67.2   Organic Disease versus Psychiatric Disorder

	ORGANIC	PSYCHIATRIC
Onset	Acute	Gradual
Dysautonomia	Present	Absent
Vitals	Abnormal	Normal
Orientation	Impaired	Intact
Memory	Impaired	Intact
Intellect	Impaired	Intact
Hallucinations	Visual	Auditory

Investigations

Consider:

- CBC, ESR, electrolytes, glucose, calcium, BUN, ammonia, LFTs, TSH
- Urinalysis
- CT and/or MRI head
- Toxicology screen

Mental Status

- Appearance, task orientation, short- and long-term memory
- Cognitive: intelligence, knowledge, ability to reason and think (locus of control)
- Activity level and age-appropriateness
- Affect: predominant feelings, nature, appropriateness (frustration tolerance and impulsivity), changes
- Thinking
  - Processes: coherence, goal-directedness, loose associations, speech without internal consistency
  - Content: themes, concerns, preoccupations, strengths, insight, capacity
- Suicidal and homicidal ideation

Social Supports

- Family structure and relationships
  - Who lives at home
  - Nature of relationships
  - Recent changes in family composition or living situation
  - Parents' level of concern
  - Ability to appreciate the child's current situation
- Parents' description of the child
  - How the child is perceived in the family
  - Parental ability to engage a withdrawn child or calm and set limits with an agitated child, and child's response
  - Encouragement of child's independent thinking and behavior
  - Ability to manage effectively at home
  - Adjustment of the child in the past and how earlier family difficulties were handled
  - Degree of coping and openness of family
- Family history of emotional difficulties

Pharmacologic Restraint

- Try benzodiazepine first; if unsuccessful, consider neuroleptic second; if still unsuccessful, consider atypical antipsychotic

Physical Restraint or Seclusion

- Five caretakers (one per limb, one for head); must avoid throat, chest, and mouth
- Requires careful explanation to patient and reassessments every 30 minutes

Indications

- Failure of verbal restraint or other means of control
- To prevent imminent harm to patient or others
- To prevent disruption of treatment plan or damage to environment
- To decrease patient stimulation (e.g., PCP, ethanol)

Table 67.3	Pharmacologic Treatment
Benzodiazepines	Lorazepam
	0.05 mg/kg PO/IM/IV q 30 min (0.5–2.0 mg usual dose)
	Diazepam
	0.1 mg/kg PO/IM/IV (2.0–10.0 mg usual dose)
Neuroleptics	
Low potency	Chlorpromazine
	0.5–1.0 mg/kg PO/IM/IV q 30 min (200 mg/day usual)
High potency	Haloperidol
	0.05 mg/kg PO/IM/IV q30min (2.5–5.0 mg usual)
Atypical antipsychotic	Olanzapine (Zyprexa®)
	2.5–5.0 mg PO/IM q 6h prn (30 mg/day max)

■ If requested by patient, secondary to their loss of control
■ Side effects may include sedation, respiratory depression, or orthostatic hypotension, acute dystonia

Acute Dystonia
■ Torticollis, oculogyric crisis, opisthotonus
■ Treatment:
  • Diphenhydramine 1–2 mg/kg (max 75 mg) PO/IV/IM, OR
  • Benztropine mesylate 0.5–2.0 mg IV/IM

Discharge Criteria
■ Safety plan
■ Nonsuicidal, medically stable, nonintoxicated, nondelirious, and nondemented

- Patient and guardian agreement with discharge plan and need to return if suicidal intent occurs, with reciprocal physician belief in patient and guardian compliance with plan
- Underlying psychiatric diagnosis treatment and removal of lethal self-harm means arranged
- Acute precipitants discussed with attempted resolution

References
Christodulu KV, et al. Psychiatric emergencies in children. *Pediatr Emerg Care.* 2002;18(4):268–270.

Fleisher GR, Ludwig S, eds. *Textbook of Pediatric Emergency Medicine.* 4th ed. Philadelphia: Lippincott Williams & Wilkins; 2000.

Goldstein AB, et al. Mental health visits in a pediatric emergency department and their relationship to the school calendar. *Pediatr Emerg Care.* 2005;21(10):653–657.

Roberge J, Walker E. The Hospital for Sick Children (personal communications), 2005.

Selbst S, Cronan K, eds. Pediatric emergency medicine secrets. Philadelphia: Hanley & Belfus; 2001.

Woolfenden S, et al. The presentation of aggressive children and adolescents to emergency departments in Western Sydney. *J Paediatr Child Health.* 2003;39(9):651–653.

Index

supplemental potassium, 143
examination, 142
history, 142
hospitalization, 145
investigations, 142–143
Atlantoaxial subluxation, 56
Atopic dermatitis, 404–405, *fig.*51.7
Atovaquone-proguanil, malaria, 268
Atropine, cardiopulmonary resuscitation, 21–22
Attention deficit disorder (ADD), 539
AVPU Scale, 44, 365
Avulsion fracture, 59f
Azithromycin (Zithromax)
otitis media, 117t
pharyngitis, 124
sexual assault, 533t

B

Bacteremia, 28
Bacteria, microscopy, 224t, 225
Bacterial pathogens
gastroenteritis, 175, 176t
meningitis, 262t
skin contaminants, urine cultures, 225
Bag-valve-mask (BVM) ventilation, 17–18
Baker Criteria, fever management, 255
Balanitis, 238
Barbiturates-pentobarbital, 516, 522t
Bazett's formula: QTc, 161
Bell-clapper deformity, 242
Benign persistent proteinuria, 228
Benign postural (orthostatic) proteinuria, 228
Benzodiazepines-Midazolam, 377t, 437t, 515, 521t, 524, 542t
Benztropine mesylate, 542
β-blocker, antidote to, 437t
Bezold-Jarisch reflex, 168
Biaxin. *See* Clarithromycin (Biaxin)
Bicarbonate, in treatment of DKA, 344
Bilious vomiting, 199
Bite wounds
antibiotic management, 476
frequency and infection rates, 478
by species, 479t
high-risk: indications for antibiotic prophylaxis, 480
low-risk: no antibiotic prophylaxis, 480
management, 479

management of infected wounds, 480–481
indications for admission, 481
intravenous antibiotic choices, 481
microbiology, 478–479
prophylactic antibiotics, 479–480
rabies
prophylaxis, 482
tetanus, 481, 481t
Bleeding. *See also* Gastrointestinal bleeding
abnormal/dysfunctional uterine bleeding
investigations, 393
management, 393–394
menarche, 392–393
after menarche, 393f
outpatient workshop, 393
vaginal, 390, 390f
Blisters, sucking, 81t
Bone injuries, child maltreatment and, 532
Bowel obstruction: malrotation
clinical presentation, 199
differential diagnosis, 199
examination, 199–200
initial management, 200
investigations, 200
Bowing fracture, 59f
Breast tissue hypertrophy, 79t
Breathing. *See also* Airway, breathing, and ventilation
cardiopulmonary resuscitation
anesthesia bags, 18
bag-valve-mask (BVM) ventilation, 17–18
impending respiratory failure, 17
self-inflating BVM device, 18
Bromage sedation score, 514t
Bronchiolitis
clinical presentation, 133
discharge instructions, 137–138
emergency care
dexamethasone, 136
epinephrine, 136
feedings, 135
salbutamol/albuterol, inhaled, 136–137
supplemental oxygen, 135
examination, 134–135
history, 134
hospitalization
absolute, 137

Procedural sedation. *See also* Analgesic
agents; Sedative agents
defined, 511
levels of sedation, 511, 512t
sedation guidelines for non-
anesthesiologists
ASA anesthesiology classification, 513t
Bromage sedation score, 514t
discharge, 515
facilities, 511–512
monitoring, 515
NPO guidelines for children
elective non-emergency procedures,
514
emergency procedures, 514–515
patient selection, 511
personnel, 512–513
preparation of patient/family, 513
presedation assessment, 513–514
Propofol, 518, 522t
Proteinuria
common causes, 228
complications, 230
diagnosis, 229
epidemiology, 229
laboratory examination, 228–229
nephrotic syndrome, 229
treatment for new-onset disease,
229–230
Proteus, UTIs, 226
Protozoan infection. *See* Malaria
Proximal humeral fracture, 62
Pseudohyponatremia, 185
Pseudokidney sign, 198
Pseudomonas
febrile neutropenia, 286
UTIs, 226
Pseudosubluxation, 54
Psilocybin, 453
pSLE. *See* Pediatric systemic lupus
erythematosus (pSLE)
Psoriatic arthritis, 309
Psychedelic street drugs
LSD, 452
management, 453
marijuana, 453
PCP, 453
psilocybin, mushrooms, mescaline,
Mexican peyote cactus, 453
Psychiatric emergencies
acute dystonia, 542

clinical assessment of
identifying complaint, 535
mood/anxiety/psychotic symptoms,
535–536
crisis, defined, 535
defined, 535
discharge criteria, 542–543
disturbed child: differential diagnosis
adjustment reaction, 539
attention deficit disorder, 539
conduct disorder, 538
depression precipitants, 538
medical considerations, 539
post-traumatic stress disorder
(PTSD), 538
psychosis
defined, 537
medical causes, 538
toxins, 538
evaluation, 539
examination, 539
features of the agitated or withdrawn
child, 537t
investigations, 540
mental status, 540
organic disease *vs.* psychiatric disorder,
540t
pharmacologic restraint, 541–542, 542t
physical restraint or seclusion, 541
social supports, 541
suicidality and homicidality assessment,
536–537
Psychiatric history, 536
Psychosis
defined, 537
medical causes, 538
toxins, 538
Psychotic symptoms, 536
Puncture wound, defined, 471
Pupillary responses, level of
consciousness, 368, 368t
Puritic eruptions
atopic dermatitis, 404–405, *fig.*51.7
contact dermatitis, 404
differential diagnosis, 403
scabies, 405, *fig.*51.8
serum sickness, 403–404
urticaria, 403
Purpura, 407–408, *fig.*51.14, *fig.*51.15
Pyelonephritis *vs.* urinary tract infection,